CONTRIBUTORS TO THE UK EDITION

Barbara Dunn, SRN, SCM, RCNT, RNT, DipN

Nurse Tutor, Nurse Education Centre, St Luke's Hospital, Guildford

Leonard Evans, BA, SRN, ONC, RCNT, RNT

Senior Tutor, Royal Orthopaedic Hospital, Birmingham

Cynthia Gilling, SRN, SCM, RNT

Assistant Director of Nurse Education, The Princess Alexandra School of Nursing, The London Hospital, London

Susan A Gowers, SRN, RCNT

Senior Nursing Officer (Capital Planning), Trent Regional Health Authority, formerly Senior Nursing Officer, Royal Marsden Hospital, London

Rosemarie Hawkins, SRN

Department of Occupational Medicine, Cardiothoracic Institute, Brompton Hospital, London

Morgan Hicks, SRN, OND, RCNT, Cert Ed, RNT

Tutor, Charing Cross Hospital School of Nursing, Charing Cross Hospital, London

Elizabeth Keighley, SRN, RSCN, RCNT, DipN

Clinical Teacher, JBCNS Course in Neuromedical/Neurosurgical Nursing, Cambridge School of Nursing, Addenbrooke's Hospital, Cambridge

Geraldine Matthison, SRN

Formerly Sister, Endocrine Unit, St Thomas's Hospital, London

Margaret Reed, SRN, DipN, Cert Ed, RNT

Tutor (Continuing and Inservice Education), Cambridge School of Nursing, Addenbrooke's Hospital, Cambridge

Lynette Stone, BA, SRN, SCM (NSW)

Nursing Officer (Outpatients), St John's Hospital for Diseases of the Skin, London

LIPPINCOTT MANUAL OF MEDICAL-SURGICAL NURSING

Volume 2

LILLIAN SHOLTIS BRUNNER,
RN, MSN, ScD, FAAN

Consultant in Nursing, Schools of Nursing: Bryn Mawr Hospital and Presbyterian-University of Pennsylvania Medical Center; formerly Assistant Professor of Surgical Nursing, Yale University School of Nursing

DORIS SMITH SUDDARTH,
RN, BSNE, MSN

Consultant in Health Occupations, Job Corps Health Office, U.S. Department of Labor; formerly Coordinator of the Curriculum, Alexandria Hospital School of Nursing

CONTRIBUTORS

Herbert H. Butler, MD

Emergency Department Physician, Underwood-Memorial Hospital, Woodbury, New Jersey; Immediate Past President, New Jersey Chapter American College of Emergency Physicians

James F. Elam, PhD

Clinical Biochemist, Pathology Department, Alexandria Hospital, Alexandria, Virginia

Joseph B. Mizgerd, MD

Director, Department of Pulmonary Medicine, Washington Adventist Hospital, Takoma Park, Maryland

Alfred Munzer, MD

Associate Director, Department of Pulmonary Medicine, Washington Adventist Hospital, Takoma Park, Maryland

THE LIPPINCOTT MANUAL
OF MEDICAL-SURGICAL NURSING

VOLUME 2

Lillian S. Brunner and Doris S. Suddarth

Harper & Row, Publishers
London

Cambridge
Mexico City
New York
Philadelphia

San Francisco
São Paulo
Singapore
Sydney

British Library Cataloguing in Publication Data

Brunner, Lillian
   Lippincott manual of medical-surgical nursing.
   Vol. 2
   1. Nursing
   I. Title   II. Suddarth, Doris
   610.73   RT41

ISBN 0-06-318208-4

Typeset by Inforum Ltd, Portsmouth
Printed and Bound by The Bath Press, Avon

NOTE:
The publishers wish to state that, whilst every effort has been made
to ensure the accuracy and correctness of the information
contained herein, the authors of the original work from which this
adaptation is taken cannot be held responsible for any changes
made to the original text in the course of the adaptation.

CONTENTS

FOREWORD

In recent years, there have been many American nursing books introduced on to the British market. Although most of these are very well presented, the differences in terminology and in some nursing practices have been great disadvantages.

The *Lippincott Manual*, which is very widely used in America, has been completely adapted for the UK by trained nurses in this country, each having a specialized knowledge in a particular field.

The information is tabulated for easy reference and we believe that these three volumes of medical-surgical nursing will form a useful source of information for both learners and trained nurses. We would like to thank our professional colleagues for their willing help and advice while we were gathering this information.

The first volume of *The Lippincott Manual of Medical-Surgical Nursing* introduces the basic nursing concepts within the framework of the nursing process. Other sections in this volume refer to conditions which are encountered in every sphere of nursing, such as the elderly patient, the cancer patient and those undergoing surgery.

The second volume introduces interrelated subjects, such as the cardiovascular system, disorders of the blood and respiratory system and, in the latter part, disorders of the digestive system, metabolism and the endocrine system. Although in the past, the emphasis may have been on the medical treatment of many of these disorders, modern investigations, a greater knowledge of physiology and improved techniques mean that surgery can now cure or alleviate many conditions. A full awareness of the physiological reasons for specialized nursing care is essential to all those concerned with caring for the patient in hospital and planning rehabilitation.

The third volume is concerned with two closely related groups of subjects. The first group consists of disorders of the nervous system itself, and the special senses of hearing and sight. Some of the disorders of the musculoskeletal system are also due to problems of nervous control. The second part of this volume has sections on the kidney, urinary tract and reproductive disorders. New techniques for treating patients with these disorders have been included and, importantly, the physiological changes which occur as a result of these problems are detailed.

Together these volumes will provide a valuable source of information, so that nurses will be able to understand fully the reasons for the decisions they make when planning the total care of their patients.

Barbara Dunn, 1982

Chapter 1

CONDITIONS OF THE CARDIOVASCULAR SYSTEM

1. Heart Disorders

2. Essentials of Basic Electrocardiography

3. Vascular Disorders

1. Heart Disorders

MANIFESTATIONS OF HEART DISEASE

The patient's symptoms of heart disease depend on (1) nature of cardiopathy and (2) resultant physiological disturbances in circulation.

Dyspnoea

Dyspnoea is undue breathlessness, an awareness of discomfort associated with breathing.

General Features

1 Cardiac dyspnoea—increased effort in breathing due to a reduction of lung capacity resulting from pulmonary venous congestion.
2 Dypsnoea due to heart disease is usually rapid and shallow.
3 The threshold (tolerance) for dyspnoea varies with the individual.

Types of Dyspnoea

1 *Exertional Dyspnoea*—breathlessness upon moderate exertion which is relieved by rest; seen in congestive heart failure, chronic pulmonary disease.
2 *Orthopnoea*—shortness of breath when lying down which is relieved by promptly sitting upright.
   a. Usually due to stasis of blood in lungs, indicating left ventricular failure, mitral disease.
   b. May be from cardiac insufficiency or pulmonary insufficiency.
3 *Paroxysmal nocturnal dyspnoea*—sudden dyspnoea at night while lying down, due to left ventricular insufficiency, pulmonary oedema, mitral stenosis.
4 *Cheyne-Stokes respiration*—periodic breathing characterized by gradual increase in depth of respiration followed by a decrease in respiration resulting in apnoea; periods of hyperpnoea alternating with periods of apnoea.
   a. Cheyne-Stokes respiration is usually considered a serious sign.
   b. Associated with left ventricular failure (severe), cerebral vascular disease.

Nursing Assessment of Dyspnoea

1 What precipitates or relieves the dyspnoea?
2 What position does the patient assume?
3 What is the skin colour? Pallor? Cyanosis?

Chest Pain

Cardiac Causes of Chest Pain

1 Usually from ischaemia caused by stimulation of afferent nerve endings in the myocardium by metabolites resulting from oxygen deficiency in heart muscle—due to coronary artery disease (angina pectoris, p. 40, myocardial infarction, p. 43).
2 Excruciating pain—due to acute dissecting aneurysms of the aorta.
3 Sharp precordial pain (over heart area) aggravated by deep breathing—indicates acute pericarditis.
4 Anxiety is a common cause of chest pain.

Nursing Assessment of Patient with Chest Pain

1 How intense is the pain—dull, sharp, boring, crushing, tearing?
2 Where is pain located? Does it radiate?
3 What are the time and mode of onset?
4 How long does the episode last?
5 What factors precipitate pain (breathing, coughing, swallowing, rapid walking, emotional stress)?
6 What factors alleviate pain (rest, change in position)?

Oedema

Oedema is an abnormal accumulation of serous fluid in the connective tissues.

General Features

1 Cardiac causes of oedema—congestive heart failure.
2 Other causes of oedema—sodium retention, liver disease, renal disease, hypoproteinaemia, venous or lymphatic obstruction.

Types

1 Ascites—excessive fluid in peritoneal cavity.
2 Pleural effusion—excessive fluid in the pleural cavity.
3 Anasarca—gross generalized oedema.

Nursing Implications

1 In heart conditions the location of oedema is influenced by gravity. Fluid collects in the lower parts of the body (dependent oedema).
    a. Assess for oedema of ankles and feet in the ambulant patient.
    b. Assess for oedema of sacral area and posterior thighs in patients confined to bed.
2 Avoid undue pressure on oedematous areas. Oedematous patients are prone to develop pressure sores.

Palpitation

Palpitation is a rapid, forceful or irregular heartbeat felt by the patient.

General Features

1 The patient complains of pounding, jumping, stopping sensations in his chest.
2 May be associated with heart disease—enlargement of heart, disturbances of rhythm.
3 Other causes—anxiety, fever, anaemia, thyroid disturbances, iatrogenic (drug induced).

Nursing Implications

1 Take electrocardiogram (ECG) during episodes of palpitation—to help establish diagnosis.
2 Count radial, carotid and apical pulses. (See Nursing the Patient with an Arrhythmia, p. 32).

Haemoptysis

Haemoptysis is the coughing up of blood.

1 Small quantities of dark, clotted blood—indicate mitral stenosis.
2 Mixture of blood and pus—indicates pulmonary suppuration.
3 Pink, frothy sputum—indicates acute pulmonary oedema.
4 Blood-streaked sputum—indicates acute pulmonary congestion.
5 Frank haemoptysis—due to lung pathology.

Fatigue

1 Fatigue associated with heart disease is produced by low cardiac output.
2 Undue fatigue related to effort—indicates advanced heart disease, congestive heart failure, mitral stenosis.

Syncope and Fainting

1 May be caused by anoxaemia or reduced cardiac output with resulting inadequate circulation.
2 Also seen in arrhythmias, atrioventricular block, carotid-sinus sensitivity.

Cyanosis

Cyanosis is a bluish discoloration of the skin and mucous membranes.

Types of Cyanosis

1 Central cyanosis—low oxygen saturation of arterial blood.
2 Peripheral cyanosis—reduction of oxyhaemoglobin in capillaries from slow circulation—results from reduced cardiac output due to mitral stenosis, pulmonary stenosis, heart failure.

Cardiac Causes of Cyanosis

1 Congenital heart disease—due to mixing of arterial stream with venous blood.
2 Congestive heart failure and pulmonary oedema—due to circulatory hypoxia resulting from circulatory failure.

Nursing Appraisal of Cyanosis

1 Look at lobes of ears, fingernail beds, cutaneous surfaces of the lips, mucous membranes.
2 Give oxygen when indicated.

Abdominal Pain or Discomfort

1 Epigastric (upper abdominal) pain—due to myocardial infarction, distension of liver capsule from congestive heart failure.
2 Severe abdominal pain—may be due to dissecting abdominal aorta, rupture of aortic aneurysm.
3 Intermittent abdominal pain (related to food intake)—indicates circulatory insufficiency of mesenteric arteries.

Other Manifestations of Heart Disease

1 Distension of neck veins—may be produced by pressure on liver (hepatojugular reflux), congestive heart failure, pericardial compression due to effusion or constrictive pericarditis.
2 Clubbing of fingers—due to cyanotic congenital heart disease, bacterial endocarditis, certain forms of lung pathology; may also be familial.
3 Jaundice—congestive heart failure associated with severe liver congestion.

DIAGNOSIS IN HEART DISEASE

This technique is performed by trained nurses working in special units, e.g. coronary care unit (CCU).

Heart Auscultation

1 Heart auscultation requires knowledge, experience and a 'listening ear' tuned to hear each event of the cardiac cycle.
2 Heart auscultation should be systematic.
3 Listen for rate and regularity of rhythm.
   a. Determine if an irregularity is related to respiratory movements.
   b. Evaluate the sequence in which an irregularity occurs.
4 During auscultation, the examiner assesses the venous pulse, feels the pulsation of the right carotid artery and the radial artery, feels precordial movement and listens to the heart (Fig. 1.1).

Cardiac Investigations

1 *Electrocardiogram*—a visual representation of the electrical activity of the heart as reflected by changes in electrical potential at the skin surface.
   a. ECG is obtained by placing leads on various body parts (Fig. 1.2) and recording the electrical impulse as a tracing on a strip of paper or on the screen of an oscilloscope.
   b. Clinical usefulness—evaluation of conditions that interfere with normal

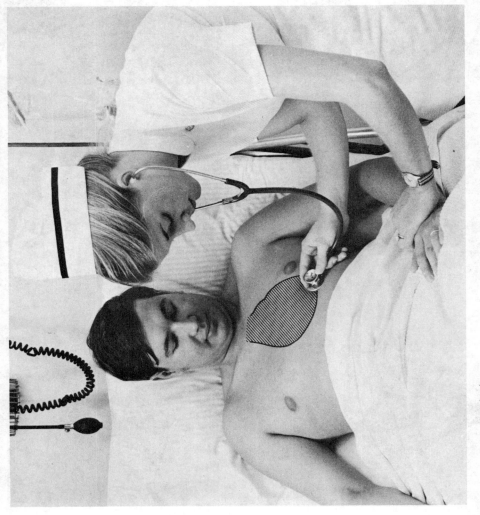

Figure 1.1. Heart auscultation.

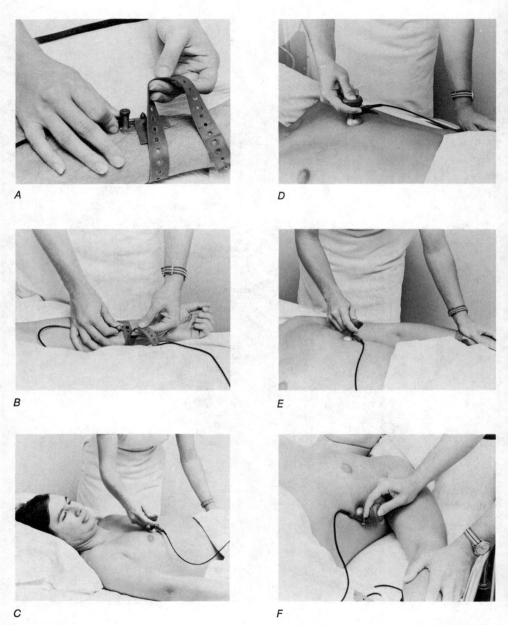

Figure 1.2. a. Lead should be attached securely but not snugly. b. Apply the limb lead to the left arm. c. V1 chest lead. d. V2 chest lead (V3 chest lead is placed slightly to the left of V2 and approximately one interspace lower). e. V4 chest lead. f. V5 chest lead (V6 chest lead would be slightly lower in the midaxillary line).

electrophysiological function—disturbances of rhythm, disorders of cardiac muscle, enlargement of chambers of heart, electrolyte disturbances.

  c. Nursing responsibilities:

    (1) Write information about patient on ECG request—age, blood pressure, symptoms, medications (especially digitalis, antiarrhythmic drugs, diuretics).

    (2; See 87 for a more detailed account of electrocardiography.

2 *Ambulatory electrocardiographic monitoring*—patient wears miniaturized tape-recording device using a single or double lead system attached to belt or worn on a shoulder device.

  a. Various systems are available which record patient's ECG continuously for up to 24 hours while he is going about his daily activities.

  b. Useful in determining the effects of stress, detecting arrhythmias, assessing response to therapy and evaluating patients after myocardial infarction.

3 *Phonocardiogram*—a graphic recording of the occurrence, timing and duration of sounds in the cardiac cycle. (An electrocardiogram may be recorded simultaneously.)

  a. Identifies and differentiates various sounds.

  b. Affords permanent record for future comparison.

  c. No patient preparation required; takes approximately 20 min.

4 *Vectorcardiography*—a method of recording the magnitude and direction of the electrical action of the heart in the form of a vector loop display on a cathode-ray oscilloscope.

5 *Echocardiography (ultrasound cardiography)*—a record of high frequency sound vibrations which have been sent into the heart through the chest wall. The cardiac structures return the echoes derived from the ultrasound. The motions of the echoes are traced on an oscilloscope and recorded on film.

  a. Patient is placed in supine position and the transducer is placed on his chest.

  b. Transducer applied (left sternal border) with ultrasonic gel to maintain airless contact between skin and transducer.

  c. This is a noninvasive, painless technique; no radiation exposure; takes 30–60 min to perform.

  d. *Clinical usefulness*

    (1) Demonstration of valvular and other structural deformities.

    (2) Detection of pericardial effusion.

    (3) Evaluation of prosthetic valve function.

    (4) Diagnosis of cardiac tumours; asymmetrical thickening of interventricular septum.

    (5) Diagnosis of cardiomegaly (heart enlargement).

6 *Exercise tolerance testing*—exercise testing on a treadmill or a bicycle-like device carried out to evaluate circulatory response to stress.

  a. Evaluates capacity for physical performance; evaluates ECG abnormalities that indicate myocardial ischaemia; useful in finding hidden heart conditions.

  b. Patient is exercised by increasing walking speed and the incline of the treadmill or by increasing the load against which he pedals.

Radiological Investigations

1 *Chest x-ray*—shows heart size, contour and position; demonstrates early interstitial pulmonary oedema.

2 *Planigraphy* (body section radiography, tomography)—identifies cardiac contour which may be obscured by regular x-ray; identifies and localizes intracardiac and vascular calcification.

3 *Fluoroscopy*—assesses unusual cardiac contours, cardiac and vascular pulsations on a luminescent x-ray screen. Also useful in verifying position of intravenous pacemaking electrodes and for guidance of catheter in cardiac catheterization.

4 *Cinefluorography*—fluoroscopic image is photographed on motion picture film.

5 *Angiocardiography*—injection of contrast medium into the vascular system (to outline the heart and blood vessels) accompanied by serial x-rays or photographed using high-speed motion picture films; provides information regarding structural abnormalities (occlusions, defects or fistulas or abnormal heart valve function).

   a. *Selective angiocardiography*—contrast medium is injected through a catheter directly into one of the heart chambers, coronary arteries or greater vessels, and the angiocardiogram is recorded by means of a rapid film changer or motion picture camera.

   b. *Aortography*—a form of angiography that outlines the lumen of the aorta and major arteries arising from it.

   In *thoracic aortography* contrast medium is introduced and the aortic arch and its great vessels are studied by means of rapid serial x-rays. The intravenous, translumbar or retrograde approach may be used.

   c. *Nursing implications:*

   (1) Keep the patient in a fasting state prior to the examination.
   (2) Limit patient's activities for approximately 12 hours after procedure.
   (3) Record blood pressure, pulse, respirations every 15 min (or more often as patient's condition indicates) until all are stable.
   (4) Check for bleeding at puncture or cutdown site.
   (5) Patient may complain of mild headache and of discomfort at puncture site.

6 *Coronary arteriography*—a radiopaque catheter is introduced into the right brachial artery via open arteriotomy (or femoral artery via percutaneous puncture), passed into the ascending aorta and manipulated into appropriate coronary artery under fluoroscopic control.

   a. Used as a diagnostic tool before coronary artery surgery or myocardial revascularization and after surgery to evaluate graft patency.

   b. Used to study suspected congenital anomalies of the coronary arteries.

7 *Cardiac catheterization*—catheter(s) is (are) introduced into the heart and blood vessels to (1) measure oxygen concentration, saturation, tension and pressure in the various heart chambers; (2) detect shunts; (3) provide blood samples for analysis; and (4) determine cardiac output and pulmonary blood flow. Angiography is usually combined with heart catheterization for coronary artery visualization.

   a. *Right-heart catheterization*—a radiopaque catheter is passed from an antecubital or femoral vein into the right atrium, right ventricle and pulmonary vasculature under direct visualization with a fluoroscope.

   (1) Right atrium and right ventricle pressures measured; blood samples taken for haematocrit and oxygen saturation.
   (2) Catheter introduced into pulmonary artery and as far as possible beyond

that point; capillary samples and capillary (wedge) pressures are then recorded.

b. *Left-heart catheterization*—may be accomplished using four sites: (1) percutaneous needle puncture of the left atrium, (2) percutaneous needle puncture of left ventricle, (3) transeptal puncture or (4) retrograde catheterization of left ventricle.

(1) Permits flow and pressure measurements (haemodynamic data) of the left heart.

(2) Useful in evaluating status of mitral and aortic valves and coronary arteries.

c. Complications of heart catheterization.

(1) Arrhythmias (ventricular fibrillation), syncope, vasospasm.

(2) Pericardial tamponade, myocardial infarction, pulmonary oedema.

(3) Thrombophlebitis of vein used for catheterization.

(4) Allergic reaction to contrast medium.

(5) Perforation of great vessels of heart; systemic emboli.

(6) Loss of pulse distal to arteriotomy and possible ischaemia of lower arm and hand.

d. *Nursing responsibilities:*

Preceding heart catheterization:

(1) Know which approach is to be used in order to anticipate possible complications.

(2) Withhold food and fluid 6 hours before procedure—to prevent vomiting and aspiration.

(3) Ascertain history of previous allergies.

(4) Explain to the patient that he will be lying on an examining table for a prolonged period and that he may experience certain sensations:

(a) Occasional thudding sensations in the chest—from extrasystoles, particularly when the catheter tip transverses right ventricle.

(b) Strong desire to cough—may occur during dye injection into right heart during angiography.

(c) Transient feeling of heat, particularly in head—from injection of contrast medium.

(5) Remove dentures.

(6) Be sure that patient has received premedication as directed.

Following heart catheterization:

(1) During the procedure the patient is attached to a cardiac monitor. Appropriate resuscitative equipment should be readily available.

(2) Record the blood pressure and apical pulse every 15 min (or more frequently), until stable after the procedure—to detect arrhythmias.

(3) Check peripheral pulses in affected extremity (dorsalis pedis, posterior tibial pulse in the lower extremity and radial pulse in upper extremity); evaluate extremity temperature and colour and complaints of pain, numbness or tingling sensation—to determine signs of arterial insufficiency.

(4) Patient rests in bed until following morning.

(5) Watch puncture (cutdown) sites for haematoma formation. Question patient about increase in pain/tenderness at site.

(6) Assess for complaints of chest pain and report occurrence immediately.

8 *Indicator dilution curves*—injection of dye into one of the heart chambers and the evaluation of its appearance in a peripheral artery.
   a. Gives information concerning presence or absence of intracardiac shunts.
   b. Is a means of calculating cardiac output.
9 *Nuclear study of cardiac output*—a radiopharmaceutical agent is injected into a vein and the appearance of radioactivity over the aorta is monitored by a detector.

Tests of Circulation Time

Circulation time measures the velocity of blood flow and helps diagnose right- and left-heart failure. Two methods are used:

1 Arm-to-tongue—rapid injection (intravenously) of dehydrocholic acid (Decholin) in a peripheral vein. Interval between time when the injection is given and time when the patient complains of a bitter taste is measured with a stopwatch.
2 Arm-to-lung—intravenous injection of either ether or paraldehyde. The end point is reached when the odour of the drug is detected on the patient's breath or when the patient begins to cough.
   a. Normal arm-to-tongue time—8 to 16 s.
   b. Normal arm-to-lung time—4 to 8 s.

Blood Studies

1 *Antistreptolysin titre*—measurement of blood antibodies against streptococcus; shows whether a patient has had a recent infection.
2 *Erythrocyte sedimentation rate*—speed of sedimentation of red cells of blood expressed in millimetres per hour. The rate is elevated when an inflammatory process is present; also used as a test for rheumatic fever. May be reduced in congestive heart failure.
3 *C-reactive protein* (CRP)—a blood test that is a sensitive (but nonspecific) indicator of inflammation of infectious or noninfectious origin.
4 *Blood culture*—test to detect presence of bacteria in circulating blood. Clinical usefulness in cardiology—indicates infective endocarditis.
5 *Blood electrolytes* (potassium, sodium, calcium—to identify patients with heart failure or renal disease (especially if treated with digitalis or diuretics).
6 *Serum enzyme tests*—heart muscle is rich in enzymes which may cause different biochemical reactions.
   a. Serum activity of enzymes increases significantly following myocardial infarction because enzymes are released by injured or dead myocardial cells.
   b. Serum activity of enzymes may also increase as the result of damage to skeletal muscles, liver, brain, kidneys and other organs.
   c. The following enzyme studies are frequently used:*
      (1) Serum lactic dehydrogenase (LDH) (100–225 mU/ml).
      (2) Serum glutamic oxaloacetic transaminase (SGOT) (7–40 mU/ml).
      (3) Serum glutamic pyruvic transaminase (SGPT) (10–40 mU/ml).
      (4) Creatine phosphokinase (CPK) (measures presence of heart muscle

---

* Normal values differ according to type of test used.

damage more specifically since it is found only in myocardium, skeletal muscle and brain tissue):
 Male: 50–325 mU/ml.
 Female: 50–250 mU/ml.
(5) Hydroxybutyric dehydrogenase (HBD) (up to 140 mU/ml).

GUIDELINES: Central Venous Pressure

Central venous pressure (CVP) is the pressure within the right atrium or in the great veins within the thorax.

Purposes

1   To serve as a guide to fluid replacement in seriously ill patients.
2   To estimate blood volume deficits.
3   To determine pressures in the right atrium and central veins.
4   To evaluate for circulatory failure (in context with total clinical picture of patient).

Vein Sites for Catheter Placement

The most commonly used sites are:
 Cephalic or basilic.
 Subclavian.
 External or internal jugular.

Equipment

Venous pressure tray
Cutdown tray
Infusion solution and infusion set
Intravenous pole; arm board; adhesive tape
ECG monitor
Carpenter's level (for establishing zero point)

Procedure (Fig. 1.3)

Doctor's/Nursing Action	Reason
Preparatory Phase	
1 Assemble equipment according to manufacturer's directions.	
2 Explain that the procedure is similar to an intravenous infusion and that the patient may move in bed as desired after the passage of the CVP catheter.	
3 Place the patient in a position of comfort. This is the baseline position used for subsequent readings.	3 Serial CVP readings should be made with the patient in the same position.

Doctor's/Nursing Action

4   Attach manometer to the intravenous pole. The zero point of the manometer should be on a level with the
patient's right atrium. The doctor will
indicate the position.

Reason

4   The right atrium is at the midaxillary line, which is about one-third of
the distance from the anterior to the
posterior chest wall (Fig. 1.3). The
midaxillary line is an external reference point for the zero level of the
manometer (which coincides with
the level of the right atrium).

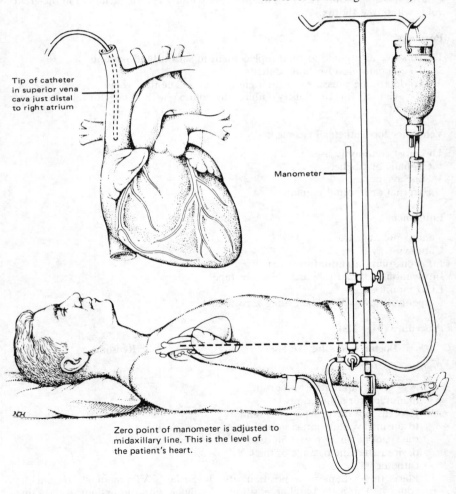

Tip of catheter
in superior vena
cava just distal
to right atrium

Manometer

Zero point of manometer is adjusted to
midaxillary line. This is the level of
the patient's heart.

Figure. 1.3.   Central venous pressure.

Doctor's/Nursing Action	Reason
5 The CVP catheter is connected to a three-way stopcock which communicates with an open intravenous infusion (saline and heparin) and with a manometer (the measuring device).	5 Or, the CVP catheter may be connected to a transducer and an electrical monitor with either digital or calibrated CVP wave readout.
6 Start the intravenous flow and fill the manometer 10 cm above anticipated reading (or until the level of 20 cm H_2O is reached). Turn the stopcock and fill the tubing with fluid.	
7 The CVP site is surgically cleansed. CVP catheter (line) is introduced percutaneously or by direct venous cutdown and threaded through an antecubital, subclavian or internal or external jugular vein into the superior vena cava just before it enters the right atrium.	7 The correct catheter placement can be confirmed by fluoroscopy or chest x-ray or by observing the fluctuations in the manometer with respirations (respiratory swing).
8 When the catheter enters the thorax an inspiratory fall and expiratory rise in venous pressure are observed.	8 The fluid level fluctuates with respiration. It rises sharply with coughing, straining.
9 The patient may be monitored by ECG during catheter insertion.	9 When the tip of the catheter contacts the wall of the right atrium (or right ventricle) it may produce aberrant impulses and disturb cardiac rhythm.
10 The catheter may be sutured and taped in place. A sterile dressing is applied.	10 Label dressing with time and date of catheter insertion.
11 The infusion is adjusted to flow into the patient's vein by a slow continuous drip.	11 The infusion may cause a significant increase in venous pressure if permitted to flow too rapidly.

To Measure the CVP

1 Place patient in the identified position (as mentioned under Preparatory Phase) and confirm the zero point.	1 The zero point or baseline for the manometer should be on a level with the patient's right atrium.
2 Turn the stopcock to open the connection between the patient and the manometer to a level 10–20 cm above the expected reading. Close the flow from the intravenous solution.	2 When the stopcock is turned to connect the manometer to the intravenous catheter, fluid in the manometer column falls until it balances the central venous pressure in the superior vena cava.

Doctor's/Nursing Action	Reason
3 Observe the fall in the height of the column of fluid in manometer. Record the level at which the solution stabilizes. This is the central venous pressure. Record CVP and the position of the patient.	3 The CVP reading is reflected by the height of a column of fluid in the manometer when there is open communication between the catheter and the manometer.
4 The CVP may range from 5–12 cm H_2O. (Absolute numerical values have not been agreed upon.)	4 The change in CVP is a more useful indication of adequacy of venous blood volume and alterations of cardiovascular function. CVP is a dynamic measurement. The normal values may change from patient to patient. The management of the patient is not based on one reading but on repeated serial readings in correlation with patient's clinical state.
5 Turn the stopcock again to allow intravenous solution to flow from solution bottle into patient's veins.	5 When readings are not being made, flow is from a very slow microdrip to the catheter, bypassing the manometer.
6 Assess the patient's clinical condition. Frequent changes in measurements (interpreted within the context of the clinical situation) will serve as a guide to detect whether the heart can handle its fluid load and whether hypovolaemia or hypervolaemia is present.	6 CVP is interpreted by considering the patient's entire clinical picture; hourly urine output, heart rate, blood pressure, cardiac output measurements. a. A CVP near zero indicates that the patient is hypovolaemic (verified if rapid intravenous infusion causes patient to improve). b. A CVP above 15–20 cm H_2O may be due to either hypervolaemia or poor cardiac contractility.
7 Observe the patient for complications. Thrombophlebitis. Sepsis. Embolus or clot at catheter tip.	7 Inspect entry site twice daily, or as directed by doctor, for signs of local inflammation/phlebitis. Inform the doctor immediately if there are any signs of infection.

GUIDELINES: Measuring Pulmonary Artery Pressure by Balloon Flotation Catheter (Swan-Ganz Catheter)

The *Swan-Ganz catheter* permits monitoring of pressure in the pulmonary artery and measurement of pulmonary artery wedge pressure. It gives useful information about intravascular filling volume and cardiac competence. It provides assessment of left heart function, determination of cardiac output and sampling of mixed venous blood.

Purposes

1   To obtain measurements of pressure in the right atrium, right ventricle and pulmonary artery, and in the distal branches of the pulmonary artery. The latter reflects the level of filling pressure in the left ventricle.
2   To permit rational selection of therapy when critical changes in cardiac dynamics occur (cardiogenic shock, heart failure, pulmonary oedema).

Underlying Considerations

1   Left atrial pressure is closely related to left ventricular end-diastolic pressure (filling pressure of the left ventricle) and is therefore an indicator of left ventricular function.
2   Swan-Ganz catheterization permits measurement of pulmonary artery pressure in an occluded vessel. This is called the wedge pressure (provides a good approximation of left atrial pressure).

Equipment

Swan-Ganz catheter set	Syringes: tuberculin; 2.5 ml syringe
ECG; monitor and display unit	Sterile saline solution
Defibrillator	Heparin
Pressure transducer; transducer holder	Lignocaine drip (for standby)
	Local anaesthetic
Cutdown tray	Skin antiseptic

Procedure for Insertion of Swan-Ganz Catheter (performed by doctor)

Preparation

1   Explain procedure to patient as condition allows.
2   Shave and prepare the skin over the insertion site. Cover with sterile towels.
3   Test the catheter under sterile water for balloon leakage.
4   A transducer/monitor for the determination of pressures will be prepared by the doctor.
5   An intravenous infusion will also be required.

Insertion

1   The Swan-Ganz catheter is inserted through an antecubital vein or through an internal jugular vein by either percutaneous puncture or intravenous cutdown. (Other vein, e.g. brachial, subclavian, femoral, may be used.)
2   The catheter is advanced to the superior vena cava. Oscillations of the pressure waveforms will indicate when the tip of the catheter is within the thoracic cavity (Fig. 1.4). (Catheter placement may be determined by fluoroscopy, by evaluation of the pressure waves and also by the markings on the catheter.)
3   When the catheter is in the superior vena cava it is inflated with air and advanced gently. The amount of air to be used is indicated on the catheter.
4   The inflated balloon at the tip of the catheter will be guided by the flowing stream of blood through the right atrium and tricuspid valve into the right ventricle. From this position it finds its way into the main pulmonary artery. (Watch ECG monitor for signs of ventricular irritability as catheter enters the right ventricle.

The balloon will flow from the right atrium to the pulmonary artery in approximately 10–20 s.)

5   The flowing blood will continue to direct the catheter more distally into the pulmonary tree. When the catheter reaches a pulmonary vessel that is approximately the same size or slightly smaller in diameter than the inflated balloon, it cannot be advanced any further. This is the wedge position.

6   The pressure is recorded with the balloon wedged in the pulmonary vascular bed.
a. Normal wedge pressure is less than 12 mmHg.
b. In patients with myocardial infarction the optimal wedge pressures are 15–18 mmHg. In these patients pressures below 15 mmHg may indicate intravascular hypovolaemia, whereas pressures over 18 indicate left ventricular failure (congestive heart failure) in the absence of mitral stenosis.

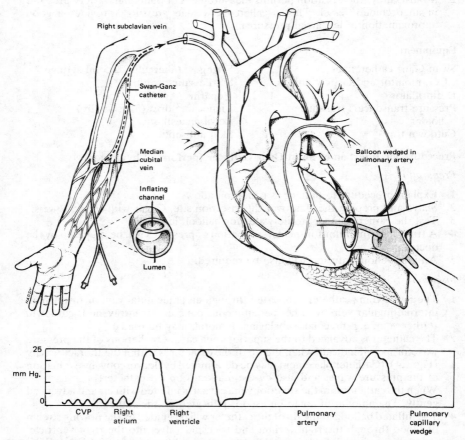

Figure 1.4.   Insertion of a Swan-Ganz catheter. The position of the catheter is reflected by the pressure tracings. Capillary wedge pressure is obtained by inflating the balloon.

7   The balloon is deflated, causing the catheter to retract spontaneously into a larger pulmonary artery. This gives the pulmonary artery pressure reading.
a. The upper limit of normal pressure in the pulmonary artery is approximately 30/12 mmHg.
b. The normal mean pulmonary artery pressure (average pressure in pulmonary artery throughout the entire cardiac cycle) is approximately 10–15 mmHg.
Increased pulmonary artery pressure readings indicate:
Pulmonary hypertension from many causes.
Chronic obstructive pulmonary disease.
Acute respiratory insufficiency.
Long-standing congenital heart disease with large shunts.
Left ventricular failure.
Mitral stenosis.
The causes for decreased pulmonary artery pressure are relatively the same as those for a low wedge pressure.

To Obtain a Wedge Pressure Reading

1   Close off the microdrip. The transducer converts the pressure wave into an electronic wave that is displayed on a screen.
2   Inflate the balloon slowly until the contour of the pulmonary arterial pressure changes to that of pulmonary wedge pressure. As soon as a wedge pattern is observed, no more air is introduced. Do not introduce more air into balloon than specified. Pulmonary capillary wedge pressure is only measured intermittently. Do not allow the catheter to remain in the wedge position for more than 1–2 min.
3   The catheter is secured in position with a ligature. Antibiotic ointment may be placed around the site and covered with a sterile dressing.
4   The catheter is flushed with heparinized saline at prescribed intervals. This prevents clotting at its tip.

For Removal of the Catheter

1   Be sure the balloon is not inflated.
2   The catheter is removed slowly; a pressure dressing is applied over the site. The site should be checked periodically for bleeding.

Complications

1   Pulmonary infarction.
2   Arrhythmias.
3   Thromboembolus.
4   Balloon rupture or knotting of catheter.

SPECIAL MEDICAL AND NURSING MEASURES

GUIDELINES: Assisting the Patient Undergoing Pericardial Aspiration (Pericardiocentesis)

Pericardial aspiration is the puncturing of the pericardial sac in order to aspirate fluid and thereby relieve cardiac tamponade.

Cardiac tamponade is compression of the heart by blood, effusion or a foreign body in the pericardial sac which restricts normal heart action.

Clinical Manifestations of Cardiac Tamponade

1 Rising venous pressure (20 cm H_2O or more).
2 Falling arterial blood pressure.
3 Small, quiet heart; muffled heart sounds (detected by fluoroscopy and chest auscultation).
4 Narrowing pulse pressure (difference between systolic and diastolic pressures).
5 Paradoxical pulse (lessening of pulse amplitude during inspiration).
6 Distension of neck veins and rise in neck veins with inspiration (Kussmaul's sign).
7 Apprehension; dyspnoea.
8 Tachypnoea; pallor or cyanosis.
9 Characteristic posture—sitting upright and leaning forward.
10 Clinical shock.

Purposes

1 To remove fluid from the pericardial sac caused by:
   a. Pericarditis.
   b. Effusion from malignant neoplasm or lymphoma.
   c. Trauma to heart or chest.
   d. Acute rheumatic fever.
   e. Uraemia.
2 To obtain fluid for diagnosis.
3 To instill certain therapeutic drugs.

Equipment

Pericardial aspiration tray
Intracath set
Skin antiseptic, e.g. chlorhexidine 0.5% in spirit
Lignocaine 1 or 2%
Sterile gloves
ECG machine for monitoring purposes
Sterile earth wire—to be connected between pericardial needle and V lead of ECG machine (use alligator clip type connectors)
Apparatus for resuscitation including thoracotomy and pacemaker equipment

Sites for Pericardial Aspiration (Fig. 1.5)

1 Subxiphoid—needle inserted in the angle between left costal margin and xiphoid.
2 Near cardiac apex, 2 cm (0·8 in) inside left border of cardiac dullness.
3 To the left of the fifth or sixth interspace at the sternal margin.
4 Right side of fourth intercostal space just inside border of dullness.

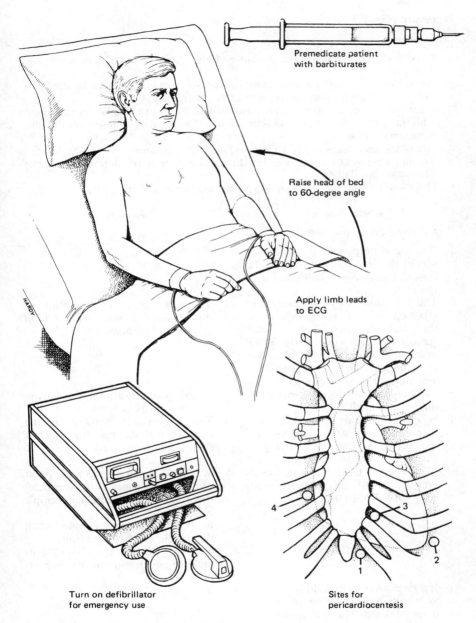

Premedicate patient
with barbiturates

Raise head of bed
to 60-degree angle

Apply limb leads
to ECG

Turn on defibrillator
for emergency use

Sites for
pericardiocentesis

Figure 1.5.   Preparing patient for pericardial aspiration.

Procedure (Fig. 1.5)

Preparation

1 Explain the procedure to the patient and give premedication as ordered, e.g. diazepam.
2 Assist the doctor with the insertion of an intravenous infusion (can be used as a route for intravenous drugs in event of an emergency).
3 Place the patient in a comfortable position with the head of the bed or treatment table raised to a 60° angle. (This position makes it easier to insert needle into pericardial sac.)
4 Apply the limb leads of the ECG machine to the patient.
5 Prepare emergency equipment as directed, e.g. turn on defibrillator, have pacemaker available.
6 Open the pericardial aspirator tray, using aseptic technique.

Nursing Action	Reason
Performance Phase (by doctor)	
1 The site is prepared with skin antiseptic; the area covered with sterile towels. Lignocaine is infiltrated into the area.	
2 The pericardial aspiration needle is attached to a 50 ml syringe by a three-way stopcock. The V lead (precordial lead wire) of the ECG machine is attached to the hub of the aspirating needle by a sterile wire and alligator clips or clamp.	2 There is danger of laceration of myocardium/coronary artery and of cardiac arrhythmias.
3 The needle is advanced slowly until fluid is obtained.	3 Fluid is generally aspirated at a depth of 2.5–4 cm (1–1.5 in).
4 When the pericardial sac has been entered, a haemostat is clamped to the needle at the chest wall just where is penetrates the skin.	4 This prevents movement of the needle and further penetration while fluid is being removed.
5 The patient's ECG monitor, blood pressure and venous pressure must be observed constantly.	5 **a.** The ST segment rises if the point of the needle contacts the ventricle; there may be ventricular ectopic beats. **b.** The PR segment is elevated when the needle touches the atrium. **c.** Large, erratic QRS complexes indicate penetration of the myocardium.
6 If a large amount of fluid is present, an Intracath may be inserted and left in the pericardial sac and attached to a drainage bottle.	

Nursing Action	Reason
7 Watch for presence of bloody fluid. If blood accumulates rapidly, an immediate thoracotomy and cardiorrhaphy (suturing of heart muscle) may be indicated.	7 Bloody pericardial fluid may be due to trauma. Bloody pericardial effusion fluid does not clot, whereas blood obtained from inadvertent puncture of one of the heart chambers *does* clot.

Follow-up Phase

1 Place patient in intensive care unit or cardiac care unit, as available.	1 Following pericardial aspiration careful monitoring of blood pressure and venous pressure will be necessary to indicate possible recurrence of tamponade. A repeated aspiration is then necessary.
2 Watch for rising venous pressure and falling arterial pressure.	2 In the presence of these signs the patient is probably experiencing cardiac tamponade.
3 Call the doctor immediately if observations vary only minimally.	
4 Be prepared for further treatment at all times.	

GUIDELINES: Cardiopulmonary Resuscitation for Cardiac Arrest*

Cardiac arrest is a sudden and unexpected cessation of the heartbeat and effective circulation.

Causes

1 Cardiac:
   a. Ventricular fibrillation.
   b. Ventricular asystole.
2 Asphyxia (drowning, carbon monoxide poisoning, drug overdose, smoke from fires).
3 Anaphylactic reaction (to insects, medications, food).
4 Accidents (electrocution, drowning, inhalation of toxic gases).
5 Surgery.
6 Acute airway obstruction.

Signs and Symptoms

1 Immediate loss of consciousness.
2 Absence of palpable carotid or femoral pulse.
3 Absence of audible heart sounds.

* Adapted from Standards for cardiopulmonary resuscitation (CPR) and emergency cardiac care (ECC), JAMA (1979) (Supplement), 227: No. 7.

4   Absence of breath sounds or air movement through nose or mouth.
5   Convulsions (may or may not be present).
6   Dilation of pupils of eyes.
7   Ashen grey colour.

Purpose

1   To establish *promptly* effective circulation and ventilation.
2   To prevent irreversible cerebral anoxic damage.

Equipment

Trained Personnel

Arrest board
Oral airway
Bag and mask device, e.g. Ambu bag

Defibrillator
Emergency cardiac drugs

Underlying Principles

1   Basic cardiopulmonary resuscitation (CPR) consists of the following ABC sequence: Airway, Breathing and Circulation.
2   Cardiopulmonary resuscitation consists of maintaining an open airway, providing artificial ventilation by means of rescue breathing and providing artificial circulation by external cardiac compression.

Procedure for Cardiopulmonary Resuscitation

Nursing Action	Reason
1 Note the time as soon as the cardiac arrest is determined. Summon help immediately. Place the patient in a horizontal position on a firm surface.	**Nursing Alert: Lack of effective circulation to the central nervous system for more than 3–5 min may result in irreversible damage.**
2 In a witnessed cardiac arrest, a precordial thump may be administered: deliver a single sharp blow over the midportion of the sternum using the fleshy portion of the fist; strike from a distance of 20.3–30.5 cm (8–12 in) above the chest (Fig. 1.6).	2 The precordial thump is useful when the pulse cannot be detected following a witnessed cardiac arrest or when dealing with a patient who is being monitored or is being paced for a known AV block. The precordial thump should be administered within the first minute after cardiac arrest.
3 If patient is not breathing, open the airway and quickly ventilate the lungs four times. (See Artificial Ventilation, which follows.)	
4 Palpate for carotid pulse.	4 Start external cardiac compression immediately if carotid pulse is absent or questionable.

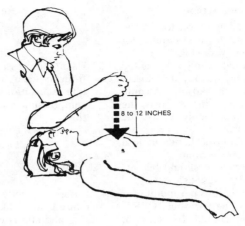

Figure 1.6. Precordial thump.

Nursing Action	**Reason**
Artificial Ventilation	
Carry out artificial ventilation and external cardiac compression *simultaneously*.	
1 Clear airway of material, e.g. saliva, vomit.	
2 Tilt the head back and pull the jaw forward.	2 This manoeuvre lifts the tongue off the back wall of the pharynx and opens the airway.
3 Insert oropharyngeal airway if available.	
4 Ventilate the patient. Inflate the patient's lungs by a forceful expiration of a full breath through a mouth-to-mouth airtight seal. Or ventilate the patient by bag and mask technique.	4 Forceful ventilation helps overcome airway obstruction by increasing the pressure gradient of air movement and dilating the upper airway. With each attempted inflation the patient's chest should rise to a visible degree. Absence of chest expansion indicates airway obstruction.
5 Keep the jaw pulled forward during ventilation to relieve obstruction.	
6 Provide 12 breaths per minute.	

External Cardiac Compression (*must be accompanied by artificial ventilation*)

1 Place the heel of one hand on the lower half of the sternum 3.8 cm (1·5 in) from the tip of the xiphoid and towards the patient's head.	1 Proper placement of the hands reduces possible complications of fractured ribs or injury to adjacent abdominal organs.

Nursing Action	Reason
2 Place the other hand on top of the first one. The fingers should not touch the chest wall (Fig. 1.7).	
3 Using your weight while keeping the elbows straight, quickly and forcefully depress the lower sternum 3.8–5 cm (1.5–2 in) towards the spine and then suddenly release the sternal pressure.	3 Each compression forces the blood from the heart into the arterial system. Relaxation immediately follows compression and is of equal duration.
a. Do not allow the hands to lose contact with the sternum.	
b. The body weight should be carried by the arm muscles.	
4 Use 60 compressions per minute for two persons performing CPR*. Compressions should be smooth, regular and uninterrupted.	4 If done correctly this rate can maintain adequate blood flow and pressure and allows cardiac refill.
5 The second person delivers one deep breath for each five cardiac compressions, without interruption of the compression cycle.	5 If only one person is available, he must give two lung inflations before each 15 chest compressions.
6 Palpate for carotid or femoral pulse periodically and note size of pupils as an indication of response.	6 The presence of a palpable carotid pulse and constriction of pupils are evidence of effective circulation and oxygenated blood. If pupils remain widely dilated and do not react to light and if the patient is deeply unconscious with absence of spontaneous respirations, serious brain damage is imminent or has occurred.
7 While resuscitation proceeds, simultaneous efforts are made to start an intravenous infusion. Have suction ready and attach ECG electrodes to the patient.	
8 The decision to terminate resuscitation is made medically and takes into consideration the cerebral and cardiac state of the patient. Cardiac compression should continue until the patient can maintain blood pres-	8 If ventricular fibrillation occurs, conversion to a normal sinus rhythm must be effected by electric countershock delivered by a defibrillator.

* This procedure is done best by two persons. If only one is available, he must perform both artificial ventilation and external cardiac compression, using a 15:2 ratio consisting of two quick lung inflations after each 15 chest compressions. The single rescuer must perform each series of chest compressions at a faster rate of 80 compressions per minute because of interruptions for lung inflation.

Nursing Action	Reason

sure, etc., or the situation becomes
hopeless.

9   Drug therapy—see Table 1.1 for
major drugs commonly used in cardiopulmonary resuscitation.

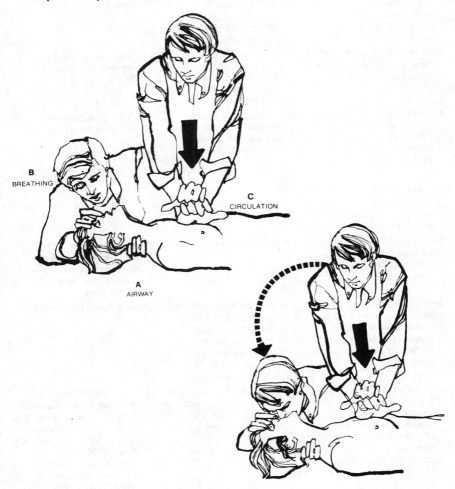

Figure 1.7.   Two-rescuer cardiopulmonary resuscitation: Five chest compressions—rate of
60/minute, no pause for ventilation; one lung inflation—after each five compressions, interposed between compressions. One-rescuer cardiopulmonary resuscitation: 15 chest compressions—rate of 80/minute.

Table 1.1. Major Drugs Commonly Used in Cardiopulmonary Resuscitation

Drugs and Dosages	Major Effects	Indications
Adrenaline: 0.5–1.0 ml of 1:1000 solution (0.5–1.0 mg) administered intravenously or intracardially; repeat every 5 min if needed	Positive inotropic, positive chronotropic and pressor effects; makes fine fibrillation coarse and thereby facilitates defibrillation	1. Ventricular asystole 2. Ventricular fibrillation (fine)
Isoprenaline: 2 mg in 500 ml dextrose 5% at 2–4μg/min (i.e., 0.5–1.0 ml/min)	Positive inotropic and positive chronotropic effects; causes vasodilation rather than vasoconstriction	1. Ventricular asystole 2. Speeds up a slow AV block
Calcium chloride: 5–10 ml (0·5–1·0 g) of 10% solution administered slowly, intravenously, over a period of 5 min or Calcium gluconate: 10–20 ml of 10% solution (1–2 g), administered slowly, intravenously	Positive inotropic and chronotropic effects; use with caution in patients receiving Digoxin	1. Ventricular asystole 2. Ventricular fibrillation (fine)
Atropine: 0.5 mg administered every 5 min, to a total of 2 mg, intravenously	Decreases vagal tone	Slow cardiac rate with supraventricular rhythm, if accompanied by hypotension or ventricular escape beats
Sodium bicarbonate: 1 mEq/kg of body weight within 2 min of cardiac arrest; repeat every 10 min in the absence of functional circulation	Combats acidosis produced by inadequate tissue perfusion; too much bicarbonate can lead to plasma alkalosis and hyperosmolality with cerebral acidosis	Absent functional circulation
Lignocaine: 1–2 mg per kg body weight in bolus doses administered intravenously; 4 g in 1000 ml (4:1 drip) as continuous intravenous drip at 2–4 mg/min for maintenance	Raises fibrillation threshold and increases the electrical stimulation threshold of the ventricle during diastole	1. Ventricular fibrillation resistant to direct current defibrillation or successful defibrillation reverting repeatedly to fibrillation 2. Control of multifocal ventricular premature beats and episodes of ventricular tachycardia
Procainamide HCl: 50–100 mg/min administered intravenously, reaching a maximum of 1 g in 15 min	Raises fibrillation threshold; slows conduction, and decreases excitability of the ventricles	Same as for lignocaine

Adapted from Vijay, N K, and Schoonmaker, F W: Major drugs commonly used in cardiopulmonary resuscitation. Published in the August 1975 issue of American Family Physician.

GUIDELINES: Direct Current Countershock Procedure for Ventricular Fibrillation

Countershock is the use of electrical discharge to patient's chest wall to terminate ventricular fibrillation.

A *defibrillator* is an instrument that delivers an electric shock to the heart to convert ventricular fibrillation to normal sinus rhythm. (Defibrillators are also used to convert other abnormal cardiac rhythms).

Purpose

To terminate ventricular fibrillation.

Equipment

DC defibrillator with paddles
Conduction jelly (electrode gel) or saline soaked 4 × 4 gauze swabs
Resuscitative equipment

NOTE: The technique of defibrillation is performed by the medical staff. Nurses working in special units, e.g. CCU or ITU, are trained to use a defibrillator and are allowed to do so.

Procedure

Nursing Action	Reason
1 Expose the patient's anterior chest.	1 This procedure should be carried out immediately after ventricular fibrillation is detected to minimize cerebral and circulatory deterioration.
2 Start cardiopulmonary resuscitation immediately.	2 Cardiopulmonary resuscitation is essential before and after defibrillation to assure blood supply to the cerebral and coronary arteries.
3 A second person should turn on the defibrillator to the prescribed setting.	3 The shock is measured in Watt seconds or joules—from 50 to 400.
4 Apply electrode paste (or saline pads) liberally to the paddle electrodes.	4 The electrode paste helps to provide better contact and prevents skin burns. Do not allow any paste on the skin between electrodes. If the paste areas touch, the current may short circuit, severely burning the patient, and may not penetrate the heart.
5 Apply one electrode just to the right of the upper sternum below the clavicle and the other electrode	5 If anteroposterior paddles are used, the anterior paddle is held with pressure on the middle sternum

Nursing Action	Reason
just to the left of the cardiac apex or left nipple (Fig. 1.8).	while the patient lies on the posterior paddle under the left infrascapular region. With this method the countershock more directly traverses the heart.
6 Grasp the paddles only by the insulated handles.	
7 GIVE THE COMMAND TO STAND CLEAR OF THE PATIENT AND THE BED.	7 If a person touches the bed, he may act as a ground for the current and receive a shock.
8 Push the discharge buttons in both paddles simultaneously.	
9 Remove the paddles from the patient *immediately* after the shock is administered.	

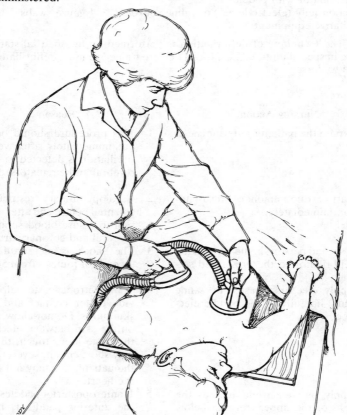

Figure 1.8. Paddle placement in ventricular defibrillation.

Nursing Action	Reason
10 Resume cardiopulmonary resuscitation efforts.	10 After discharge of the countershock, CPR efforts should be resumed. Total delay should be no more than 5 s in order to oxygenate the patient and restore circulation.
11 Further shocks may be necessary either immediately or after appropriate drug therapy.	

GUIDELINES: Application of Rotating Tourniquets

Rotating tourniquets refers to a technique whereby tourniquets are systematically rotated on the extremities to remove a volume of blood from the central circulation in order to decrease venous return and reduce acute pulmonary oedema.

Purpose

To pool the blood temporarily in the extremities in order to reduce venous return to the heart.

Underlying Principles

1 Three of the four extremities are compressed while one extremity is usually free at all times.
2 No single extremity should be compressed continuously for more than 45 min.
3 Tourniquets may have to be rotated at 5-min intervals on the elderly patient to prevent gangrene and other complications.
4 These principles are important since they can reduce the risks of phlebothrombosis and fatal pulmonary embolism.

Equipment

Equipment for extremity compression
   4 sphygmomanometer cuffs or
   4 tourniquets, 61 cm (2 ft) long with outside diameter 0.8–3.8 cm (0.312–1.5 in)
   or
   equipment designed to inflate and deflate blood pressure cuffs automatically (Danzer apparatus)
Small towels
Watch—to note time interval
Work sheet

Procedure

Nursing Action	Reason
Performance phase (Fig. 1.9)	
1 Explain to the patient (if his condition permits) the purpose of the	1 To relieve anxiety.

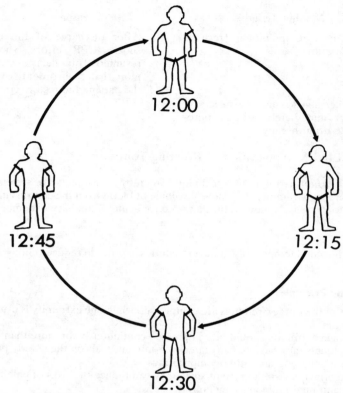

Figure 1.9.   One method of rotating tourniquets. This illustration shows a clockwise pattern.

Nursing Action	Reason
compression and that the skin of the extremities may become discoloured.	
2 Take the blood pressure.	2 Initial blood pressure reading serves as a baseline for future comparison.
3 Apply the four blood pressure cuffs (or Danzer apparatus if available) to extremities and inflate three to a pressure less than the systolic blood pressure.	3 Venous flow must be occluded but arterial flow must not be impeded.
4 Apply tourniquets as high as possible on three extremities. Place tourniquets over gown or small towel in a definite rotation pattern.	4 Tourniquet should be placed in such a way that the arterial pulse can be palpated. One extremity should be free of a tourniquet during each time interval.

Nursing Action	Reason
5 Release one tourniquet every 15 min. Then apply a tourniquet to the previously free extremity.	5 The venous outflow in any one extremity will be occluded for 45 min and unoccluded for 15 min. The time interval may be shorter if the patient's condition indicates.
6 Rotate tourniquets in a definite clockwise pattern.	
7 Monitor blood pressure every few minutes after tourniquets have been applied.	7 Application of tourniquets may precipitate hypotension in some patients.
8 Measure urinary output at frequent intervals. Usually an indwelling catheter is used.	8 Watch for sudden reduction in plasma volume with hypotension and oliguria after administration of rapid-acting diuretics, e.g. ethacrynic acid, frusemide.
9 Remove one tourniquet at a time according to the specified time interval (usually 15 min) at the completion of the rotation.	9 Releasing the tourniquets one at a time prevents a sudden increase in circulatory blood volume and thus prevents circulatory overload.

Follow-up Phase

Record starting time of procedure, rotation intervals, clinical response, medications given and the time tourniquets were discontinued.

CARDIAC ARRHYTHMIAS

Arrhythmia is a clinical disorder to the heart beat; it may include a disturbance of rate, rhythm (sequence), or both. Arrhythmias are derangements of heart function and not of heart structure.

Aetiology

1 Arrhythmias due to organic heart disease:
   a. Inflammatory heart disease.
   b. Degenerative heart disease (atherosclerosis).
   c. Congenital heart disease.
   d. Hypertensive heart disease.
2 Arrhythmias due to disturbances of other organ systems:
   a. Disease of central nervous system—from sympathetic and vagal stimulation.
   b. Pulmonary disease.
   c. Endocrine disorders (hyper- and hypothyroidism, hypoglycaemia, diabetic ketoacidosis).
   d. Gastrointestinal disorders (fluid and electrolyte imbalance).
   e. Renal disorders (renal failure).

3   Arrhythmias from other causes:
   a. Drugs (digitalis intoxication, quinidine, procainamide).
   b. Infection.
   c. Disturbances of electrolyte balance.
   d. Anaemia.
   e. Following cardiac surgery.

Classification of Arrhythmias Based on Disturbed Physiology

1   Disturbance of impulse formation—heartbeat activated for one or more beats by a pacemaker other than the SA node.
2   Disturbances of conduction—due to delayed transmission of impulse, the failure of some impulses to be conducted or to a block at the affected site.
3   Combined disorders—combination of abnormally rapid impulse formation and decreased ability to conduct the impulses.

Clinical Manifestations

Depends on ventricular rate, condition of heart and patient's psychological reaction.

1   Symptoms and signs of rapid arrhythmias:
   a. Palpitation.
   b. Dizziness and fainting.
   c. Throbbing in head and neck.
   d. Shortness of breath.
   e. Precordial discomfort and pain.
   f. Anxiety.
2   Symptoms and signs of slow heart action (bradyarrhythmia/bradycardia)
   a. Shortness of breath.
   b. Fatigue on exertion.
   c. Dizziness and fainting—may indicate syncopal attacks, leading to convulsive seizures.

Clinical Effects

1   Some arrhythmias are relatively harmless while others are forerunners of cardiac arrest.
2   Cardiac arrhythmias can reduce cardiac output, lower the blood pressure and decrease blood perfusion of the brain, heart, kidneys, gastrointestinal tract, muscles and skin.
3   Cardiac arrhythmias often produce attacks of transient cerebral ischaemia with complete stroke.
4   Arrhythmias can precipitate congestive heart failure or angina pectoris in certain patients.
5   Bradyarrhythmias/bradycardia (rate below 60) predispose to electrical instability of the heart.
6   A marked degree of disability may accompany an arrhythmia.

Nursing Assessment

1   How does the patient describe his symptoms?
2   What is the duration and frequency of the arrhythmia?
3   Evaluate the patient's general appearance: pallor, cyanosis, sweating—may indicate peripheral arteriolar constriction.
4   Observe carotid pulsation: Rapid and vigorous? Irregular with varying amplitude?
5   Listen to the heartbeat with a stethoscope.
   a. Listen for rate, presence of irregularity, increase in intensity of first heart sound.
      (1) 30 beats or lower—complete AV block, partial AV block or sinus bradycardia.
      (2) 40–60 beats/min—varying degrees of AV block, sinus bradycardia.
      (3) 60–110 beats/min—sinus arrhythmia, premature beats, AV heart block, atrial fibrillation, atrial flutter, atrial tachycardia with block.
      (4) 140–180 beats/min—atrial tachycardia, atrial flutter, junctional or ventricular tachycardia.
   b. If possible have an ECG taken during an episode of arrhythmia.
   c. Take the blood pressure and pulse—distal pulses give clue to heart's ability to perfuse the periphery.
6   Take respiratory rate: note depth and effort.
7   Evaluate for:
   a. Mental confusion with arrhythmia—indicates cerebral ischaemia.
   b. Presence of signs and symptoms of congestive heart failure—may indicate arrhythmia causing serious effect.
   c. Chest pains with arrhythmia—due to myocardial ischaemia.
   d. Weakness.
8   Use portable cardiac monitoring for persons with suspected arrhythmias (patients with dizzy spells, palpitations, chest pain) and to evaluate antiarrhythmic therapy.
   a. One lead sensor is taped to patient's chest and connected to portable recording equipment. Recorder is started.
   b. Patient goes about his daily routine while keeping a diary of times and activities during which he feels his symptoms.
   c. After 8–24 hours the tape is put through a scanner for oscilloscope reading (computer scanning now available).
9   See p. 95–118 for a complete discussion of the most common arrhythmias and their treatment.

Cardiac Pacing

A *pacemaker* is an electronic device that provides repetitive electrical stimuli to the heart muscle for the control of heart rate. It initiates and maintains the heart rate when the natural pacemakers of the heart are unable to do so.

Underlying Principles

1   Pacemakers consist of two component parts: (1) the pacemaker pulse generator (the power source) and (2) the pacemaker electrodes (the transmitter of the pacing impulse).
2   For temporary pacing, the pulse generator is outside the body (Fig. 1.10). For permanent pacing, the pulse generator is implanted within the body (Fig. 1.11).
3   The stimuli from the pacemaker travel through catheter electrodes (wire) that are threaded through a vein into the right ventricle or are introduced by direct penetration of the chest wall or via a subcutaneous tunnel from implanted units.

Clinical Indications

1   Heart block (especially those complicated by Stokes-Adams syndrome).
2   Bradycardias; tachycardias.
3   Arrhythmias and conduction defects following acute myocardial infarction.
4   Following open heart surgery; during coronary arteriography.

Types of Pacemakers

1   *Demand (standby; noncompetitive)*—most commonly used; has the advantage of working only when the heart rate goes below a certain level. Therefore it does not compete with the heart's basic rhythm. It stimulates the heart when a normal ventricular depolarization does not occur or if heart rate drops below a specified rate.
2   *Fixed rate (asynchronous; competitive)*—this unit stimulates the ventricle at a preset constant rate that is independent of the patient's rhythm. However, it can compete with the patient's own rhythm. May be used in patients with complete and unvarying heart block.

Approaches to Pacemaker Implantation

1   *Temporary transvenous pacing*—insertion of catheter electrode threaded through a vein into the apex of the right ventricle under the guidance of an image intensifier; the distal electrode is connected to a negative terminal of a battery-powered external pacemaker (Fig. 1.10).
   a. The catheter electrode is secured in the vein with suture.
   b. Antibiotic ointment is applied around the incision and catheter.
   c. Catheter electrode position confirmed by x-ray.
   d. Patient placed in cardiac care unit for monitoring.
      (1) Temporary pacing may be done for hours, days or weeks; it is continued until patient improves or a permanent pacemaker is implanted.
      (2) Improves cardiac output and coronary, cerebral and renal blood flow.
      (3) Controls ventricular tachycardia and fibrillation.
      (4) Allows complete control of heart rate during surgery.
      (5) Permits observation of effects of pacing on heart function so that optimum pacing rate for the patient can be selected before permanent pacemaker is implanted.
2   *Permanent pacemakers:*
   a. *Transvenous*—electrodes (unipolar or bipolar) are threaded through cephalic

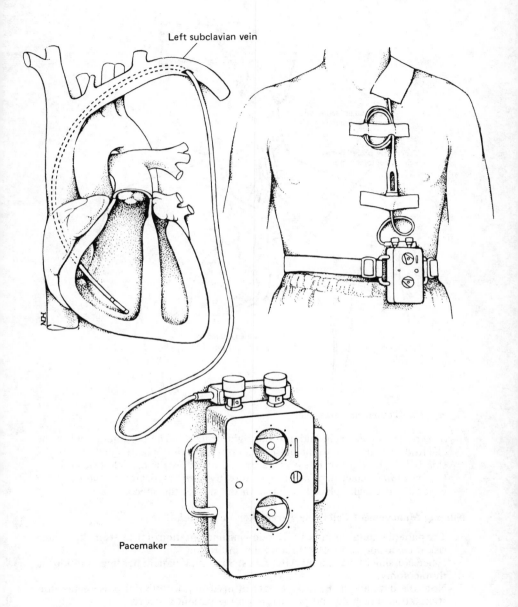

Figure 1.10.   Temporary pacemaker: the transvenous catheter electrode is attached to a battery-powered external pacemaker. The catheter is wedged in the apex of the right ventricle.

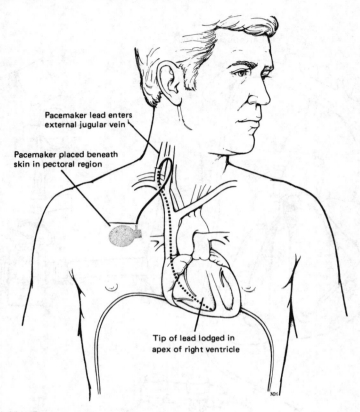

Pacemaker lead enters
external jugular vein

Pacemaker placed beneath
skin in pectoral region

Tip of lead lodged in
apex of right ventricle

Figure 1.11.   Permanent pacemaker.

or external jugular vein and into the right ventricle. The peripheral end of the electrode is connected to the pulse generator which is implanted underneath the skin below the right or left pectoral region or below the clavicle (Fig. 1.11).
b. *Epicardial*—electrodes are applied directly to the myocardium and the pulse generator is usually placed underneath the skin of the subcostal area.

Nursing Management Following Pacemaker Implantation

1   The patient is monitored by ECG following implantation of the pacemaker—high risk if electrode is displaced soon after insertion.
    See Nursing Management After Chest Surgery, if patient has implantation via thoracotomy.
2   Note the data about the model, date of insertion, location of pulse generator, stimulation threshold and pacer rate on the patient's record.
    a. Place a card at the head of the bed indicating that the patient has a pacemaker.
    b. Make sure the preset pacemaker rate remains constant.

3   Keep the intravenous infusion running—to have a readily accessible vein in the event of an arrhythmia and to combat dehydration.
4   Make sure all equipment is earthed with three-pronged plugs inserted into a proper outlet—improperly earthed equipment can generate currents capable of producing ventricular fibrillation.

NOTE: A clinical engineer, electrician or other qualified person should make certain that the patient is in an electrically safe environment.

5   Inspect the incision site under the pressure dressings for bleeding and haematoma.
6   Observe the vein through which the pacing catheter has been placed for evidence of phlebitis.
7   Give analgesic drugs to relieve pain.

Complications

1   *Complications arising from the presence of the pacemaker within the body:*
    a. Local infection (sepsis or haematoma formation)—occurs at the site of venous cutdown or subcutaneous pacemaker placement.
    b. Arrhythmias; ventricular ectopic activity—from irritation of the ventricular wall by the electrode. (Pacemakers can create baffling arrhythmias).
    c. Perforation of myocardium or right ventricle by catheter.
    d. High ventricular threshold—may cause abrupt loss of pacing.
2   *Complications from pacemaker malfunction:*
    a. Failure in one or more components of the pacing system.
    b. Battery exhaustion.
    c. Breakage or dislocation of the electrode catheter(s).

Health Teaching

1   Physical activity does not usually have to be curtailed because of an implanted pacemaker.
2   Inform the patient that the present conventional pacemakers must be surgically removed and replaced approximately every 4–5 years* because the batteries wear out and must be replaced. The procedure usually requires a local anaesthetic.
3   Give the patient the manufacturer's instructions (for his particular pacemaker) and help him to become familiar with his pacemaker.
4   Encourage patient to have regular pacemaker checkup (preferably at a pacemaker clinic) for monitoring function and integrity of his pacemaker.
5   Teach the patient to check his own pulse rate daily. Report *immediately* any sudden slowing of pulse greater than 4–5 beats/min or any increase in pulse rate.
6   Report signs and symptoms of dizziness, fainting, palpitation, chest pain to doctor immediately—indicative of pacemaker failure.
7   See that the patient has a copy of his ECG tracing (according to policy of doctor)—for future comparisons so that rate changes and decreases in amplitude may be noted.

8   Advise patient to avoid working with faulty electrical equipment, poorly earthed equipment or devices that may cause electrical interference (diathermy, electrocautery, radar, ignition systems of motors).
9   Advise patient to wear loose-fitting clothing around the area of pacemaker implantation until healing has taken place.
10   Encourage patient to wear identification bracelet that lists his pacemaker type, rate, doctor's name and the hospital where the pacemaker was inserted.

ATHEROSCLEROTIC HEART DISEASE

Angina Pectoris

Angina pectoris is a clinical syndrome characterized by paroxysms of pain or oppression in the anterior chest produced as a result of insufficient blood flow and myocardial hypoxia.

Altered Physiology

Atherosclerosis of major vessels → CRITICAL OBSTRUCTION WITH DIMINUTION OF CORONARY BLOOD FLOW → decreased myocardial oxygen delivery in response to myocardial oxygen demand → anginal pain. Disparity between myocardial oxygen supply and demand.

Aetiology

1   Usually due to atherosclerotic heart disease—is almost invariably associated with a significant obstruction of a major coronary artery.
2   May be from severe aortic stenosis or insufficiency, aortitis, hyperthyroidism, anaemia, tachycardia.

Clinical Manifestations

Pain—probably caused by metabolic changes produced by ischaemia.

1   *Location*—behind middle or upper third of sternum (retrosternal) felt deep in chest. Patient may make a fist over site of pain.
2   *Radiation*—usually radiates to neck, jaw, shoulders and upper extremities (on left side more often than on right).
     a. Frequently may be localized.
     b. Patient often experiences tightness, choking or a strangling sensation.
3   *Character*—constrictive, oppressive, strangling, vice-like, insistent.
     a. May be mild to severe.
     b. May produce numbness or weakness in arms, wrist, hands.
     c. Accompanied by severe apprehension and feeling of impending death.
4   *Duration*—attack usually lasts less than 3 min.
     Attacks occurring when patient is at rest—persist 5–15 min.

Nursing Alert: Suspect an impending myocardial infarction if anginal pain lasts more than 20–30 min.

5 *Factors precipitating pain:*
   a. Exertion.
   b. Exposure to cold.
   c. Eating a heavy meal.
   d. Emotion and excitement.

Treatment and Nursing Management

Objectives

To reduce the discrepancy between myocardial oxygen demands and the available supply of oxygen.
To relieve pain.
To prevent myocardial infarction.

Activity Considerations

1 Reduce activity to below the point where anginal pain occurs.
2 Remove precipitating or contributing factors that cause symptoms.
3 Reduce walking speed; take more time for dressing; eat lighter meals, etc.
4 See Health Teaching, p. 42.

Drug Therapy to Prevent Myocardial Ischaemia

1 *Glyceryl trinitrate (GNT):*
   a. GNT (mainstay of treatment) produces coronary artery dilatation, peripheral artery dilatation and peripheral vein dilatation—reduces myocardial oxygen consumption and myocardial work.
   b. GNT should be taken *before* pain develops. The patient regulates the drug usage, taking the smallest dose that relieves pain.
   c. GNT is usually given sublingually (under tongue).
      (1) Pain relief begins in 1–3 min; prompt response to GNT usually distinguishes cardiac from noncardiac pain.
      (2) Dosage may be repeated at 5-min intervals for a total of three doses. Call doctor immediately if no relief is obtained.
      (3) Note how long it takes for relief of pain. A record should be kept of number of tablets taken to evaluate any change in anginal pattern.
      (4) GNT should be used prophylactically to avoid pain known to occur with certain activities (stair climbing, sexual intercourse, exposure to cold).
      (5) Side-effects: hypotension, dizziness, syncope, pounding headache; these symptoms usually subside after drug has been taken for an extended period.
2 *Other sublingual nitrates:*
   a. Isosorbide dinitrate (Isordil).
   b. Erythrityl tetranitrate (Cardilate).
3 *Beta-adrenergic blocking drugs*—to decrease myocardial oxygen need:
   a. Propranolol hydrochloride (Inderal)—reduces oxygen consumption by blocking sympathetic impulses to the heart. This produces a reduction in heart rate, systemic blood pressure and myocardial contractility which is associated with a

decrease in myocardial oxygen consumption. This allows patient to work or exercise while requiring less myocardial oxygen delivery.

b. Given daily in divided doses; dosage variable according to patient's cardiac status.

c. Side-effects: fatigue, hypotension, severe bradycardia, mental depression; may precipitate congestive heart failure.

d. Take blood pressure and heart rate with patient in upright position 2 hours after administration to assess for postural hypotension.

e. Do not give if pulse rate drops below 50/min.

f. Propranolol also used in conjunction with sublingual isosorbide dinitrate for anti-anginal and anti-ischaemia prophylaxis.

g. Exercise ECG testing may be used to determine when optimal therapy has been achieved.

4 *Sedatives and tranquillizers*—may be used to prevent attacks precipitated by aggravation, excitement, or tension, e.g. diazepam.

Other Considerations

1 Correct other problems in order to decrease oxygen demands of myocardium—hypertension, hyperthyroidism, aortic stenosis, anaemia.

2 Evaluate for development of unstable angina (recurrent crescendo patterns of pain).

a. Bed rest—patient may be admitted to CCU for monitoring for impending infarction.

b. Combined administration of propranolol and sublingual isosorbide dinitrate may be effective.

c. Support patient having coronary arteriography to decide if surgical intervention is advisable.

3 Prepare for surgical intervention (revascularization by vein or artery bypass procedure to bring a new blood supply to ischaemic myocardium when symptoms cannot be controlled). (See p. 78.)

Health Teaching

Instruct the patient as follows:

1 Use moderation in all activities.

a. Participate in a normal daily routine whose activities do not produce chest discomfort, shortness of breath and undue fatigue.

b. Avoid activities known to cause anginal pain—sudden exertion, walking against the wind, extremes of temperature, high altitude, emotionally stressful situations; may accelerate heart rate, raise blood pressure and increase cardiac work.

c. Avoid overeating. Refrain from engaging in physical activity for 1 hour after meals. Rest after each meal if possible.

d. Do not undertake activities requiring heavy effort (carrying heavy objects).

e. Try to avoid cold weather if possible; dress warmly and walk more slowly. Wear scarf over nose and mouth when in cold air.

f. Reduce weight if necessary to reduce cardiac load.

g. Avoid caffeine-containing drinks (coffee)—can produce arrhythmias in susceptible persons.

h. Stop smoking—inhaled carbon monoxide decreases the blood's oxygen-carrying ability and increases severity of anginal attacks.

i. Engage in a regular graded programme of prescribed exercise; keep exercise below level of pain threshold—improves exercise tolerance, produces decrease in blood lipids, improves feeling of well-being.

j. Modify attitudes and living habits to adapt to life stresses.

2   Use prescribed GNT effectively.

   a. Carry GNT at all times.

     (1) GNT is volatile and is inactivated by heat, moisture, air, light and time.

     (2) Keep GNT in original dark glass container, tightly closed—to prevent absorption of drug by other pills or pillbox.

     (3) Do not carry GNT in a plastic or metal pillbox or mixed with other pills.

     (4) Renew supply every 3 months (nonstabilized) and every 6–12 months (stabilized form).

     (5) GNT should cause a slight burning sensation under the tongue when it is potent.

   b. Place GNT under tongue at first sign of chest discomfort.

     (1) Stop and rest until all discomfort subsides—relief should be obtained within a few minutes.

     (2) Do not swallow saliva until tablet is dissolved.

     (3) Bite the tablet between front teeth and slip under tongue to dissolve if quick action is desired.

     (4) Repeat dosage in a few minutes for total of three tablets if relief is not obtained.

     (5) Keep a record of number of tablets taken—to evaluate any change in anginal pattern.

     (6) Take GNT prophylactically to avoid pain known to occur with certain activities.

3   If taking propranolol HCl (Inderal), do not interrupt therapy without first consulting the doctor—abrupt withdrawal can produce exacerbation of angina; myocardial infarction.

4   Call doctor immediately if chest pain becomes more intense or prolonged and if it is brought on more easily.

Myocardial Infarction (MI)

Myocardial infarction refers to the process by which myocardial tissue is destroyed in regions of the heart that are deprived of their blood supply after closure of the coronary artery or one of its branches, either by a thrombus or by obstruction of the vessel lumen by atherosclerosis. There is an imbalance between myocardial oxygen supply and demand.

Incidence of Cardiovascular Disease in the UK

In the past three decades the incidence of cardiovascular disease in the UK has risen at a steady rate and now accounts for 250 000 deaths per annum. Approximately

180 000 (70%) of these deaths are attributable to the effects of coronary artery disease, and of this number, 50% are sudden deaths (MI). Almost half the number of deaths occur in people who have had no recognizable manifestations of ischaemic heart disease.

Causes

1   Atherosclerotic heart disease—coronary artery disease with proximal obstruction to coronary flow in one or more major vessels.
2   Coronary artery embolism.
3   Decreased coronary blood flow with shock/haemorrhage.

Clinical Manifestations

1   Chest pain—steady, constrictive pain (central portion of chest and epigastrium) not relieved by rest or nitrates; pain may radiate widely; may produce arrhythmias, hypotension, shock, cardiac failure.
2   Profuse perspiration; moist, clammy skin with pallor.
3   Drop in blood pressure.
4   Dyspnoea, weakness and fainting.
5   Nausea and vomiting.
6   Anxiety and restlessness.
7   Tachycardia or bradycardia.

Nursing Alert: Many patients do not have symptoms; these are the 'silent coronaries'. Nevertheless there is still resultant damage to the myocardium.

Diagnosis

1   Clinical history and findings from physical examination.
2   ECG changes; abnormal Q waves, ST segment and T wave changes—*some patients have no changes on initial ECG tracing*.
3   Serum enzyme or isoenzyme alterations—certain enzymes in the heart muscle are released into blood when myocardium is infarcted; the larger the infarct the greater the enzyme response.
    a. Serial estimations of creatinine phosphokinase (CPK) and lactic dehydrogenase (LDH)—infarct size can be estimated by increases in these enzymes.
    b. SGOT and HBD may also be increased (see p. 13).

Treatment and Nursing Management (Fig. 1.12)

Objectives

To prevent death from arrhythmia, asystole and cardiogenic shock.
To limit the size of the infarct.
To provide healing for the myocardium.
To facilitate rehabilitation.

To Provide Constant Nursing Surveillance During the Critical Stage of the Illness

1   Admit patient to cardiac care unit for constant monitoring and aggressive early

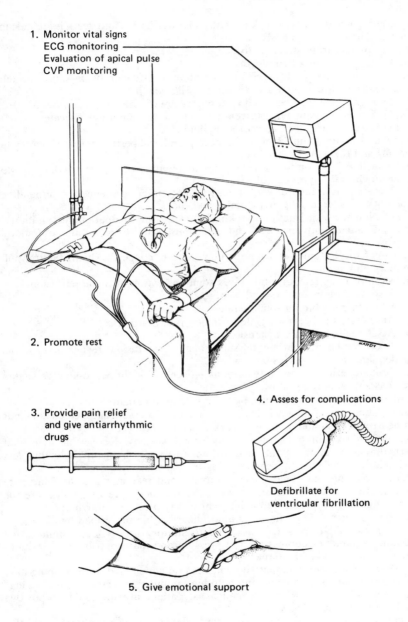

1. Monitor vital signs
   ECG monitoring
   Evaluation of apical pulse
   CVP monitoring

2. Promote rest

3. Provide pain relief
   and give antiarrhythmic
   drugs

4. Assess for complications

Defibrillate for
ventricular fibrillation

5. Give emotional support

Figure 1.12.   Myocardial infarction.

treatment of arrhythmias—risk of ventricular fibrillation and death is greatest in first few hours following MI.

a. Lift patient from stretcher to bed.

b. Place in position of comfort.

c. Be vigilant for occurrence of premature ventricular beats—may foretell ventricular tachycardia and ventricular fibrillation.

(1) Lignocaine may be given to suppress premature ventricular beats.

(2) Prepare patient for transvenous pacing if his condition indicates.

(3) See p. 32 for discussion of arrhythmias.

2 Provide continuing nursing assessment of peripheral perfusion (blood supply to organs and tissues).

a. Attach ECG monitoring electrodes to monitor the heart rhythm and to confirm clinical impression of MI.

b. Measure and record vital signs—to determine presence of impending complications, especially arrhythmias and shock.

(1) Note on record method of taking blood pressure (palpation/auscultation).

(2) Evaluate both apex beat and radial pulse rates. Note strength of femoral pulse.

c. Count respirations—tachypnoea may indicate congestive heart failure, pulmonary embolism.

d. Monitor body temperature—gives some indication of tissue perfusion.

e. Assess skin temperature and colour.

f. Auscultate for breath sounds, rales.

g. Auscultate the heart for gallop, friction rub, murmurs.

h. Assess neck veins for distension.

i. Assess for changes in mental state (apathy, confusion, restlessness)—from inadequate cerebral perfusion.

j. Evaluate urine output (30 ml/hour)—decrease in urine volume reflects a decrease in renal blood flow.

3 Utilize haemodynamic monitoring for critically ill patient.

4 Place patient at rest—to lower heart rate and blood pressure and oxygen demands of heart and to maintain cardiac work at its lowest level.

5 Administer oxygen by nasal cannula or mask—may decrease incidence of arrhythmias by allowing the myocardium to be less ischaemic and thus less irritable; reduces pain by decreasing tissue hypoxia.

6 Relieve patient's pain and anxiety—anxiety and fear increase the heart rate (which puts heart under more stress), raise the blood pressure and cause the adrenal glands to release adrenaline which may produce an arrhythmia.

a. Give analgesic (morphine or diamorphine) within prescribed limits.

b. Monitor blood pressure, pulse and respiratory rate before administering narcotics—narcotics depress arterial pressure and may contribute to development of shock and arrhythmias.

c. Discuss CCU environment and what can be anticipated in the coming days with patient—to allay anxiety and help him mobilize his resources for coping.

d. Give intelligent reassurance and assist patient in establishing a positive attitude toward his illness.

(1) Most persons use the mechanism of denial during initial stages of MI.

(2) Depression is commonly encountered on about the third day in coronary

care unit although it may not surface until the patient returns home.

(a) Depression following MI is normal; patient is grieving over his losses—health, confidence, independence.

(b) Patient may feel pressure from having to alter his life-style; i.e. eating, drinking, smoking.

e. Review the facts of his illness with patient; reassure him that life can be relatively normal after a heart attack.

7 Prepare for the insertion of an intravenous infusion—to keep vein open for administration of intravenous medications in event of arrhythmia.

To Provide Nursing Surveillance and Support of Patient's Activities

1 Diet (as prescribed by doctor). Many variations of diet are in use.

a. Liquids, progressing to soft low calorie diet, for first few days—to lessen cardiac work.

b. Restrict sodium if signs and symptoms of congestive heart failure are present.

c. Restrict coffee (substitute decaffeinated coffee)—can affect heart rate, rhythm, coronary circulation and blood pressure.

2 Activities: Patient management is individualized and activities must be specified by doctor.

a. Apply antiembolism stockings.

b. Patient is usually allowed out of bed to use bedside commode—requires less cardiovascular work than using bedpan.

(1) Use laxatives.

(2) Avoid straining at stool—this form of isometric exercise can strain coronary reserve.

c. Chair rest (after 24 hours) if free of pain, arrhythmias, failure and shock—work of heart is less when patient is sitting than when he is recumbent.

d. Usually permitted light reading, transistor radio for diversion.

e. Start physical activities as directed. Avoid exercise for at least 1 hour after meals.

f. Monitor pulse and patient response during and after exercise.

g. Instruct patient to avoid sudden effort.

h. Gradually increase patient's physical activity (walk around room, in hall, etc.)—to enable him to achieve the activity level required for self-care by the time he returns home.

i. Graduate to progressive cardiac care unit, as available.

To be Alert for Complications

1 Cardiogenic shock (see p. 49).

a. Falling arterial blood pressure.

b. Reduced urinary volume (30 ml/hour or less).

c. Cool, moist skin; may be peripheral cyanosis—due to systemic vasoconstriction caused by reduction in cardiac output.

d. Restlessness, apathy, lessening of responsiveness—from systemic vasoconstriction.

e. See p. 49 for management of cardiogenic shock. A patient with cardiogenic shock should ideally be transferred to cardiac centre with haemodynamic monitoring capabilities.

2   Arrhythmias—occur frequently in first few days after infarction. The reduction in myocardial oxygenation produces myocardial ischaemia. Ischaemic muscle is electrically unstable and produces arrhythmias.
   a. Assess, prevent and treat conditions which may initiate an arrhythmia—congestive heart failure, pulmonary embolus, inadequate pulmonary ventilation, electrolyte disturbances, underoxygenation of blood.
   b. Draw arterial blood for blood gas analysis.
   c. Watch for ventricular fibrillation, ventricular tachycardia, AV block, asystole.
   d. See p. 32 for management of arrhythmias.
3   Congestive heart failure—myocardial infarction reduces ability of left ventricle to eject blood, diminishes cardiac output, produces an elevation of left ventricular end pressure with ensuing pulmonary vascular complications.
   a. Assess for tachycardia and gallop rhythm, dyspnoea, orthopnoea, oedema, hepatomegaly.
   b. Watch for development of pulmonary oedema (see p. 76)—represents extreme left ventricular failure. Assess for extreme dyspnoea, frothy, blood-stained mucus, tachycardia, distended neck veins and diffuse rales.
   c. See p. 66 and p. 76 for treatment of congestive heart failure and acute pulmonary oedema.
4   Other complications:
   a. Papillary muscle rupture, ventricular septal defect, ventricular aneurysm, ventricular rupture.
   b. Cerebral and peripheral emboli; pulmonary emboli.

Prepare for Myocardial Revascularization Procedure if Indicated

(See nursing management of patient undergoing heart surgery, p. 78.

Health Teaching

Objectives

To restore patient to his optimal physiological, psychological, social and occupational level.
To aid in restoring confidence and self-esteem.
To prevent progression of underlying disease (atherosclerosis).

1   Inform the patient about what has happened to his heart and explain that myocardial healing starts early but is not complete for 6–8 weeks.
2   A myocardial infarction usually requires some modification of life-style.
3   Exercise tolerance testing will be done after myocardial healing to determine how much function has been lost and to plan rehabilitation programme.
4   A programme of exercise training will be prescribed at this time to improve cardiovascular functional capacity.
5   Physical limitations are usually only temporary. The following guidelines usually apply until the patient is re-evaluated after complete myocardial healing:
   a. Walk daily, slowly increasing the distance and time.
   b. Avoid doing anything that tenses the muscles (weight lifting, straining, lifting heavy objects, pushing/pulling heavy loads)—may place strain on coronary reserve.

   c. Rest after meals and before doing any exercise.

   d. Space activities throughout the day to alternate rest and work.

     (1) Stop as soon as tired.

     (2) Avoid tenseness and rushing.

   e. Avoid working with arms above shoulder level.

   f. Shorten work hours when first returning to work.

6 Advise the patient to eat three to four meals daily (each containing about the same amount of food).

   a. Avoid large meals.

   b. Avoid hurrying while eating.

   c. Limit coffee drinking (unless doctor orders otherwise).

   d. Stay with prescribed diet (modifications in calories, fats and sodium).

7 Extremes of temperature and walking against the wind should be avoided.

   a. Stop immediately for shortness of breath.

   b. Sit down and take GNT for chest pain.

8 Sexual relations may be resumed upon advice of doctor, usually after exercise tolerance is assessed.

   a. If patient can walk briskly he can usually resume sexual activity; resumption of sexual activity parallels resumption of usual activities.

   b. Sexual activity should be avoided after eating a heavy meal, after drinking alcohol or when tired.

9 Instruct patient to notify the doctor when the following symptoms appear:

   a. Chest pressure or pain not relieved in 15 min by GNT.

   b. Shortness of breath.

   c. Unusual fatigue.

   d. Swelling of feet and ankles.

   e. Fainting.

   f. Slow or rapid heart beat.

Cardiogenic Shock

Cardiogenic shock (power failure), the end stage of left ventricular dysfunction, occurs when the left ventricle is extensively damaged by myocardial infarction. The heart muscle loses its contractile power and there is marked reduction in cardiac output with decreased perfusion (lack of blood and oxygen) to vital organs (heart, brain and kidneys). The degree of pump dysfunction is related to the extent of damage to the heart muscle.

Cardiogenic shock now accounts for the majority of hospital deaths in myocardial infarction and has a high mortality rate.

Clinical Manifestations

1 Low systolic pressure (90 mmHG or 30 mmHg less than previous levels).

2 Oliguria—urine output less than 30 ml/hour.

3 Cold, clammy skin—from peripheral vasoconstriction.

4 Mental lethargy, confusion—from poor cerebral perfusion.

Treatment and Nursing Management

Objectives

To maintain perfusion to vital organs while preserving the borderline areas of myocardium and limiting infarct size.
To improve the ability of the heart to pump blood throughout the body.
To determine effectiveness of treatment.

1   Start haemodynamic monitoring at the *first* indication of deterioration of patient's condition—haemodynamic monitoring is necessary for continuing patient evaluation and serves as a guideline for therapy.
2   Measure left ventricular pressure—oxygen demands of ischaemic myocardium are determined by left ventricular pressure and heart rate, myocardial contractility, size, shape and wall thickness of left ventricle.
   a. Measurement of left ventricular pressure accomplished by pulmonary arterial wedge pressure or left ventricular end-diastolic pressure.
   Pulmonary arterial wedge pressure measurement (Swan-Ganz) (see pp. 16–19).
   (1) Balloon tipped flow-directed catheter introduced via antecubital vein into superior vena cava.
   (2) When balloon is distended with small amount of air, the force of the venous blood flowing around the balloon tip propels the catheter through the right atrium and right ventricle and into the pulmonary artery.
   (3) Balloon is inflated to wedge it firmly in place in the pulmonary artery, where pressures are measured.
   (4) Optimum wedge pressure—15–18 mmHg.
   (5) Pulmonary artery catheters are also used to evaluate cardiac output.
   b. Measurement of left ventricular pressure.
   Pulmonary artery end-diastolic pressure (PAEDP).
   (1) Passage of catheter to pulmonary artery.
   (2) Optimum PAEDP pressure—15–18 mmHg. (This may not be a true reflection of PAEDP in patients with chronic obstructive pulmonary disease.)
3   Measure intra-arterial pressure by direct arterial cannulation.
   a. This is a more accurate measurement of blood pressure than is cuff pressure.
   b. Provides an arterial line for measuring blood gases and lactate.
4   Administer intravenous fluids (according to left ventricular pressure measurements, keeping wedge pressure low enough to prevent pulmonary oedema).
5   Give appropriate drug therapy if patient is still in shock—to lessen ischaemia and limit size of infarct, causing the heart to pump more effectively.
   Drug therapy is selected and guided by cardiac output and mean arterial blood pressure.
   a. Dopamine (Intropin):
   (1) Acts directly on renal and mesenteric vessels, causing them to dilate.
   (2) Remainder of systemic arteries constrict in response to alpha-adrenergic effects of dopamine.
   b. Sodium nitroprusside (Nipride); phentolamine (Regitine):
   (1) Given in an attempt to reduce myocardial oxygen consumption and to limit infarct size; can give controlled reduction of arterial pressure ('impedance

reduction') so that improved cardiac output and tissue perfusion and reduction in left ventricular filling pressure are achieved.

(2) Frusemide (a diuretic)—to free fluid in the lungs of patient with pulmonary oedema; lowers pulmonary blood volume and left ventricular filling pressure.

(3) Sodium bicarbonate—to treat metabolic acidosis due to accumulation of lactic acid; used only in severe shock.

    c. Other combinations of pressor drugs or catecholamines may be tried.

6   Measure urine volume via indwelling catheter every 30–60 min—urine flow reflects renal blood flow and the status of central circulation.

7   Take arterial blood gases to assess for hypoxia and metabolic acidosis.

8   Utilize counterpulsation to decrease ventricular work load of patient with severe shock. (See description of method, which follows.)

9   Prepare patient for surgical intervention to correct defects that are interfering with pump function and to reperfuse the heart.

Counterpulsation (Mechanical Cardiac Assistance)

Counterpulsation (diastolic augmentation) is a method of assisting the failing heart and circulation by mechanical support that may be accomplished by (1) external counterpulsation pressure or (2) intra-aortic balloon pump.

External counterpulsation pressure (ECP) is a noninvasive method of assisting the circulation; it is designed to boost the heart temporarily during a period of pump failure. It helps maintain adequate perfusion of vital organs and tissues until the heart is able to resume its function (Fig. 1.13).

1   The counterpulsation apparatus is positioned around the patient's legs; the legs are encased in two rigid troughs lined with water bags. The feet are left free and the system is closed to make an airtight seal.

2   The pump is positioned between the patient's ankles. The legs are used as a pumping chamber.

3   Water is pumped into the bags during diastole (positive pressure pulse) in response to an electronic signal triggered by the ECG. This raises the diastolic pressure.

4   The pressure is released (application of negative pressure) during cardiac systole, which lowers the systolic pressure (and thus the peak left ventricular pressure).

5   In cardiogenic shock, ECP increases the coronary blood flow by raising diastolic pressure, which may improve cardiac function; compression of the legs also increases venous return to the heart and thus increases cardiac output. Left ventricular work is thus reduced.

Intra-aortic balloon pump—introduction of a balloon catheter via the femoral artery into the descending thoracic aorta; it is inflated and deflated in sequence with the cardiac cycle and acts as an auxiliary pump assisting forward blood flow (Fig. 1.14).

1   Using synchronization with the patient's ECG the balloon is inflated at the onset of diastole, which results in increased aortic pressure and thus encourages the increase of coronary blood flow (termed 'diastolic augmentation').

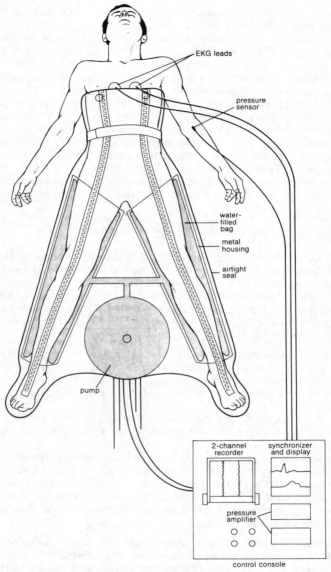

Figure 1.13.   External counterpulsation pressure, a pressure sensor is threaded into a radial artery (right). Bags contained in rigid cylinders that encase both legs are filled with water on diastole and emptied on systole with a pump—placed between the patients ankles—which is triggered by ECG signals. (From: Putting the counterpressure on, Emergency Medicine, August 1975.)

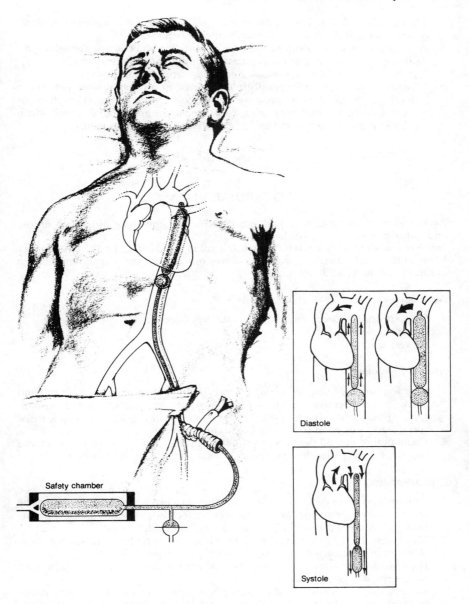

Diastole

Systole

Safety chamber

Figure 1.14.   Intra-aortic balloon pump. (From: Lewis, R P, Russell, R O, and Williams, D O (1976) Therapies to brighton post-MI prospects, Patient Care, 1 Jan. Copyright 1976, Miller and Fink Corp., Darien, Ct. All Rights reserved.)

2   The balloon is deflated at the onset of cardiac systole to lower the aortic blood pressure so that the work of the left ventricle is reduced.
3   A bedside console provides gas for balloon inflation and controls the inflation// deflation cycle to accommodate variations in the patient's heart rate.
4   It is timed by the ECG and monitored by the arterial pulse wave.
5   It augments diastole, which results in an increase in coronary blood flow, and it reduces left ventricular-end pressure (by causing a more complete emptying of the left ventricle). This decreases the resistance in the arterial tree against which the heart must pump and reduces myocardial oxygen requirements.

ENDOCARDIAL DISEASE

Endocarditis is an exudative and proliferative inflammatory alteration of the endocardium (inner lining of the heart).
Infective endocarditis (bacterial endocarditis) is an infection of the valves and inner lining of the heart caused by direct invasion of bacteria or other organisms; leads to deformity of the valve leaflets.

Aetiology

1   Bacteria (streptococci, pneumococci, staphylococci).
2   Fungi.
3   Rickettsiae.

Altered Physiology

1   Characterized by bacteria lodging on endocardium of valves (usually mitral and aortic). The bacteria multiply—fibrin and platelet thrombi are deposited, forming vegetations (verrucae). The vegetations on the affected endocardial surface may embolize to various organs and tissues.
2   Formation of emboli may occur in spleen, kidney, central nervous system and lungs. Observe patient for petechiae of skin and mucous membranes.

Characteristics

1   Although infective endocarditis may develop on a heart valve already injured by other disease (rheumatic fever, congenital defects) or on abnormally vascularized valves, normal heart valves can become infected.
2   May follow cardiac surgery, especially when prosthetic heart valves are used. (Foreign bodies, such as prosthetic valves, predispose to infection.)
3   High incidence among heroin addicts in whom the disease affects, for the most part, normal valves.
4   Hospitalized patients with indwelling catheters, those on prolonged intravenous therapy or prolonged antibiotic therapy, and those on immunosuppressive drugs or steroids may develop fungal endocarditis.
5   Rapid valvular destruction may lead to death.

Clinical Manifestations

General

1 Fever, chills, sweats (fever may be absent in elderly or in patients with uraemia).
2 Anorexia, weight loss.
3 Cough; back and joint pain.
4 Splenomegaly.

Skin and Nails

1 Splinter haemorrhages in nail beds.
2 Petechiae—conjunctiva, mucous membranes.
3 Roth's spots (haemorrhages with pale centres in the fundi of eyes).
4 Osler's nodes (painful red nodes on pads of fingers and toes).
5 Janeway's lesions (purplish macules on palms or soles).

Heart

Murmur—appearance of a new murmur or change in an old one.

Central Nervous System

Headaches, transient cerebral ischaemia, focal neurological lesions, cerebrovascular accidents, encephalopathy, meningitis.

Embolic Phenomena

Lung (recurrent pneumonia); kidney (haematuria); spleen; heart (myocardial infarction); brain (stroke); or peripheral vessels.

Diagnosis

1 Blood culture—serial blood cultures are drawn to document the presence of continuous bacteraemia and to determine aetiological agent.
2 Sensitivity studies—to determine the antibiotic for treatment.
3 Elevated erythrocyte sedimentation rate; anaemia; mild leucocytosis.
4 ECG.
5 Echocardiography—to follow ventricular dimensions, progressive cardiomegaly.

Treatment and Nursing Management

Objectives

To eradicate the invading organisms by adequate doses of appropriate agent to kill every organism in every vegetation.
To prevent development of endocarditis in susceptible persons.

1 Determine the causative organism by obtaining serial blood cultures.
2 Treat with bactericidal (capable of destroying bacteria) or other appropriate drugs based on proven sensitivity to causative agent.
   a. Bactericidal serum levels of selected antibiotic are monitored by titrating it against the causative organism; if the serum does not have adequate bactericidal activity more antibiotic or a different antibiotic is given.
   b. Blood cultures are taken periodically—to monitor adequacy of therapy.

    c. Intravenous route usually used for long-term administration of parenteral antibiotics.

        (1) Apply antibiotic ointment at needle entry site and cover with sterile dressing.

        (2) Note the date of needle or cannula insertion on nursing care plan.

    d. Adequate dosages are necessary to kill every organism in every vegetation.

    e. Combinations of drugs may be used if adequate serum levels are not achieved with one drug.

    f. Treatment with amphotericin B and surgery usually required for patient with fungal endocarditis.

3   Take temperature at regular intervals—course of fever is evaluated as one determinant of effectiveness of treatment.

4   Place patient in cardiac monitoring unit if patient is in congestive heart failure or to detect cardiac arrhythmias (secondary to involvement of heart conduction system or myocarditis).

5   Prepare for surgical intervention for:

    a. Congestive heart failure secondary to perforation of aortic valve or to ruptured chordae tendinae or papillary muscle.

        (1) Onset of congestive heart failure carries a grave prognosis and is a major indication for surgery.

        (2) Aortic valve predominantly involved.

    b. Excision of infected valves—for patients refractory to antibiotic therapy (particularly if resistant organisms involve either mitral or aortic valves).

    c. Excision of tricuspid valves—encountered with drug abusers

    d. Removal of prosthetic valve or patch for patient with prosthetic valve endocarditis. (Be alert for new or changing murmurs.)

    e. Formation of emboli.

    f. Drainage of abscess/empyema—for patient with localized abscess or empyema.

    g. Repair of peripheral or cerebral mycotic aneurysm.

Preventive Management and Health Teaching

1   Give prophylactic antibiotic (penicillin, erythromycin, etc.) to patients with known valvular, rheumatic or congenital heart disease or to patients with previously documented infective endocarditis who are undergoing diagnostic or surgical procedures that can cause transient bacteraemia:

    a. Dental procedures (including cleaning of teeth).

    b. Oral Surgery.

    c. Intubation procedures.

    d. Bronchoscopy.

    e. Instrumentation of genitourinary tract.

    f. Barium enemas; sigmoidoscopy.

    g. Surgery of lower intestinal tract.

    h. Childbirth.

2   Patients with prosthetic valves should report febrile episodes.

3   Ask the patient to report for long-term follow-up for valvular deformities caused by infection and scarring and for possible surgical correction of valve lesions.

RHEUMATIC HEART DISEASE

Rheumatic heart disease is damage done to the heart, particularly the valves, by one or more attacks of rheumatic fever. There is valvular deformity with associated compensatory changes in the size of the heart chambers and in the thickness of their walls.

Role of Streptococcal Infection

Rheumatic fever is a disease which is sequela of Group A streptococcal respiratory infection. Rheumatic fever is probably a sensitivity reaction precipitated by streptococci.

Symptoms of Haemolytic Streptococcal Infection

1 Sudden onset of sore throat; throat reddened with exudate.
2 Swollen, tender lymph nodes at angle of jaw.
3 Headache and fever 38.9–40°C (101–104°F).
4 Abdominal pain (children).

NOTE: Some cases of streptococcal throat infection are relatively asymptomatic.

Diagnosis

Throat culture—to determine presence of streptococcal organisms

Treatment of Streptococcal Infection

1 Benzathine penicillin (single dose intramuscularly) or oral penicillin for full 10 days—to eradicate streptococci.
2 Erythromycin for patients sensitive to penicillin.

Clinical Manifestations of Rheumatic Fever

1 Polyarthritis; warm and swollen joints.
2 Carditis.
3 Chorea (irregular, jerky, involuntary, unpredictable muscular movements).
4 Erythema marginatum (wavy, thin red-line skin rash on trunk and extremities).
5 Subcutaneous nodules.
6 Fever.
7 Prolonged PR interval demonstrated by ECG.
8 Friction rub; mitral systolic murmur; aortic diastolic murmur.

Laboratory Tests

1 Increased erythrocyte sedimentation rate; white blood cell and differential and C-reactive protein—increase during acute phase of infection.
2 Positive antistreptolysin O (ASO) titre.

Treatment and Nursing Management of Rheumatic Fever

Objective

To protect the heart.

1   Limit physical activity during the acute phase—patient should rest in bed as long as signs of active carditis are present.
2   Utilize penicillin therapy—to eradicate haemolytic streptococcus; erythromycin or lincomycin may be used if patient is allergic to penicillin.
3   Give salicylates or corticosteroids to suppress rheumatic activity by controlling toxic manifestations, to relieve joint pain and to reduce fever.
   a. Salicylates:
     (1) Give after meals—to reduce gastric irritation.
     (2) Give vitamins K and C—to prevent haemorrhage if large doses of salicylates are continued for a long period.
     (3) Assess for toxic signs of salicylates—nausea and vomiting, gastric distress, tinnitus, headache.
   b. Corticosteroid therapy—given for very ill patients with carditis:
     (1) Steroids are started with large doses and decreased according to patient's clinical response.
     (2) Steroids must be withdrawn gradually—to prevent reappearance of signs and symptoms of acute rheumatic fever.
     (3) Sodium is restricted—retention of sodium and fluids and loss of potassium are apt to occur with steroid therapy.
4   Give liquid high carbohydrate diet during acute febrile period; normal diet is resumed after fever subsides.

Health Teaching for Prevention of Recurrent Rheumatic Fever

It will be necessary to have *continuous* penicillin prophylactic therapy (or other suitable antibiotic) to prevent streptococcal infections and the possibility of recurrent attacks of rheumatic fever.

Sequelae of Rheumatic Fever (Complications)

Chronic rheumatic heart disease is a complication of rheumatic fever which frequently produces progressive disability and a shortened life span.

1   Although the patient is symptom-free for a time, the damage to the valves (rigidity and deformity, thickening and fusion of the commissures, or shortening and fusion of chordae tendinae) will produce heart sounds that are characteristic of valvular stenosis, regurgitation, or both.
2   The myocardium will compensate for these valvular defects for a while, but in time it fails to compensate and the patient develops symptoms of congestive heart failure.
3   See p. 62 for treatment of valvular heart disease and p. 68 for treatment of congestive heart failure.
4   *Health Teaching.*
   Persons with rheumatic heart disease should have prophylactic penicillin therapy before undergoing dental procedures or surgery of genitourinary tract and lower intestinal tract. See also p. 56.

MYOCARDITIS

Myocarditis is an inflammatory process involving the myocardium.

Aetiology

Follows infection:
Bacterial—beta-haemolytic streptococcus.
Viral—Coxsackie group, influenza, viral pneumonia, mumps, infectious mono-nucleosis.
Mycotic—blastomycosis, moniliasis.
Parasitic—trichinosis.
Protozoal—trypanosomiasis (Chagas' disease), malaria
Spirochaetal—syphilis.

Clinical Manifestations

Symptoms

1 Depend on type of infection, degree of myocardial damage, capacity of myocardium to recover and host resistance.
2 Fatigue and dyspnoea.
3 Palpitations.
4 Occasional precordial discomfort.

Clinical Findings

5 Cardiac enlargement.
6 Cardiac murmur—abnormal heart sound; sounds like fluid passing an obstruction.
7 Pericardial friction rub.
8 Gallop rhythm—a tripling or quadrupling of heart sounds (resembling the galloping of a horse) heard upon auscultation.
9 Pulsus alternans—a pulse in which there is regular alternation of weak and strong beats.
10 Fever with tachycardia.
11 Evidence of development of congestive heart failure.

Treatment and Nursing Management

Objective

To reduce the work of the heart.

1 Give specific therapy for underlying disease (e.g. antibiotic for haemolytic streptococci).
2 Place patient on bed rest to reduce heart rate, stroke volume, blood pressure and heart contractility—tends to reduce heart size.
   a. Prolonged bed rest may be required—until there is reduction in heart size and improvement of function.
   b. Assess for clinical evidence that disease is subsiding—evaluate pulse, heart sounds, temperature, etc.

3   Treat the symptoms of congestive heart failure (see p. 66).
   a. Restrict activity—to reduce systemic oxygen requirements.
   b. Give digitalis—augments myocardial contractility and slows heart rate.

Nursing Alert: Patients with myocarditis are sensitive to digitalis–assess for toxic symptoms (see p. 70).

   (1) Evaluate patient's pulse and apex beat for signs of tachycardia and gallop rhythm—indications that congestive heart failure is recurring.
   (2) Evaluate for evidence of arrhythmia—*patients with myocarditis are prone to develop arrhythmias.*
      (a) See p. 95 for management of arrhythmias.
      (b) Place patient in unit with continuous cardiac monitoring if signs of an arrhythmia develop.
      (c) Have equipment for resuscitation, cardiac defibrillation and cardiac pacing available in event of life-threatening arrhythmia.
4   Watch for evidence of embolic phenomena—emboli from venous thrombosis and mural thrombi occur frequently.
   a. Use elastic stockings; passive and active leg exercises.
   b. Long-term anticoagulant therapy may be required.

Health Teaching

Instruct patient as follows:

1   There is usually some residual heart enlargement; physical activity may be *slowly* increased; begin with chair rest for increasing periods of time; follow by walking in the room and then outdoors.
2   Report any symptom involving rapidly beating heart.
3   Avoid competitive sports, alcohol and other myocardial toxins (daunorubicin, adriamycin).
4   Pregnancy is not advisable for women with cardiomyopathies (diseases which affect structure and function of myocardium).

PERICARDITIS

Pericarditis is an inflammation of the pericardium, the membranous sac enveloping the heart. It is a manifestation of a more generalized disease.
   Pericardial effusion is an outpouring of fluid into the pericardial cavity.
   Constrictive pericarditis is a condition in which a chronic inflammatory thickening of the pericardium compresses the heart so that it is unable to fill normally during diastole.

Aetiology

1   Nonspecific:
   Usually occurs secondarily or as a complication of some other disease— uraemia, metastatic tumours, etc.
2   Infection:
   a. Bacteria—staphylococcus, meningococcus, streptococcus, pneumococcus,

gonococcus, *Mycobacterium tuberculosis* (commonly follows rheumatic fever and pneumonia)

   b. Virus.

   c. Fungus.

3   Disorders of connective tissues and allergies—lupus erythematosus, periarteritis nodosa.

4   Myocardial infarction; early, 24–72 hours; or late, 1 week to 2 years (Dressler's syndrome)

5   Neoplastic processes; following irradiation of mediastinal tumours.

6   Chest trauma, particularly after heart surgery.

7   Drugs

Clinical Manifestations

1   Pain in anterior chest, aggravated by thoracic motion—may vary from mild to sharp and severe; located in precordial area (may be felt beneath clavicle, neck, scapular region)—may be relieved by leaning forward.

2   Pericardial friction rub—scratchy, grating or creaking sound.

3   Dyspnoea—from compression of heart and surrounding thoracic structures.

4   Fever, sweating, chills—due to inflammation of pericardium.

5   Arrhythmias.

Diagnosis

1   Echocardiogram—most sensitive method for detecting pericardial effusion.

2   Chest x-ray—may show heart enlargement.

3   ECG—to evaluate for myocardial infarction.

4   White blood cell and differential.

5   Antinuclear antibody serological tests and lupus erythematosus cell preparation—to rule out lupus erythematosus.

6   Purified protein derivative test—for tuberculosis; ASO titres—for rheumatic fever.

7   Pericardial aspiration for examination of pericardial fluid for aetiological diagnosis.

8   Serum urea nitrogen (SUN)—to evaluate uraemia.

Nursing Alert: Normal pericardial sac contains less than 25–30 ml of fluid; pericardial fluid may accumulate slowly without noticeable symptoms. However, a rapidly developing effusion can produce serious haemodynamic alterations.

Treatment and Nursing Managment

Objectives

To determine the cause.

To administer therapy for the specific cause (when known).

To be on the alert for the complication of cardiac tamponade.

1   Be alert for the possibility of cardiac tamponade. Intervention with pericardial aspiration is indicated immediately (see p. 19). Watch for falling arterial pressure, rising venous pressure and quiet heart sounds.

2 Encourage patient to remain on bed rest when chest pain, fever and friction rub occur.
   Nursing assessment. Pericardial pain is aggravated by breathing, turning in bed and twisting the body.
3 Give specific therapy when the cause is known.
   a. Bacterial pericarditis—penicillin, methicillin and other antibiotic agents.
   b. Rheumatic fever—procaine penicillin, prednisone.
   c. Tuberculosis—antituberculosis chemotherapy (combinations of isoniazid, ethambutol, streptomycin). (There is a high incidence of constriction in tuberculosis pericarditis).
   d. Fungal pericarditis—amphotericin B.
   e. Disseminated lupus erythematosus—adrenal steroids.
   f. Uraemic pericarditis—dialysis (peritoneal or haemodialysis), Indomethacin, renal transplantation.
4 Prepare patient for surgical intervention (direct pericardial decompression)—for patient with cardiac embarrassment associated with constrictive pericarditis.

Health Teaching

1 The patient should increase his activities gradually.
2 Bed rest should be resumed if fever, pain or friction rub appear.

ACQUIRED VALVULAR DISEASE OF THE HEART

Causes

1 Rheumatic fever.
2 Congenital aortic stenosis.
3 Traumatic lesions of aortic valve.
4 Syphilis.

Altered Physiology

1 Inflammatory process→thickening and retraction of valve cusps→fusion and shortening of chordae tendinae→inadequate closure of valve.
2 Mitral valve most commonly involved, followed by aortic, tricuspid and pulmonary valves.
3 Patients with valvular disease usually develop congestive heart failure in time.

Diagnosis

1 Chest x-ray—to determine size and shape of heart.
2 ECG—to detect atrial and ventricular hypertrophy, myocardial infarction; to diagnose disturbances of rhythm.
3 Fluoroscopy—to detect intracardiac calcification.
4 Echocardiography—can visualize abnormal valves (mitral, aortic) and chamber enlargement.
5 Cardiac catheterization.
   a. To observe and record intracardiac pressure and oxygen saturation of blood in each heart chamber.

b. To receive information regarding presence of shunts.

c. To calculate cardiac output.

6   Angiography—used as part of diagnostic cardiac catheterization and to confirm diagnosis.

Aortic Stenosis

Aortic stenosis is a narrowing of the orifice between the left ventricle and the aorta. The obstruction to the aortic outflow places a pressure load on the left ventricle that results in hypertrophy and failure. It is often caused by rheumatic fever or arteriosclerosis, or it may be congenital.

Clinical Manifestations

1   Exertional dyspnoea and fatigue.
2   Dizziness and fainting—from reduced blood supply to brain.
3   Angina pectoris.
4   Low blood pressure and low pulse pressure—from diminished blood flow.
5   Arrhythmias
6   Symptoms of congestive heart failure.

Diagnosis

1   Chest x-ray—usually shows left ventricular enlargement.
2   Cardiac catheterization ⎱ will reveal the pressures in the
3   Angiocardiography ⎰ left ventricle and aorta.

Treatment

1   Surgical replacement of aortic valve—prosthetic device or aortic valve homograft. See p. 78 for care of patient undergoing heart surgery.
2   Treat angina and congestive heart failure as dictated by patient's condition.

Aortic Insufficiency

Aortic insufficiency (regurgitation) is caused by inflammatory lesions that deform the flaps so that they fail to completely seal the aortic orifice during diastole and thus permit a backflow of blood from the aorta into the left ventricle.

It may be caused by rheumatic endocarditis, bacterial endocarditis or congenital malformation, or from diseases which cause dilation or tearing of the ascending aorta (syphilitic disease, rheumatoid spondylitis, dissecting aneurysm).

Clinical Manifestations

1   Dyspnoea: exertional dyspnoea, paroxysmal nocturnal dyspnoea.
2   Chest pain.
3   Palpitations; patient is aware of overactivity of heart.
4   Diastolic murmur.
5   Symptoms of congestive heart failure.

Diagnosis

1 ECG—shows pattern of left ventricular hypertrophy.
2 Chest x-ray—reveals varying degrees of cardiomegaly from left ventricular enlargement.
3 Echocardiography—estimates size and thickness of left ventricle.
4 Cardiac catheterization and angiography.

Treatment

Surgical intervention—replacement of damaged aortic valve. See p. 78 for nursing management of patient undergoing heart surgery.

Mitral Stenosis

Mitral stenosis is the progressive thickening and contracture of valve cusps with narrowing of the orifice and progressive obstruction to blood flow. It is a late manifestation of rheumatic damage to the endocardium.

Clinical Manifestations

1 Dyspnoea; excessive fatigue.
2 Pulmonary congestion, haemoptysis, cough, orthopnoea.
3 Characteristic murmurs—increased first heart sound, opening snap and low pitched rumbling diastolic murmur heard at the apex.
4 Arrhythmias—palpitations during exercise; atrial fibrillation.
5 Angina pectoris.
6 Systemic embolism.

Diagnosis

1 ECG—shows evidence of left atrial enlargement, right ventricular hypertrophy.
2 Echocardiography—can demonstrate mitral valve thickening, calcification and abnormal, slowed diastolic valve excursion.
3 Cardiac catheterization and angiocardiography.

Treatment

1 Medical treatment.
   a. Prevent rheumatic recurrences with antibiotic therapy.
   b. Treat the developing congestive failure—digitalis, sodium restriction, limitation of activity (see p. 68).
   c. Control atrial fibrillation.
2 Surgical intervention may be accomplished by:
   a. Closed mitral valvotomy—introduction of dilator through left ventricular apex into valve to split its commissures.
   b. Open mitral valvotomy—direct incision of the commissures.
   c. Mitral valve replacement.
   d. See p. 78 for the management of the patient undergoing heart surgery.

Mitral Insufficiency

Mitral insufficiency (regurgitation) is the result of incompetence and distortion of the mitral valve so that the free margins can no longer come into apposition during systole. The chordae tendinae may become shortened, preventing complete closure of the leaflets.

Clinical Manifestation

1   Shortness of breath on exertion, fatigue, cough.
2   Arrhythmias.
3   Systolic murmur—heard in left axilla.
4   Cardiac enlargement.

Diagnosis

1   Chest x-ray—shows enlarged left atrium.
2   ECG—may reveal evidence of both left ventricular and left atrial enlargement.
3   Angiocardiography and cardiac catheterization—confirm diagnosis.

Treatment

Surgical intervention—replacement with prosthetic device, either ball valve or disc type. This procedure is done when there is extensive calcification and destruction of the chordae tendinae.

Tricuspid Stenosis

Tricuspid stenosis is restriction of the tricuspid valve orifice due to commissural fusion and fibrosis usually following rheumatic fever. It is commonly associated with diseases of the mitral valve.

Clinical Manifestations

1   Dyspnoea, nocturnal dyspnoea, orthopnoea.
2   Haemoptysis.
3   Visible pulsations of neck veins.
4   Murmurs—similar to those of rheumatic mitral disease; blowing diastolic murmur along left sternal border.
5   Symptoms of right-sided heart failure (late).

Diagnosis

1   ECG—may reveal atrial fibrillation.
2   Cardiac catheterization and angiocardiography—to confirm diagnosis.

Treatment

1   Patient may have mitral and aortic disease which must be corrected.
2   Surgical treatment of accompanying tricuspid valve disease may be carried out at the time of operation after correction of mitral valve disease.

Tricuspid Insufficiency

Tricuspid insufficiency allows the regurgitation of blood from the right ventricle into the right atrium during ventricular systole.

Clinical Manifestations

1 Right-sided heart failure—from overload of right ventricle.
2 Oedema—with congestion of liver and hepatic malfunction, ascites, hydrothorax.
3 Elevated venous pressure.

Treatment

1 Surgical treatment of mitral valve disease or combined mitral and aortic valve disease—may reverse pulmonary hypertension and produce disappearance of tricuspid regurgitation.
2 Replacement of tricuspid valve may be indicated.

CONGESTIVE HEART FAILURE

Heart failure is the inability of the heart to pump the amount of oxygenated blood necessary to effect venous return and to meet the metabolic requirements of the body.

   Congestive heart failure is the occurrence of circulatory congestion due to decreased myocardial contractility; as a result, cardiac output is inadequate to maintain the blood flow to body organs and tissues. This ultimately causes sodium and water retention and elevation of left atrial pressure, which results in pulmonary vascular congestion.

Causes

1 Secondary to heart disease: coronary atherosclerosis, hypertension, valvular heart disease, congenital heart disease, diffuse myocardial disease, arrhythmias.
2 Pulmonary embolism; chronic lung disease.
3 Haemorrhage and anaemia.
4 Anaesthesia and surgery.
5 Transfusions or infusions.
6 Thyrotoxicosis.
7 Pregnancy.
8 Infections.
9 Physical and emotional stress.
10 Excessive sodium intake.

Clinical Manifestations

Initially there may be either left or right ventricular failure, but in time the other ventricle fails because of the additional workload. The patient usually has a combination of symptoms; any system may be involved.

Left-sided Heart Failure

1 Congestion occurs mainly in the lungs from damming back of blood into pulmonary veins and capillaries.
   a. Shortness of breath, dyspnoea on exertion, paroxysmal nocturnal dyspnoea (due to reabsorption of dependent oedema that has developed during day), orthopnoea.
   b. Cough—may be dry, unproductive; often occurs at night.
2 Fatigue—from insomnia, nocturia, dyspnoea, cough, low cardiac output.
3 Insomnia.
4 Tachycardia—S_3 ventricular gallop.
5 Restlessness.

Right-sided Heart Failure

Signs and symptoms of elevated pressures and congestion in systemic veins and capillaries:

1 Oedema of ankles; unexplained weight gain.
   Pitting oedema—is obvious only after retention of at least 4.5 kg (10 lb) of fluid.
2 Liver congestion—may produce upper abdominal pain.
3 Distended neck veins.
4 Abnormal fluid in body cavities (pleural space, abdominal cavity).
5 Anorexia and nausea.
6 Nocturia—diuresis occurs at night with rest and improved cardiac output.
7 Weakness.

Complications

1 Intractable or refractory heart failure—patient becomes progressively refractory to therapy (not yielding to treatment).
2 Cardiac arrhythmias.
3 Myocardial failure.
4 Digitalis toxicity—from decreased renal function, potassium depletion, etc.
5 Myocardial failure.
6 Pulmonary infarction; pneumonia.

Diagnostic Findings

1 Cardiovascular findings.
   a. Cardiomegaly (hypertrophy of heart)—detected by physical examination and chest x-ray.
   b. Ventricular gallop—evident on auscultation; ECG.
   c. Rapid heart rate.
   d. Development of pulsus alternans.
   e. Distended neck veins.
   f. Hepatomegaly (enlargement of the liver).
2 ECG.
3 Chest x-ray—to evaluate heart size; show lung fields (for pleural effusion) and vascular congestion.

4   Arterial blood gas studies.
5   Liver function studies—may be altered due to hepatic congestion.

Treatment and Nursing Management

Objective

To reduce the cardiac load by (a) reducing circulatory demands and improving tissue oxygenation and (b) eliminating factors that stimulate heart action.

Cause of Decompensation

Determine the cause of decompensation (inability of heart to maintain circulation)—history, physical examination, laboratory studies and appropriate special studies (cardiac fluoroscopy, pulmonary function tests, serum enzymes, thyroid function studies, cardiac catheterization, angiography)

Rest Provisions

Place the patient at rest—to reduce the work of the heart, increase the cardiac reserve, diminish blood pressure, decrease work of respiratory muscles and slow the heart rate.

1   Ascertain the amount of activity that can be done without producing discomfort.
   a. Provide bed rest in semirecumbent position or in armchair in air-conditioned room—this position reduces venous return to the heart and lungs, increases lung volume and vital capacity, alleviates pulmonary congestion and reduces pressure on the diaphragm by the liver.
   b. Assess the patient's response to rest; are his symptoms alleviated?
2   Provide for rest and sleep—patients with congestive heart failure have a tendency to be restless at night because of cerebral hypoxia with superimposed nitrogen retention.
   a. Give oxygen during acute stage—to diminish work of breathing and increase the comfort of the patient.
b. Give appropriate sedation—to relieve insomnia and restlessness.
   (1) Give small doses of morphine as prescribed for extreme dyspnoea
   (2) Give mild sedation as needed for sleep.
   c. Raise head of bed 20–25 cm (8–10 in) on blocks.
   d. Keep a night-light on in the room.
3   Increase the patient's activities gradually.
   a. Alter or modify patient's activities—to keep within the limits of his cardiac reserve.
   b. Observe the pulse response to increased activity.
4   Observe for the complications of bed rest—phlebothrombosis and pulmonary embolism.
   a. Encourage patient to do deep breathing and leg exercises—improves muscle tone, aids in venous return to the heart.
   b. Use bedside commode—to avoid straining at stool, which may precipitate a pulmonary embolism.
   c. Use sedatives carefully—to prevent respiratory depression, immobility of patient and delayed detoxification of drugs due to hepatic congestion.

5   Provide for psychological rest—emotional stress may produce changes in pulse rate, stroke volume, cardiac output, peripheral resistance, salt and water metabolism.
   a. Offer careful explanations and answers to patient's questions.
   b. Give intelligent and reasonable reassurance.

Digitalis Therapy

Administer digitalis (a cardiac glycoside) as prescribed—to increase the force of myocardial contraction and produce a stronger systolic contraction of the heart and to slow the heart rate. This results in increased cardiac output; decreased heart size, venous pressure and blood volume; diuresis and relief of oedema. Digitalis is also used to slow the ventricular rate in the treatment of supraventricular arrhythmias.

1   A loading (digitalizing) dose may be given in order to induce the full therapeutic effect of the drug.
2   The patient is then given a daily dose just adequate to replace the drug that is destroyed or excreted—to maintain digitalis effect without toxicity.
3   Some clinicians are digitalizing patients without a loading dose for slow digitalization; a maintenance dose is started and continued daily.
4   *Digitalis preparations* (choice of drug depends on speed of onset and duration of cardiac action):
   a. Digitoxin (Digitaline Nativelle)
   b. Digoxin (Lanoxin).
   c. Deslanoside (Cedilanid) (injection)
   d. Lanatoside (Cedilanid) (tablet).
   e. Ouabain (injection).
5   *Clinical uses of digitalis:*
   a. Congestive heart failure.
   b. Atrial fibrillation.
   c. Atrial flutter.
   d. Supraventricular tachyarrhythmias.
   e. Before cardiac surgery.
6   Factors that may cause increased sensitivity to digitalis:
   a. Myocardial infarction, particularly ischaemia.
   b. Potassium depletion.
   c. Kidney or hepatic disease.
   d. Diuretic therapy.
   e. Diarrhoea
   f. Loss of appetite
   g. Advancing age
   h. Hypoxia and hypercapnia in pulmonary disease
   i. Acidosis; alkalosis
7   Serum concentration of digitalis (digitalis assay) may be measured (by laboratory) for therapeutic guidance and to assess for toxicity.
8   Serum potassium levels are followed in patients receiving digitalis, especially in patients receiving both digitalis and diuretics.
9   *Nursing responsibilities in administration of digitalis.*
      Assess clinical response of patient with respect to relief of symptoms (lessening dyspnoea, orthopnoea, râles, hepatomegaly, peripheral oedema).

a. The optimal dosage is the amount that relieves the patient's signs and symptoms of congestive heart failure or slows the ventricular response to arrhythmias *without causing toxicity*.

b. Watch for toxic effects—*arrhythmias* (most important toxic effect), *anorexia*, nausea, vomiting, diarrhoea, bradycardia, headache, malaise, behavioural changes, increasing congestive failure.

Nursing Alert: The incidence of digitalis toxicity is high because of the narrow margin between therapeutic and toxic doses. Toxic effects do not always appear in a predictable manner. Digitalis toxicity has a high mortality rate.

c. Record pulse and apex beat rate before administering each dose of digitalis.

d. Withhold digitalis and notify doctor if following is noted:
   (1) Slowing of rate.
   (2) Change in rhythm—bradycardia, premature ventricular contractions, bigeminy (two pulse beats following in rapid succession), atrial fibrillation.*
   (3) Dangerous cardiac arrhythmias require immediate treatment (see p. 95)

e. Assess for symptoms of electrolyte depletion—lassitude, apathy, mental confusion, anorexia, decreasing urinary output, azotaemia (excess urea in blood).

f. Watch carefully patient who is being treated simultaneously with diuretics and digitalis—*there is a predisposition to arrhythmias if the state of potassium balance is not evaluated and corrected.*

Diuretics

Administer prescribed diuretic (agent which increases the rate of urine flow)—acts primarily by blocking reabsorption of sodium; used to enhance excretion of sodium and water in congestive heart failure.

1   Type and dosage of diuretic administered depends on degree of heart failure and state of renal function.
2   Dosage also determined by patient's daily weight, clinical signs and symptoms.
3   See Table 1.2 for most commonly used diuretics.
4   *Nursing responsibilities in administration of diuretics*
   a. Give diuretic early in the morning—night-time diuresis disturbs sleep.
   b. Keep input and output record—patient may lose large volume of fluid after a single dose of diuretic
   c. Weigh patient daily—to determine if oedema is being controlled; weight loss should not exceed 1–2 lbs (0.45–0.9 kg) per day.
   d. Assess for weakness, malaise, muscle cramps—diuretic therapy may produce hypovolaemia and electrolyte depletion, namely *hypokalaemia*.
   e. Give oral potassium as prescribed.
   f. Be aware that problems associated with diuretic administration include disorders of potassium balance, hyperuricaemia, volume depletion and hyponatraemia, hyperglycaemia, and diabetes mellitus.

* Regularization of the rate in patient with chronic atrial fibrillation should be a warning that digitalis intoxication may be present.

Table 1.2. Frequently Used Diuretics

Definition
Diuretics are agents which increase rate of urine flow.
Action
    Dependent on functionally active kidneys; most diuretics decrease the reabsorption of electrolytes (principally sodium) by the kidneys and promote water loss as a secondary action.
    In the treatment of hypertension the naturetic (sodium excretion) effect is probably the action of importance.
    In oedema states the salt and water effects are both important.
Dosage Determination
    (1) Patient's daily weight; (2) Clinical signs and symptoms; (3) Physical examination; (4) State of renal function.

Diuretic	Action	Nursing Implications
Thiazides (Benzothiazine derivatives)		
Chlorothiazide (Saluric) Hydrochlorothiazide (Hydrosaluric) Hydroflumethiazide (Hydrenox) Bendrofluazide (Aprinox)	Increases renal excretion of sodium (naturesis), potassium, chloride, bicarbonate (alkaline urine) with accompanying 'osmotic' water loss Most widely used for prolonged administration	Watch for side-effects from electrolyte imbalance; hypokalaemia (weakness and fatigue), hyperuricaemia, hyperglycaemia, nausea and vomiting diarrhoea, abdominal cramps, dizziness, paraethesias Give supplementary potassium
Potassium-Sparing Diuretics		
Spironolactone (Aldactone)	Inhibits action of aldosterone in distal tubule and reduces reabsorption of sodium and chloride Gives gradual diuretic effect Used in treatment of cirrhosis and oedema when other diuretics are toxic or ineffective	Usually used in combination with thiazide diuretic Watch for side-effects—skin rash, gynaecomastia
Triamterene (Dytac)	Appears to interfere with exchange of sodium for potassium and H+ in the distal tubule	Usually used as an adjunct to thiazide therapy May cause elevation in blood urea levels Watch for nausea, vomiting, diarrhoea, weakness, headache and skin rash

(continued)

Table 1.2 (*cont.*)

Diuretic	Action	Nursing Implications
Potent Diuretics Frusemide (Lasix) Ethacrynic Acid (Edecrin)	Usually reserved for patients who do not respond to classical thiazide diuretics Blocks the reabsorption of sodium and water in proximal renal tubule and interferes with reabsorption of sodium in ascending limb of loop of Henle and in the most proximal portion of the distal tubule Associated with sodium, potassium, chloride and hydrogen on loss (acid urine) Frusemide has an almost immediate action when given intravenously Ethracrynic acid; maximum activity is reached in 2 hours and diuresis persists 6–8 hours	Potent and rapid-acting Especially useful in acute pulmonary oedema *May produce profound diuresis* with elevation of BUN (prerenal azotaemia) Watch for nausea, vomiting, diarrhoea, skin rash, pruritis, blurring of vision, postural hypotension, vertigo, hearing loss Frusemide is chemically related to sulphonamides; consider cross allergies Administer early in the day to avoid nocturia and consequent loss of sleep
Osmotic Diuretics Urea Mannitol (most commonly used)	Substances given in hypertonic solution by vein, excreted by the kidneys; because of limitation of kidney to reabsorb or concentrate them, water loss is obligatory Substances given by vein in hypertonic solutions that slowly cross the blood-brain barrier; thus the osmotic gradient across the blood-brain barrier results in an outward translocation of water from the brain tissue	May be used to treat oedema of the brain, especially in acute head injury with rapid swelling of the brain

Diet

Assist the patient in adapting to the prescribed diet—usually low sodium to rid the body of extracellular fluid retention.

1 Diet may be limited in both calorie and sodium content initially.
2 Advise patient to avoid using table salt. The patient with renal disease must avoid salt substitutes.
3 Teach the patient the importance of adhering to the low sodium diet.
   a. Sodium is present in all foods in varying amounts.
   b. Moderate sodium restriction—about 3 g of sodium daily.
   c. Severe sodium restriction—about 0.5–1.5 g of sodium daily.
4 Make the diet as palatable as possible.
   a. Use flavourings, spices, herbs and lemon juice.
   b. Avoid salt substitutes in the presence of renal disease.
5 Offer small, frequent feedings—to avoid excessive gastric filling and abdominal distension with subsequent elevation of diaphragm that causes decrease in lung capacity.
6 Teach the patient to rinse the mouth well after using tooth cleansers and mouthwashes—some of these contain large amounts of sodium. Water softeners are to be avoided.
7 Teach the patient that sodium is present in antacids, cough remedies, laxatives, pain relievers, oestrogens, etc.
8 Give the patient written dietary instructions. See Table 1.3 for example.

Health Teaching

1 Explain the disease process to the patient; the term 'failure' may have terrifying implications
   a. Explain the pumping action of the heart—'to move blood through the body to provide nutrients and aid in the removal of waste material'.
   b. Explain the difference between 'heart attack' and congestive heart failure.
2 Teach the signs and symptoms of recurrence.
   a. Ask patient to recall how he felt when he first became ill.
   b. Watch for
   (1) Gain in weight—report weight gain of more than 2–3 lb (0.9–1.4 kg) in a few days. Weigh at same time daily to detect any tendency toward fluid retention.
   (2) Swelling of ankles, feet or abdomen.
   (3) Persistent cough.
   (4) Tiredness; loss of appetite.
   (5) Frequent urination at night.
3 Review medication regimen.
   a. Label all medications.
   b. Given written instructions concerning digitalis and diuretic therapy.
   (1) Make sure patient has a system that will show that he has taken his medications.
   (2) Teach patient to take and record his pulse rate.
   (3) Tell the patient the signs and symptoms of digitalis toxicity and potassium depletion.

Table 1.3. Sodium-restricted Diet* (500 mg; 1800 calories)†

Category	Allowed	To Be Avoided
Dairy Products		
Milk	2 glasses	Salt or monosodium glutamate
Cheese	¼ cup unsalted cottage cheese	Ice cream
	1 oz low sodium dietetic cheese	Sherbet
Fat	Unsalted butter or margarine	Malted milk
	Unsalted cooking fat or oil	Milk shakes
	Unsalted French dressing	Chocolate milk
	Unsalted mayonnaise	Condensed milk
	Unsalted nuts	Regular butter or margarine
	Heavy or light cream	Commercial salad dressing
Eggs	1 egg daily	Bacon or bacon fat
		Olives
		Salted nuts
		Party spreads and dips
Meat, Fish, Fowl	Fresh, frozen or dietetic canned meat or poultry; beef, lamb, pork, veal, fresh tongue, liver, chicken, duck, turkey, rabbit Fresh or dietetic canned (not frozen) fish	Brains or kidneys Canned, salted or smoked meat (bacon, salami, corned or chipped beef, frankfurters, ham, meats koshered by salting, luncheon meats, salt pork, sausage, smoked tongue) Frozen fish fillets; canned, salted or smoked fish; canned tuna or salmon Shellfish—clams, crabs, lobsters, oysters, scallops, prawns, shrimps, etc.
Vegetables	Fresh, frozen or canned dietary vegetables (except those listed)	Canned vegetables or vegetable juices unless they are low sodium dietetic Frozen vegetables if processed with salt Artichokes, beet greens, beets, carrots, celery, chard, dandelion greens, kale, mustard greens, spinach, white turnips
Fruits	Any fruit or fruit juice (if sugar has not been added)	Fruits canned or frozen in sugar (because of the extra calories)
Breads, Cereals, Cereal Products	Low sodium bread, rolls, crackers Dry cereals (puffed rice, puffed wheat, shredded wheat) Unsalted melba toast Macaroni or noodles Spaghetti, rice, barley Unsalted popcorn Flour	Regular breads, crackers Commercial mixes Cooked cereals containing a sodium compound Dry cereals other than those listed or those having more than 6 mg of sodium in 100 g of cereal Self-raising flour

(continued)

Table 1.3 (*cont.*)

Category	Allowed	To Be Avoided
		Potato chips Pretzels Salted popcorn
Miscellaneous	Coffee, tea, coffee substitutes, lemons, limes, plain unflavoured gelatine, vinegar, cream of tartar, potassium bicarbonate, sodium-free baking powder, yeast	Instant cocoa mixes; other beverage mixes, including fruit-flavoured powders; malted milk; soft drinks (both regular and low calorie); any kind of commercial bouillon (cubes, powders or liquids); sodium cyclamate and sodium saccharin; commercial sweets; commercial gelatine desserts; regular baking powder; baking soda (sodium bicarbonate); rennet tablets; molasses; pudding mixes

* From Sodium-restricted Diet, 500 mg, American Heart Association.
† For a 250-mg sodium diet, use low sodium milk (either low sodium whole milk or low sodium powdered milk) instead of regular milk.
For 1000 mg sodium diet, follow 500-mg sodium diet, plus one of the following for the additional 500 mg of sodium.

$\frac{1}{4}$ teaspoon salt (scant)	Average serving of cooked cereal, rice,
$\frac{3}{4}$ teaspoon monosodium glutamate	spaghetti, noodles, etc., seasoned with salt
$\frac{1}{2}$ bouillon cube	1 cup drained sauerkraut
1 cup tomato juice	1 average frankfurter
	$1\frac{1}{2}$ oz ham

(4) If patient is taking oral potassium solution, it may be diluted with juice and taken after a meal.
4 Review activity programme.
Instruct the patient as follows:
a. Increase walking and other activity gradually, provided they do not cause fatigue and dyspnoea.
b. In general, continue at whatever activity level you can maintain without the appearance of symptoms.
c. Avoid excesses in eating and drinking.
d. Undertake a weight reduction programme until optimum weight is reached.
e. Avoid extremes in heat and cold—cardiac stress is increased by environmental heat or cold.
f. Keep *regular* appointment with doctor or clinic.
5 Restrict sodium as directed
a. Give patient written diet plan with list of permitted and forbidden foods.
b. Advise patient to look at all labels to ascertain sodium content (antacids, laxatives, etc.).
c. Advise patient to accept the fact that restricting sodium and taking digitalis will be a permanent part of his way of life.

ACUTE PULMONARY OEDEMA

Acute pulmonary oedema refers to the presence of excess fluid in the lung, either in the interstitial spaces or in the alveoli. It usually follows acute left ventricular failure.

Nursing Alert: Acute pulmonary oedema is a true medical emergency since it is a life-threatening condition.

Causes

1   Heart disease: acute left ventricular failure, myocardial infarction, aortic stenosis, severe mitral valve disease, hypertension, congestive heart failure.
2   Circulatory overload—transfusions and infusions.
3   Drug hypersensitivity; allergy; poisoning.
4   Lung injuries—smoke inhalation, shock lung, pulmonary embolism or infarct.
5   Central nervous system injuries—stroke, head trauma.
6   Infection and fever.

Clinical Manifestations

1   Coughing and restlessness during sleep (premonitory symptoms).
2   Extreme dyspnoea and orthopnoea—patient usually uses accessory muscles of respiration with retraction of intercostal spaces and supraclavicular areas.
3   Cough with varying amounts of white- or pink-tinged frothy sputum.
4   Extreme anxiety and panic.
5   Noisy breathing—inspiratory and expiratory wheezing and bubbling sounds.
6   Cyanosis with profuse perspiration.
7   Distended neck veins.
8   Tachycardia.

Treatment and Nursing Management

Objective

To reduce pulmonary congestion. Take steps to reduce the right atrial inflow of systemic venous blood (retard venous return).

1   Place patient in upright position, head and shoulders up, feet and legs hanging down—to favour pooling of blood in dependent portions of body by gravitational forces; to decrease venous return.
2   Give morphine in small titrated intermittent doses (intravenously) until dyspnoea lessens—to allay the acute anxiety and decrease respiratory effort, allowing better oxygen exchange and inducing sleep.
    a. Morphine is *not* given if pulmonary oedema is caused by cerebral vascular accident or occurs in the presence of chronic pulmonary disease or cardiogenic shock.
    b. Watch for excessive respiratory depression.
    c. Monitor blood pressure since morphine may intensify hypotension.
    d. Have morphine antagonist available—naloxone hydrochloride (Narcan).
3   Give oxygen in high concentration—to relieve hypoxia and dyspnoea.
    a. Oxygen may be given with high enough pressure to provide blood

oxygenation and to overcome the pressure barrier of the oedema fluid.

b. This is accomplished by giving oxygen by mask or by oropharyngeal catheter.

4 Administer aminophylline—relaxes bronchospasm; increases renal blood flow and enhances diuresis; decreases pulmonary arterial pressure; decreases peripheral venous pressure and peripheral resistance.

a. Give aminophylline *very slowly* intravenously—arrhythmias, syncope and sudden death may follow too rapid administration.

b. Watch for falling blood pressure—may be a dangerous complication.

5 Give injections of diuretic (ethacrynic acid; frusemide) intravenously—to reduce blood volume and pulmonary congestion by producing prompt diuresis.

a. Insert an indwelling catheter (if patient is in shock or has retention of urine).

b. Profuse diuresis may result soon after administration.

c. *Watch for falling blood pressure, increasing heart rate, and decreasing urinary output—indications that the total circulation is not tolerating diuresis and that hypovolaemia may develop.*

d. Watch for signs of urinary obstruction in patients with prostatic hypertrophy.

6 Use rotating tourniquets (see p. 31)—to produce venous stasis in extremities; reduces venous return to the heart and thus helps the congestion in the lungs. This treatment is not used very often.

a. Apply tourniquets to extremities.

b. Rotate tourniquets every 15 min (or more often it patient has circulatory impairment).

c. Do not use tourniquets if patient is in shock.

7 Use phlebotomy (rapid withdrawal of blood from a peripheral vein)—to decrease venous return and produce a corresponding decline in right ventricular output.

a. Phlebotomy is usually done to reduce intravascular pressure when attack is precipitated by overadministration of blood or infusion fluids.

b. Save the blood since it may be needed in the treatment of shock if there has been extension of infarction. Packed cells may be returned to patient if need arises.

8 Stay with the patient and display a confident attitude—the presence of another person is therapeutic since the acute anxiety of the patient may tend to intensify the severity of his condition. (Arterial vasoconstriction diminishes as anxiety is relieved.)

9 Administer digitalis (intravenously) to undigitalized patient if pulmonary oedema is of cardiac origin—to increase left ventricular output and thus relieve symptoms and prevent pulmonary oedema from recurring.

10 Assess renal and electrolyte status of patient.

11 Give appropriate drugs for severe, sustained hypertension.

Health Teaching

During convalescence instruct the patient as follows in order to prevent recurrences of pulmonary oedema.

1 Ask: What symptoms did you have before the attack? (He should be aware of these.)

2   If coughing develops (a wet cough), sit with legs dangling over side of bed. If this does not help, call the doctor.
3   Restrict sodium.
4   Take diuretics and digitalis exactly as prescribed.
5   Sleep with head elevated (use 25 cm [10-in] blocks at head of bed.)
6   Avoid excessive and sudden physical exertion.
7   Weigh daily—to determine need for additional diuresis.
8   Treat all infections promptly with antibiotics.
9   See Health Teaching (congestive heart failure), p. 73

HEART SURGERY

Cardiac Conditions Requiring Surgery

Surgical procedures have been established for the following conditions:*

Congenital Disease of the Heart and Great Vessels

Patent ductus arteriosus†
Coarctation of aorta†
Atrial septal defect (secundum)
Atrial septal defect (primum)
Ventricular septal defect
Endocardial cushion defect
Tetralogy of Fallot
Valvar pulmonic stenosis
Valvar aortic stenosis
Subvalvar aortic stenosis

Transposition of great vessels
Tricuspid atresia
Truncus arteriosus
Aortic septal defect
Aortic vascular ring†
Mitral stenosis
Mitral insufficiency
Congenital origin of left coronary artery from pulmonary artery
Coronary arteriovenous fistula

Acquired Disease of the Heart and Great Vessels

Mitral stenosis
Mitral regurgitation
Aortic stenosis
Aortic regurgitation
Constrictive pericarditis†
Heart block†
Coronary artery occlusive disease
Ventricular aneurysm
Acute ventricular septal defect

Direct myocardial trauma
Traumatic rupture of aorta
Saccular thoracic aneurysm
Fusiform thoracic aneurysm
Dissecting aortic aneurysm
Aorto-coronary sinus fistula
Tricuspid stenosis
Aneurysm sinus of Valsalva
Massive pulmonary embolism

Preoperative Nursing Management

Objective

To bring the patient to the peak of his physical and psychological capabilities.

* Adapted from Report of Inter-society Commission for Heart Disease Resources. Circulation, 44: 228, Sept. 1971. By permission of the American Heart Association.
† Ordinarily, cardiopulmonary bypass is not required.

1 Support the patient undergoing diagnostic studies to determine type and severity of specific lesions; tests also provide a baseline for postoperative evaluation.
  a. Cardiac catheterization and angiography.
  b. Pulmonary function studies.
  c. ECG, echocardiogram, phonocardiogram.
  d. Exercise tolerance testing.
  e. Chest x-ray.
2 Assess laboratory studies.
  a. Complete blood count, serum electrolytes, lipid profile, nose, throat, sputum and urine cultures.
  b. Antibody screen.
  c. Preoperative coagulation survey (prothrombin time, fibrin degradation products, fibrinogen test, clotting time)—extracorporeal circulation will affect certain coagulation factors.
  d. Renal and hepatic function tests.
3 Evaluate patient's emotional state and try to reduce his anxieties—patients undergoing heart surgery are more anxious and fearful than other surgical patients.
  a. Give support by being present, by listening and by showing interest—patient is called upon to deal with a stressful and life-threatening crisis.
  b. Encourage the patient to express what he feels and thinks—giving vent to feelings relieves sense of isolation and facilitates a growing and supportive relationship.
  c. Help the patient to mobilize his defences and cope with his fears.
  d. Clarify the information given him previously by the cardiovascular surgeon.
  e. Anticipate and answer the patient's questions.
    (1) Ask the patient what he wants to know.
    (2) Establish a relationship of trust.
  f. Reinforce and accelerate education of patient as day of operation approaches.
  g. Expect some patients to have psychological and psychiatric problems from prolonged illness.
4 Prepare the patient for events in the postoperative period.
  a. Take patient and family on tour of intensive care unit—lessens anxiety about being in intensive care unit.
    (1) Introduce him to staff personnel who will be caring for him.
    (2) Give family a schedule of visiting hours and times for phone contact.
  b. Teach chest physical therapy procedures—to optimize pulmonary function.
    (1) Have patient practice with IPPR (assisted ventilation) machine.
    (2) Show and practise diaphragmatic breathing techniques.
    (3) Have him practise effective coughing, leg exercises.
  c. Prepare patient for presence of monitors, chest tubes, intravenous infusions, blood transfusion, endotracheal tube, etc.
5 Assess the patient's reactions to medications—these patients are usually on multiple drugs.
  a. Digitalis:
    (1) Patient may be receiving large doses to improve myocardial contractility.
    (2) Drug may be stopped several days before surgery—to avoid digitoxic arrhythmias from cardiopulmonary bypass.

b. Diuretics:

(1) Assess patient for potassium depletion and volume depletion (weakness, postural hypotension)—diuretics may produce potassium loss, and severe diuresis may cause a decrease in blood volume.

(2) Give potassium supplement if patient is on prolonged diuretic therapy—to replenish body stores.

(3) Diuretics may be omitted several days preoperatively to avoid electrolyte imbalance and consequent arrhythmias postoperatively. Salt and water restriction may be advised.

c. Beta blockers (propranolol); withdraw drug gradually before surgery—sudden cessation of propranolol can precipitate status anginosus or myocardial infarction.

d. Determine if patient has taken corticosteroids within the year prior to surgery—patients on steriods are given supplemental doses to cover stress of surgery.

e. Prophylactic antibiotics may be given preoperatively.

f. Determine whether patient has any drug sensitivities.

6   Be aware of the preoperative conditions which predispose to postoperative respiratory complications.

a. Pulmonary hypertension.

b. Pulmonary congestion or oedema.

c. Pre-existing lung disease.

d. Pulmonary sepsis.

e. Elderly or debilitated patient.

7   Encourage the patient to stop smoking—smoking increases incidence of postoperative respiratory complications.

Postoperative Surgical Care and Nursing Management

Objective

To evaluate patient closely and continuously to prevent complications.

1   Secure all connections for lines and tubes (arterial, central venous pressure, chest tubes, urinary catheter to collecting bottle, endotracheal tube to ventilator, ECG to monitoring system, pacing wires, etc.)

2   Assure adequate oxygenation in early postoperative period; respiratory insufficiency is common following open heart surgery.

3   Employ physiological monitoring* during immediate postoperative period, especially for cardiovascular state, respiratory state and fluid and electrolyte balance.

4   Monitor cardiovascular state to determine effectiveness of cardiac output. Serial readings of blood pressure and arterial pressure, heart rate, central venous pressure and left atrial pressure from monitors are observed, correlated with patient's condition and recorded.

a. Assess arterial pressure every 15 min until stable and as directed there-

---

* Monitoring equipment is valuable only when it is understood and used correctly. The clinical assessment of the patient by the nurse is indispensable to patient care.

after—blood pressure is one of the most important physiological parameters to follow.

(1) Measure by catheter (usually in femoral or radial artery) connected to a transducer and oscilloscope—more accurate than cuff pressure. Residual vasoconstriction following extracorporeal circulation makes blood pressure auscultation unreliable.

(2) Heparin flushing system may be interposed between the arterial line and transducer to prevent clotting.

(3) Arterial pressure may be 10–20 mmHg higher than cuff pressure.

(4) Watch diastolic measurement in patient with aortic valve prosthesis; decrease may show valve is slipping.

b. Auscultate the heart for evidence of cardiac tamponade (muffled distant heart sounds), precordial rub (pericarditis), etc.

(1) Check peripheral pulses (pedal, tibial, radial) as a further check on heart action.

(2) Palpate the carotid, brachial, popliteal and femoral pulses; if these pulses are absent it may be due to recent catheterization of the extremity.

c. Take central venous pressure readings hourly (see p.13) indicate blood volume, vascular tone and pumping effectiveness of the heart.

(1) High central venous pressure reading may result from hypervolaemia, heart failure, cardiac tamponade, vasoconstriction. Ventilator may elevate central venous pressure.

(2) If blood pressure drop is due to low blood volume, central venous pressure will show corresponding drop.

(3) *Changes* in values are more important than isolated readings.

d. Measure left atrial pressure or pulmonary artery wedge pressure—to determine the left ventricular end-diastolic volume and to assess cardiac output (see p. 16).

Rising pressures may indicate congestive heart failure or pulmonary oedema.

e. Watch ECG monitor—cardiac arrhythmias frequently occur after heart surgery.

(1) Premature ventricular contractions occur most frequently following aortic valve replacement and coronary bypass surgery. May be treated with pacing, lignocaine, potassium.

(2) Arrhythmias also apt to occur with ischaemia, hypoxia, alterations in serum potassium, oedema, bleeding, acid-base or electrolyte disturbances, digitalis toxicity, myocardial failure.

(3) Observe other parameters in correlation with monitor information—a low serum potassium makes the heart susceptible to ventricular arrhythmias.

(4) See p. 32 for discussion of cardiac arrhythmias.

f. Check urine output every 30–60 min (from indwelling catheter)—urine output is an index of cardiac output and peripheral perfusion.

g. Continue with ongoing patient assessment.

(1) Observe buccal mucosa, nail beds, lips, ear lobes and extremities for duskiness/cyanosis—signs of low cardiac output.

(2) Feel the skin; cool, moist skin reveals lowered cardiac output. Note temperature and colour of extremities.

(3) Note fullness and tone of superficial veins of feet.

5   Evaluate respiratory state of patient.
  a. Employ assisted or controlled ventilation (p. 300)—respiratory support is used during first 24 hours to provide airway in the event of cardiac arrest, to decrease work of heart, to maintain effective ventilation.
    (1) Adequacy of ventilation is assessed by patient's clinical state and by direct measurement of tidal volume and arterial blood gases.
    (2) Check endotracheal tube placement.
    (3) Auscultate chest for breath sounds—crepitations indicate pulmonary congestion; decreased or absent breath sounds indicate pneumothorax.
    (4) Chest x-ray taken immediately after surgery and daily thereafter—to evaluate state of lung expansion and to detect atelectasis.
    (5) Arterial blood gas analysis usually performed first hour postoperatively and as necessary thereafter to assess respiratory function.
    (6) Sedate patient adequately—to help him tolerate endotracheal tube and cope with ventilatory sensations.
    (7) Use chest physiotherapy for patients with lung congestion to prevent retention of secretions and atelectasis.
      (a) Check chest x-ray and auscultate chest to determine problems areas.
      (b) Use percussion and vibrating techniques to loosen secretions.
      (c) Promote coughing, deep breathing and turning—to keep airway patent, prevent atelectasis and facilitate lung expansion.
    (8) Suction tracheobronchial secretions carefully—prolonged aspiration leads to hypoxia and possible cardiac arrest.
    (9) Restrict fluids (per request) for first few days—danger of pulmonary congestion from excessive fluid intake.
6   Maintain fluid and electrolyte balance—metabolic acidosis and electrolyte imbalance can occur after use of pump oxygenator.
  a. Fluids may be limited to avoid overloading.
  b. Keep input and output flow chart as a method of determining positive or negative fluid balance and patient's fluid requirements.
    (1) Intravenous fluids (including flush solutions through arterial and venous lines) considered as input.
    (2) Assess hydration state of patient—weight, electrolyte levels, haematocrit readings, distension of neck veins, tissue oedema, liver size, breath sounds.
    (3) Record urine output every 30–60 min.
    (4) Measure postoperative chest drainage—should not exceed 200 ml/hour for first 4–6 hours.
      (a) Watch for sudden cessation of chest drainage—from kinked or blocked chest tube.
      (b) See p. 358 Management of Patient with Water-seal Drainage.
7   Be alert to changes in serum electrolytes—a specific concentration of electrolytes is necessary in both extracellular and intracellular body fluids in order to sustain life.
  a. *Hypokalaemia* (low potassium):
    (1) May be caused by inadequate intake, diuretics, vomiting, excessive nasogastric drainage, stress from surgery.
    (2) Effects of low potassium—arrhythmias, digitalis toxicity, metabolic alkalosis, weakened myocardium, cardiac arrest.

(3) Give intravenous potassium replacement as directed.

b. *Hyperkalaemia* (high potassium):

(1) May be caused by increased intake, red cell breakdown from the pump, acidosis, renal insufficiency, tissue necrosis and adrenal cortical insufficiency.

(2) Effects of high potassium—mental confusion, restlessness, nausea, weakness and paraesthesia of extremities.

(3) Be prepared to administer an ion-exchange resin, sodium polystyrene sulphonate (Resonium A), which binds the potassium, or give intravenous sodium bicarbonate or intravenous insulin and glucose to drive the potassium back into the cells from the extracellular fluid.

c. *Hyponatraemia* (low sodium):

(1) May be due to reduction of total body sodium or to an increased water intake causing a dilution of body sodium.

(2) Effects of low sodium—weakness, fatigue, confusion, convulsions and coma.

d. *Hypocalcaemia* (low calcium):

(1) May be due to alkalosis (which reduces the amount of Ca^{2+} in the extracellular fluid) and multiple blood transfusions.

(2) Signs and symptoms of reduced calcium levels—numbness and tingling in the fingertips, toes, ear and nose, carpopedal spasm, muscle cramps and tetany.

(3) Give replacement therapy as directed.

e. *Hypercalcaemia* (high calcium):

May cause arrhythmias imitating those caused by digitalis toxicity.

8 Relieve patient's pain—cardiac surgical patients experience pain caused by severance of intercostal nerves and irritation of pleura by chest tubes.

a. Record nature, type, location and duration of pain—pain and anxiety increase pulse rate, oxygen consumption and cardiac work.

b. Medicate patient as often as prescribed—to reduce amount of pain and to aid patient in performing deep breathing and coughing exercises more effectively.

c. Differentiate between incisional pain and anginal pain.

d. Watch for restlessness and apprehension—may be from hypoxia or a low-output state; analgesics or sedatives do not correct this problem.

9 Assess neurological state—the brain is dependent on a continuous supply of oxygenated blood and must rely on adequate and continuous perfusion by the heart.

a. Low arterial pressure during perfusion and prolonged bypass may produce CNS damage after heart surgery.

b. Observe for symptoms of hypoxia—restlessness, headache, confusion, dyspnoea, hypotension and cyanosis.

c. Assess patient's neurological state hourly in terms of:

(1) Level of responsiveness.

(2) Response to verbal commands and painful stimuli.

(3) Pupillary size and reaction to light.

(4) Movement of extremities; handgrasp ability.

d. Treat postoperative convulsive seizures.

10 Give medications according to therapeutic directives—coronary vasodilators (Isordil, GNT), antibiotics, analgesics, anticoagulants (patients with prosthetic valves).

11   Offer reassurance, orientation to time and place; and attention to patient's needs to avoid postcardiotomy psychosis (see p. 85).

Complications Following Cardiac Surgery

1   *Hypovolaemia* (decreased circulating blood volume).
   a. Low central venous pressure is an indication of hypovolaemia.
   b. Observe for arterial hypotension, low central venous pressure, increasing pulse rate.

2   *Persistent bleeding*—from tissue fragility, trauma to tissues, clotting defects; blood clotting disturbances usually transitory following cardiopulmonary bypass; however, a significant platelet deficiency may be present.
   a. Watch for steady and continuous drainage of blood; watch central venous pressure and left atrial pressures.
   b. Treatment: protamine sulphate; aminocaproic acid, vitamin K, fresh blood or blood components (packed cells, albumin, platelets).
   c. Prepare for potential return to surgery for bleeding persisting (over 300 ml/hour) for 4–6 hours or if there is measurable clotting defect.

3   *Cardiac tamponade*—results from bleeding into the pericardial sac or accumulation of fluids in the sac, which compresses the heart and prevents adequate filling of the ventricles.
   a. Assess for signs of tamponade—arterial hypotension, rising central venous pressure, muffled heart sounds, weak, thready pulse, neck vein distension, falling urinary output.
   b. Check for diminished amount of drainage in the chest-collection bottle; may indicate that fluid is accumulating elsewhere.
   c. Prepare for pericardial aspiration (see p. 19).

4   *Cardiac failure* (low-output syndrome)—causes deficient blood perfusion to different organs.
   a. Observe for falling mean arterial pressure, rising venous pressure and increasing tachycardia; patient may exhibit signs of restlessness and agitation, cold and blue extremities, venous distension, laboured respirations, tissue oedema and ascites.
   b. Treatment may include diuretic therapy and rapid digitalization to avoid acute failure; oxygen therapy/mechanical ventilation (for respiratory insufficiency); sodium bicarbonate to correct acidosis.

5   *Myocardial infarction.*
   a. Symptoms may be masked by the usual postoperative discomfort.
   (1) Watch for fall of mean arterial pressure in the presence of normal circulating volume and a normal venous pressure.
   (2) Obtain serial ECGs to determine extent of myocardial injury.
   (3) Assess pain to differentiate myocardial pain from incisional pain.
   b. Postoperative activity level may be reduced to allow heart adequate time for healing.

6   *Renal failure*—urine output depends on cardiac output, blood volume, state of hydration and condition of kidneys.
   a. Renal injury may be caused by deficient perfusion, haemolysis, low cardiac output prior to and following open heart surgery; use of vasopressor agents to increase blood pressure.

b. Measure urine volume; less than 20 ml/hour can indicate hypovolaemia.

c. Carry out specific gravity tests to determine kidneys' ability to concentrate urine in renal tubules.

d. Watch BUN and serum creatinine levels as well as urine and serum electrolyte levels.

e. Give rapid-acting diuretics and/or inotropic drugs (digitalis, dopamine, isoproterenol) to increase cardiac output and renal blood flow.

f. Prepare patient for peritoneal dialysis if indicated. (Renal insufficiency may produce serious cardiac arrhythmias.)

7 *Hypotension*—may be caused by reduction in circulating blood volume which can occur after patient has been removed from cardipulmonary bypass.

a. Monitor vital signs, left atrial pressure, central venous pressure and arterial pressure.

b. Note chest tube drainage—hypotension may be caused by excessive bleeding.

c. Give blood as directed to maintain left atrial pressure at a level which will provide an adequate circulating volume for good tissue perfusion.

8 *Formation of emboli*—may result from injury to the intima of the blood vessels, dislodgement of a clot from a damaged valve, venous stasis aggravated by certain arrhythmias, loosening of mural thrombi and coagulation problems.

a. Common embolic sites are lungs, coronary arteries, mesentery, extremities, kidneys, spleen and brain.

b. Symptoms of emboli formation (vary according to site):

(1) Midabdominal or midback pain.

(2) Pain, cessation of pulses, blanching, numbness, coldness of extremity.

(3) Chest pain and respiratory distress with pulmonary embolus or myocardial infarction

(4) One-sided weakness, pupil changes, as in stroke.

c. Initiate preventive measures: antiembolic stockings; omit pressure on popliteal space (leg crossing); start passive and active exercises.

9 *Postperfusion syndrome*

a. Signs and symptoms—fever, splenomegaly, atypical lymphocytes and maculopapular rash

b. Prepare to help doctor to take blood for culture—postperfusion syndrome can mimic bacterial endocarditis or hepatitis.

c. Give medication as prescribed for fever and rash.

d. Reassure patient that this is only a temporary setback in his convalescence.

10 *Febrile complications*—fever almost always follows extracorporeal circulation; places an undesirable demand on heart.

a. Control higher degrees of fever by use of hypothermia mattress.

b. Evaluate for atelectasis, pleural effusion or pneumonia if fever persists.

c. Evaluate for urinary tract infection/wound infection.

d. Bear in mind the possibility of infective endocarditis if fever persists (see p. 54)

11 *Postcardiotomy psychosis*—may appear after a brief lucid period.

a. Signs and symptoms include delirium (impairment of orientation, memory, intellectual function, judgement), transient perceptual distortions, visual and auditory hallucinations, disorientation and paranoid delusions.

b. Symptoms may be related to sleep deprivation, prolonged inability to speak due to endotracheal intubation, age, preoperative cardiac state, etc.

c. Keep patient orientated to time and place; notify of procedures and expectations of patient's co-operation. Give repeated explanations of what is happening.

d. Establish rapport with patient preoperatively; have patient visit intensive care unit *before* surgery.

e. Encourage family to come in at regular times—helps patient regain sense of reality.

f. Plan care to allow rest periods and day-night pattern.

g. Keep the patient's surroundings as quiet as possible. Prevent bodily injury.

h. Reassure patient and his family that psychiatric disorders following cardiac surgery are usually transient.

i. Remove patient from intensive care unit as soon as possible.

j. Allow patient to discuss events of his psychotic episode—helps him deal with and assimilate experience.

Health Teaching Following Cardiac Surgery

1 Begin discussing long-range plans with patient during convalescence in order to help him make modifications in his life-style.

2 Give written guidelines:

    a. *Activities:*

        (1) Increase activities gradually within limits. Avoid strenuous activities and contact sports.

        (2) Participate in activities that do not cause pain or discomfort.

        (3) Increase walking time each day.

        (4) Stairs (1–2 times daily) the first week; increase as tolerated.

        (5) Avoid large crowds at first.

        (6) Driving: Avoid driving until after first postoperative checkup. At this time ask doctor when you may drive.

        (7) Sexual relations: resumptions of sexual relations parallels ability to participate in other activities.

        (8) Return to work—after first postoperative checkup as advised by doctor.

    b. *Diet:*

        (1) Some patients will require fluid restriction.

        (2) Most patients are placed on minimum salt restriction, e.g., no added salt at table.

        (3) Give a list of low sodium foods.

    c. *Medications:*

        (1) Label all medications; give purposes and side-effects.

        (2) Patients with prosthetic valves may continue warfarin indefinitely.

3 Patients with prosthetic valves:

    a. Pregnancy usually discouraged in women with prosthetic valves.

    b. Caution patient about need for antibiotic coverage following dental and surgical procedures.

    c. Patients on anticoagulants should watch for bleeding and should avoid use of aspirin (and many other drugs)—interferes with action of warfarin.

4   Advise patient to carry an identification card stating cardiac condition and medications being taken.
5   Patient may be placed on rehabilitation and exercise programme after exercise tolerance testing.

2. Essentials of Basic Electrocardiography*

THE ECG AND HEART PHYSIOLOGY

The Electrocardiogram (ECG)

1   A recording of the heart's electrical impulse.
2   The heart is stimulated to contract and thus pump blood to the body organs by the electrical pulsation which originates at the top of the heart and travels downward.
3   To record the impulse, electrodes do not have to be placed directly on the heart, but can be placed on the extremities, where the heart's activity can be sensed (Fig. 1.15).

Clinical Use of ECG

An electrocardiogram can be helpful in diagnosing the following:

1   Myocardial infarction and arteriosclerotic heart disease.
2   Cardiac arrhythmias.
3   Cardiac enlargement.
4   Electrolyte abnormalities (especially potassium and calcium).
5   Pericarditis (inflammation of the pericardial sac which surrounds the heart).
6   Pericardial effusion (fluid in the pericardial sac which can restrict the heart's pumping ability).

Heart Anatomy and Physiology (Fig. 1.16)

1   The normal electrical impulse of the heart, which causes the heart to contract, begins in the SA node (also called sinoatrial node, sinus node or normal physiological pacemaker).
2   The SA node occupies the superior aspect of the right atrium.
3   The impulse, after beginning in the SA node, travels across the atria causing them to contract and pump blood into the ventricles.
4   The impulse then hits the AV node (atrioventricular node) which lies between the atria and ventricles.
5   The impulse is somewhat delayed in the AV node and then travels down the ventricles, causing them to contract and thus pump blood to the body organs.
6   Both the SA and AV nodes are connected to two main nerve systems which control the rate at which the heart beats.
    a. Sympathetic nerves—cause the heart rate to increase.
    b. Parasympathetic nerves (vagus nerve)—slow the heart rate.

* Illustrations in this section are from RN magazine. Butler, H (1973) How to read an ECG, RN, 36, (reproduced with permission).

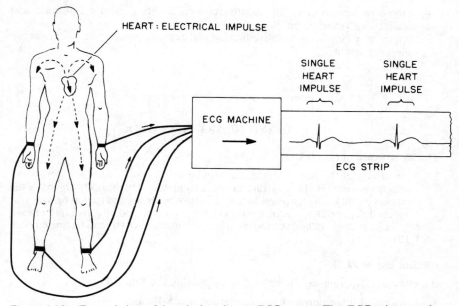

Figure 1.15.   Transmission of heart's impulse to ECG paper. The ECG wires on the extremities sense the electrical impulse as it travels from the top of the heart to the bottom. The impulse is sent through the ECG machine where a picture of the heart's activity is recorded.

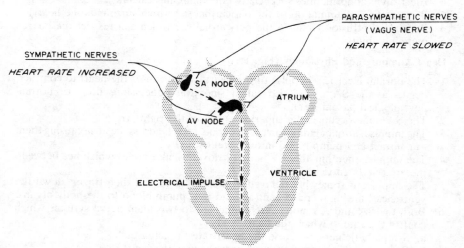

Figure 1.16.   Heart physiology. Pictured is the pathway of the normal electrical impulse which inscribes the ECG and causes the heart to contract and pump blood. Also shown are the nerves which regulate the heart rate.

Normal ECG

1　Figure 1.17 represents a normal ECG.
2　Each heart beat manifests as three major deflections:
  a. P wave.
  b. QRS complex.
  c. T wave.
3　The QRS complex is composed of three parts:
  a. Q wave—the first downward deflection.
  b. R wave—the first upward deflection.
  c. S wave—the first downward deflection after the R wave.
4　Beats come at regular intervals (normal sinus rhythm), indicating that the impulse is originating properly from the sinus node.

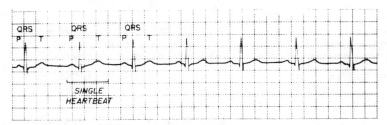

Figure 1.17.　A normal ECG.

ECG Waves Related to Heart Anatomy (Fig. 1.18)

1　*The P wave*—begins in the SA node and can be thought of as representing the cardiac electrical impulse travelling through the *atria*.
2　*QRS complex*—represents the impulse going through the *ventricles*. It begins in the AV node which lies above the ventricular chambers.
3　*T wave*—does not represent an impulse going through any specific chamber but is a purely electrical phenomenon and signifies recovery of the electrical forces (*repolarization*).

ECG Paper (Fig. 1.19)

1　Vertical lines—measure the *magnitude* of the electrical impulse.
2　Horizontal inscriptions—represent the *time* it takes for an impulse to travel over cardiac tissue.
3　In vertical axis—each small block is 1 mm and one darker large block is 5 mm.
4　In horizontal axis one small block represents 0.04 s and one darker large block represents 0.20 s.

Determination of Cardiac Rate on ECG Paper

1　Cardiac rate can be obtained by dividing the number of heavily lined large blocks that lie between every two QRS complexes into 300.
2　The number 300 is used because 300 large blocks represent 1 min on the ECG paper.

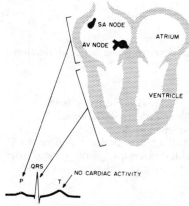

Figure 1.18.   ECG waves related to heart anatomy. The electrical impulse is shown travelling through the chambers of the heart and thus inscribing the normal ECG of one heart beat. The P wave represents atrial activity and the QRS complex is derived from ventricular stimulation.

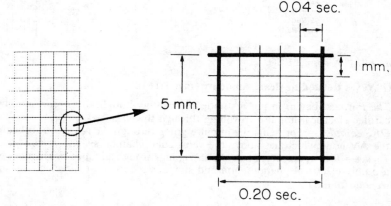

Figure 1.19.   Meaning of blocks on ECG paper. All one really needs to remember is that one small block is 1 mm tall and 0.04 s wide.

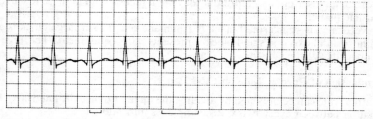

Figure 1.20.   Determination of rate. There are three large blocks between every two QRS complexes. By dividing 300 by 3 the rate is 100 beats/min.

Examples:
>   If there are three large blocks between every two QRS complexes, the rate
>   would be 100 beats/min (300 divided by 3 = 100). (See Fig. 1.20.)
>   If there are two and one-half blocks between every two QRS complexes, the
>   rate would be 120 beats/min.

ECG Leads

1 Standard ECG machines have a dial which turns to 1 to 12 leads (I, II, III, AVR,
   AVL, AVF, V1, V2, V3, V4, V5, V6).
2 Each lead receives and records the heart's electrical impulse from a different
   anatomical position relative to the heart's surface.
3 Letter designations can be confusing; thus position of each lead must be
   memorized.
4 The area of the heart represented by each lead is shown in Fig. 1.21.
5 Location of leads helps to localize cardiac pathology.

Significance of Each ECG Wave and Interval

P Wave (Fig. 1.22a)

1 P wave represents the atrial contraction.
2 Enlargement of the P-wave deflection indicates enlargement of the atrium such
   as might occur in mitral stenosis. (The atrium enlarges in mitral stenosis because
   the mitral opening between the atrium and ventricle is small, causing blood to
   dam back, which in turn forces the atrial wall to expand.)
3 P wave is considered enlarged if it is over 3 mm tall (three small blocks) or 0.12 s
   wide (three small blocks).

PR Interval (Fig. 1.22b)

1 Starts at the beginning of the P wave and extends to the onset of the Q wave.
2 At normal rates, the PR intervals should not exceed 0.20 s (five small blocks).
3 This interval increases in length in arteriosclerotic heart disease and in rheumatic
   fever.
4 The PR interval is prolonged because the area of heart tissue represented by the
   PR interval (namely the atrium and AV node area) is scarred or inflamed and the
   impulse is forced to travel at a slower rate.

The QRS Complex (Fig. 1.22c)

1 Q wave (first downward stroke)—when enlarged it is indicative of an old
   myocardial infarction.
2 The R wave (first upward deflection).
   a. Increases in amplitude when the ventricle enlarges, as in most types of heart
   disease. (Overwork of a specific part of the heart causes enlargement).
   b. May become small when the heart is compressed by fluid, as in a pericardial
   effusion

The ST Segment (Fig. 1.22d)

1 Begins at the end of the S wave (the first downward deflection after the R wave)
   and terminates at the beginning of the T wave.

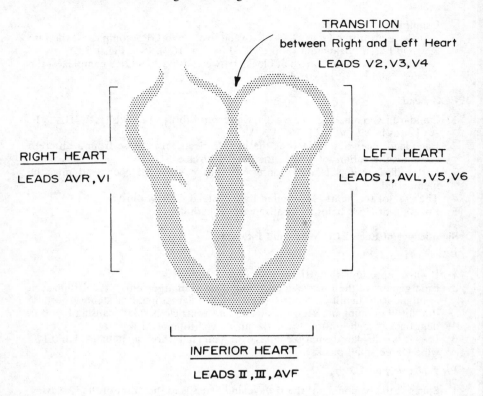

Figure 1.21.   ECG leads related to heart anatomy.

2   Is elevated above the baseline on the ECG strip in an acute myocardial infarction or in pericarditis.
3   Becomes depressed when the heart muscle is getting a decreased supply of oxygen or when a patient is taking digitalis.
4   Becomes long in hypocalcaemia. (Hypocalcaemia occurs most commonly in chronic renal disease because the scarred kidneys cannot excrete phosphate. Since phosphate and calcium maintain a reciprocal balance in the body fluid, the elevated phosphate causes a depression in the calcium level.)
5   Becomes shorter in hypercalcaemia, which is most commonly seen in metastatic carcinoma because the tumour erodes the bones and spills calcium into the serum.

The T Wave (Fig. 1.22e)

1   Represents no cardiac activity, but reflects the electrical recovery of the ventricular contraction. (An electrical impulse is the flow of electrons; the T wave is inscribed when these electrons migrate back to their resting position after traversing the heart muscle to make it contract.)

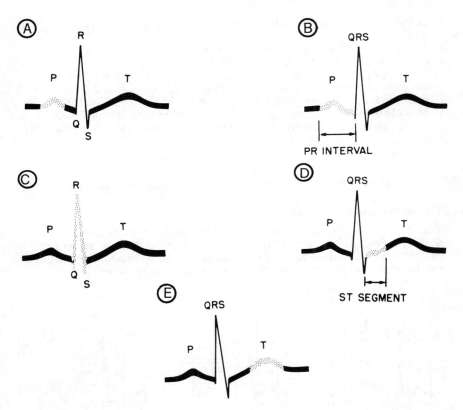

Figure 1.22. Parts of a heart beat. a. The P wave. b. The PR interval (extends from the beginning of the P wave to the onset of the Q wave). c. The QRS complex. (Even when the complex does not have a discrete Q or S wave it is still referred to as the QRS complex to denote a ventricular impulse and to provide simplicity and uniformity.) d. The ST segment begins at the termination of the S wave and ends at the beginning of the T wave. e. The T wave.

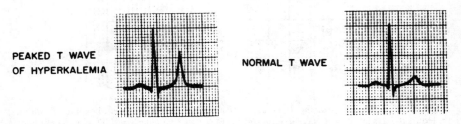

PEAKED T WAVE OF HYPERKALEMIA

NORMAL T WAVE

Figure 1.23. The ECGs show the difference between the tall peaked T wave of hyperkalaemia and the normal rounded T wave.

2   Is flat when the heart is not receiving enough oxygen (arteriosclerotic heart disease).
3   May be inverted in a myocardial infarction.
4   May be made tall by an elevated serum potassium.

The most common cause of elevated serum potassium levels is renal disease; the most frequent ECG finding is a tall, peaked, narrow-based T wave which begins to form when the potassium reaches levels of about 6 mEq/l (Fig. 1.23).

5   Should not be over 10 mm (10 small blocks) high in the precordial leads (those that are placed on the chest) and should not be over 5 mm in the remaining leads.

ECG INTERPRETATION OF MYOCARDIAL INFARCTION

ECG Interpretation (Fig. 1.24)

NOTE: The ECGs of some patients suffering myocardial infarctions may show *no specific changes* on the initial tracing. Therefore, if a person has symptoms compatible with a heart attack and has a normal ECG, he should nevertheless be admitted to the hospital for observation and further electrocardiograms.

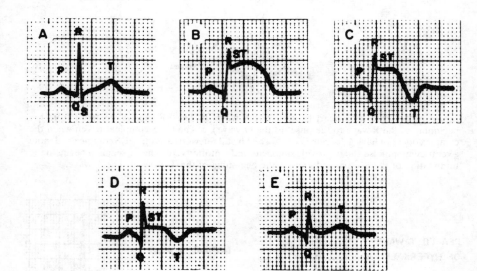

Figure 1.24.   a. Normal tracing. b. Hours after infarction, the ST segment becomes elevated. c. Hours to days later the T wave inverts and the Q wave become larger. d. Days to weeks later the ST segment returns to near-normal. e. Lastly, the T wave becomes upright again, but the Q wave may remain permanently large.

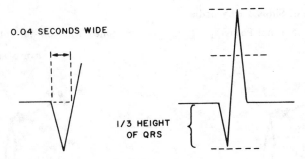

Figure 1.25.   Abnormal Q wave. A Q wave is considered abnormal when it is over 0.04 s (one small block on the ECG paper) or over one-third the height of the QRS complex. This usually indicates an old myocardial infarction.

1 Elevation of ST segment is first finding.
2 T wave inversion follows.
3 Then a large Q wave appears
   a. As infarct heals, Q wave may remain as the only sign of an old coronary occlusion. (In AVR a large Q wave is normal.)
   b. Q wave can be considered abnormal if it is over 0.04 s wide (one small block is 0.04 s) or if it is greater in depth than one-third the height of the QRS complex (Fig. 1.25).

ECG INTERPRETATION OF CARDIAC ARRHYTHMIAS

NOTE: The lower the ectopic focus resides in the heart, the more lethal the arrhythmia becomes.

Sinus Tachycardia

Sinus tachycardia can be defined as a cardiac rate of over 100 beats/min. All the complexes are normal, but their rate is excessive.

Altered Physiology

The impulse begins normally in the SA node but comes at a faster rate secondary to increased sympathetic nerve stimuli.

Causes

1 Exercise.
2 Anxiety.
3 Fever.
4 Shock.

Mechanism of Sinus Tachycardia

Normal Pathway   Sinus Tachycardia Pathway

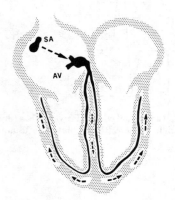

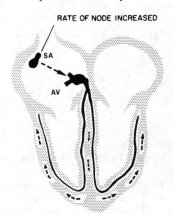

The pathway of sinus tachycardia is the same as that of a normal sinus rhythm, but the number of impulses per minute is greater in sinus tachycardia.

ECG of Sinus Tachycardia

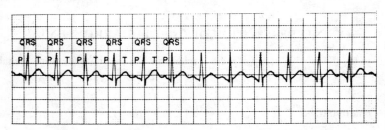

The P wave, the QRS complex and the T wave are all normal. The only abnormality is a rate of over 100 beats/min.

Treatment

Since sinus tachycardia is usually a compensatory rhythm, treatment is directed at the primary causes, which usually are not cardiac.

Sinus Bradycardia

Sinus bradycardia is defined as a heart rate below 60/min. All the complexes are normal.

Aetiology

1 Seen *normally* in well-trained athletes.
2 May be secondary to certain drugs, such as digitalis and morphine, or from processes involving the SA node, such as arteriosclerosis.
   a. When the SA node is severely diseased it may not respond to stimulant drugs such as atropine—'sick sinus syndrome'.
   b. A tachycardia can so exhaust a diseased SA node that when the tachycardia ceases the SA node fails to take up the rhythm at a respectable rate and the patient is left with a severe bradycardia.
   c. When this occurs, the 'sick sinus syndrome' is called the 'tachycardia-bradycardia syndrome.'
3 Also seen in myocardial infarction in which instance it could be detrimental to the patient, who is already in a compromised cardiac state.

Complications

Slow rate and low cardiac output can cause:
   Fainting (Stokes–Adams syndrome) or
   Congestive heart failure. (Heart cannot pump all the fluid presented to it, resulting in stasis or 'congestion' of the blood in the lungs and other body tissues.)

Mechanism of Sinus Bradycardia

Normal Pathway   Sinus Bradycardia Pathway

RATE OF NODE DECREASED

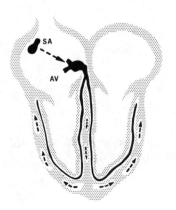

ECG of Sinus Bradycardia

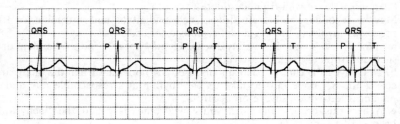

The only abnormality is a rate below 60 beats/min.

Treatment

1   Rarely has to be treated.
2   If congestive failure or fainting occurs, treatment should be initiated immediately to increase the heart rate.
    a. Give 0.5–1 mg of atropine intravenously (inhibits the vagal or 'slowing' nerve and therefore makes the heart go faster).
    b. If patient becomes resistant to atropine, the rate can be increased by adding 1 mg of isoprenaline hydrochloride to 250 ml of 5% glucose in water and initially running the solution at about 10 drops/min. (Stimulates the sympathetic or 'fast' nerve of the heart.) (Atropine can be prepared more quickly and is less toxic to the heart than isoprenaline hydrochloride.)
    c. The heart rate can be increased or decreased by adjusting the rate of fluid administered.
    d. An electrical pacemaker may be necessary in unresponsive cases or when the fluid load becomes excessive.

Sinus Arrhythmia

Sinus arrhythmia is normally found in children and young adults and is characterized by a heart rhythm that is normal in every way except for irregularity.

Aetiology

1   On inspiration the heart rate increases and on expiration the heart rate decreases.
2   Inspiration tends to inhibit the vagus nerve (slows the heart) and causes an acceleration of the cardiac rate.

Mechanism of Sinus Arrhythmia

Normal Pathway

Sinus Arrhythmia Pathway

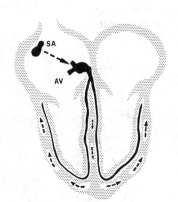
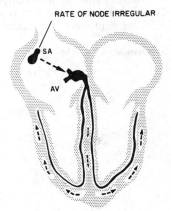

The pathway of sinus arrhythmia is the same as that of the normal sinus rhythm; the only difference being the regularity of the impulses.

ECG of Sinus Arrhythmia

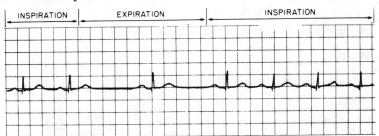

All the complexes are normal; only the rate is irregular—varying with respiration. The rate increases with inspiration and decreases with expiration.

Treatment

Since sinus arrhythmia is usually normal, no treatment is necessary.

Premature Atrial Contractions (PACs)

PACs constitute a very common rhythm disturbance and are seen in both normal and abnormal hearts. They rarely cause symptoms and are felt to be of little consequence except when they occur frequently, at which time they may tend to deteriorate into other more serious arrhythmias.

Altered Physiology

1   Beats occur *early* in the cycle; they begin in the atrium, but *outside* the sinus node where normal impulses originate.
2   Since the atrial pathway is abnormal, the P wave is distorted.
3   Since ventricular activation is undisturbed, the QRS is normal.

Mechanism of a PAC

Normal Pathway   PAC Pathway

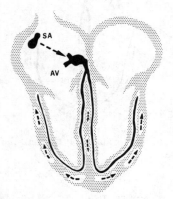 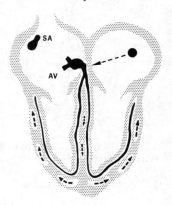

The PAC begins in the atrium outside the SA node.

ECG of a PAC

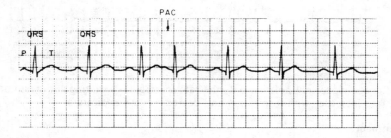

1   PAC comes early in the cycle.
2   P wave is abnormally shaped.
3   QRS complex is normal.

Treatment

1   Most of the time PACs do not need to be treated.
2   Quinidine, which is a good suppressant of atrial ectopic beats, may be used when the patient requires therapy.

Paroxysmal Atrial Tachycardia (PAT)

PAT is a common arrhythmia in young adults; it is usually found in normal hearts. There is a rapid heart rate which ranges from 140–250 beats/min with an average of about 180 beats/min.

Clinical Manifestations

Patient will complain of a pounding or fluttering in the chest associated with shortness of breath and fainting—due to rapid heart rate.

Altered Physiology

1   Begins in an ectopic focus of the atrium outside the sinus node.
2   Its pathway over the heart is similar to that of a PAC. Thus PAT may be thought of as a rapid succession of PACs.
3   The P wave (atrial wave) is distorted because the pathway over the atrium is abnormal. (Most of the time the rate is so fast that the P wave is buried in the previous complex and is not seen).
4   The QRS complex (ventricular wave) is normal because the route of the cardiac impulse after penetrating the AV node is undisturbed.

Mechanism of PAT

Normal Pathway   PAT Pathway

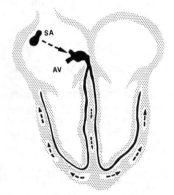
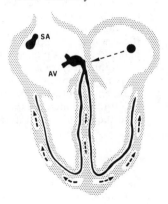

An impulse travelling along the abnormal PAT pathway (right) produces an abnormal P wave and a normally shaped QRS complex (ventricular wave). Notice that the focus of the PAT is the same as that of a PAC.

ECG of PAT

1   The rate is very rapid—over 140/min (higher than in sinus tachycardia).
2   P waves cannot be seen since they are superimposed within the T wave of the

preceding beat. If the P waves were seen they would be abnormal in configuration.

3   The QRS complex is normal.

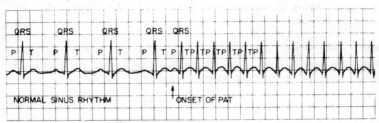

Treatment

1   Since cardiac arrest can occur with any mode of treatment for PAT, an ECG machine should remain attached to the patient, an intravenous infusion should be started, and appropriate resuscitation equipment, including a defibrillator, should be at hand.

2   If the patient is relatively asymptomatic and stable, with a normal blood pressure, giving a simple sedative and waiting 5–10 min may result in spontaneous conversion of PAT.

3   Start by stimulating the right carotid sinus (an area of dense nerve supply) of the carotid artery for several seconds or gagging the patient with a tongue depressor in an effort to terminate the arrhythmia. These manoeuvres work by stimulating the vagus nerve, which puts a 'brake' on the heart.

4   If the above procedure is not effective and if the blood pressure is low (many patients with PAT have a systolic pressure of about 90 mmHg), a slow drip of metaraminol (Aramine), intravenously, can be started.
   a. Add 100 mg of Aramine to 500 ml of 5% glucose in water and run the intravenous infusion initially at 10 drops/min.
   b. Gradually increase the rate of the infusion until the PAT terminates, at which time the intravenous infusion should be stopped (usually a matter of seconds). (See Fig. 1.26).

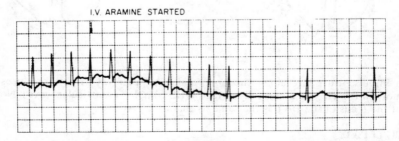

Figure 1.26. Termination of PAT. The ECG illustrates PAT being terminated with an intravenous infusion of Aramine.

c. Do not raise the systolic blood pressure above 180. This drug increases the blood pressure, which in turn stimulates the vagus nerve to inhibit the ectopic focus of the atrium.

d. If the patient is already hypertensive (rare), Aramine should not be used.

e. Some authorities do not use a vasopressor such as Aramine because of the occasional report of a cerebral vascular accident, but this complication has usually occurred when the drug is used in bolus form. Instead of Aramine, they prefer a fast-acting digitalis preparation which works in part by stimulating the vagal nerve.

5   In an unusual case, in which the preceding steps are ineffective or contra-indicated, 1–3 mg of propranolol (Inderal)—a sympathetic nerve blocker—may be given by intravenous infusion at a rate no greater than 1 mg/min.

5   In the extreme case when the patient is in congestive heart failure, DC synchronized electrical shock (cardioversion) should be instituted (instead of giving Inderal).

a. Initial shock—can be 50–100 W/s (Joules).

b. Electrical shock stops the heart and allows the heartbeat to begin again normally at the SA node.

Atrial Flutter

Atrial flutter is a rapid, regular 'fluttering' of the atrium.

Altered Physiology

1   P waves take on a 'sawtooth' appearance because they are coming from a focus other than the sinus node and are coming at a very rapid rate.

2   As in PAC or PAT, the impulse comes from *one* ectopic focus in the atrium, but the *atrial* rate (not the pulse or ventricular rate) is between 250 and 350/min for atrial flutter.

The following oversimplified arbitrary rule may be used to distinguish the atrial arrhythmias from each other:

Atrial rate in sinus tachycardia goes up to 140/min.

Atrial rate in PAT is between 140 and 250/min.

Atrial rate in atrial flutter is between 250 and 350/min.

3   Atrial flutter generally occurs in a pathological heart (usually arteriosclerotic or rheumatic), as contrasted with PAT, which in many cases is associated with a normal heart.

4   Since the abnormality is above the AV node, the QRS complex (ventricular wave) is normal in configuration.

5   Since the P waves come so rapidly, the AV node cannot accept and conduct each one; therefore there is some degree of 'blockage' at the AV node.

Example: If the atrial rate is 300, the ventricular rate (which is the same as the pulse rate) might be 150, since the AV node is not able to conduct every atrial impulse because of the excessive rapidity. In this instance, the 'block' is said to be 2:1 since there are two atrial impulses per venticular response.

6   The 2:1 block is the most common block in atrial flutter.

7   Most cases of PAT do not exhibit a block since P waves do not occur as fast as in atrial flutter. Thus in PAT all the impulses are transmitted by the AV node to the ventricles.

Mechanism of Atrial Flutter

Normal Pathway   Atrial Flutter Pathway

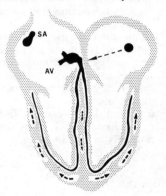

The pathways for atrial flutter are the same as for PAC and PAT, but in atrial flutter the ectopic impulse fires at a faster rate.

ECG of Atrial Flutter

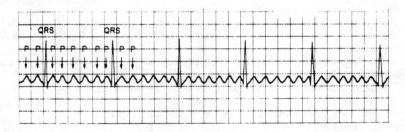

1   The arrows indicate the P waves generated by the fast-firing ectopic focus in the atrium.
2   Notice that not every P wave stimulates a QRS complex (ventricular wave).
3   Since the abnormality present in the heart is above the AV node, the QRS complexes that appear are normal in configuration.

Treatment

1   Classic initial treatment is digitalis, which partially blocks the AV node; this allows fewer P waves to pass through the ventricles and thus slows the pulse rate.

2 The fast pulse rate must be slowed down (ventricular rate) because the heart is not given enough time to fill itself with blood when it is contracting rapidly; this causes the blood to dam back in the body tissues, leading to congestive failure.
3 Cardioversion:
   a. Tried when the patient is not tolerating the arrhythmia well.
   b. Atrial flutter responds well to cardioversion at a relatively low wattage (50–100 W/s).

Nursing Alert: When a patient is taking digitalis, cardioversion can be dangerous since a lethal arrhythmia may be precipitated.

Atrial Fibrillation

Atrial fibrillation is an atrial arrhythmia occurring at an extremely rapid and unco-ordinated rate. The atria produce impulses so rapidly that the ventricles are not capable of responding to every atrial beat; therefore, only a small percentage of atrial stimuli excite the ventricles. Since the atrial rate is irregular, the ventricular rate (pulse rate) will also be irregular.

Aetiology

Usually seen in patients with arteriosclerotic or rheumatic heart disease.

Altered Physiology

1 Arteriosclerosis leads to scarring of the atrium and thus to disruption of the normal course of the P wave (atrial wave).
2 P waves are replaced by irregular, rapid waves each of which is different in configuration from the other.
3 P waves (often called fibrillatory waves) assume different shapes because they come from different foci in the atrium. (In atrial flutter the P waves are very regular and uniform since they come from one focus.)
4 Because P waves occur at variable intervals, the QRS complexes assume an irregular rhythm, and thus the patient's pulse is irregular. (The configuration of the QRS is normal since the conduction tissue beyond the AV node has not yet become critically involved with the arteriosclerotic process.)
5 Since the P waves come so fast, all of them do not pass on to the ventricles, because of normal refraction of the AV node. Thus the atrial rate is usually much faster than the ventricular rate.
6 Occasionally, the ventricular rate is very fast because the AV node is blocking relatively fewer beats than is normal. If this is the case, atrial activity may not be seen, because the QRS complexes are so close together (since their rate is so rapid) that it is difficult to define the arrhythmia.

NOTE: General rule: If *normal* QRS complexes are present at a very rapid rate, so that atrial activity cannot be seen and the rhythm is *irregular*, the probable diagnosis is atrial fibrillation.

Mechanism of Atrial Fibrillation

Normal Pathway   Atrial Fibrillation Pathway

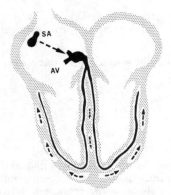
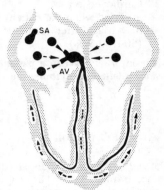

1   In atrial fibrillation many ectopic foci are present in the atrium (right).
2   Since each small atrial wave comes from a different focus and travels a different route, the shape of each atrial wave (P wave) is different.

ECG of Atrial Fibrillation

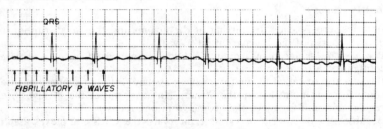

1   Note the small, irregular fibrillating P waves (arrows).
2   As with atrial flutter, only an occasional P wave travels through the AV node to form a QRS complex, but since these complexes come at irregular intervals in atrial fibrillation, the ventricular rate is irregular.
3   Each P wave is different in shape because it comes from a different focus in the atrium.

Treatment

1   Depends on patient's clinical condition, cardiac rate and drug therapy.
2   For the average patient who is not critical and not on digitalis, the following treatment is common:
    a. Intravenous digoxin (0.5 mg) given over a 5-min period under ECG control.
    b. After 2 hours, an additional 0.25–0.5 mg is given, depending on the ECG and

the patient's condition. (Total intravenous dose before oral maintenance therapy is 0.75–1.5 mg)

3   If atrial fibrillation is an imminent, life-threating emergency (rare):

a. Cardioversion may be started with 100 W/s.

b. As with atrial flutter, cardioversion becomes somewhat of a risk when the patient is taking digitalis.

c. In contrast to atrial flutter, atrial fibrillation is more difficult to correct to normal sinus rhythm with electric countershock.

AV Block

AV block means that the AV node is diseased and has difficulty conducting the atrial waves (P waves) into the ventricles. Common causes are congenital and arteriosclerotic heart disease.

Types of AV Block

1st degree
2nd degree
3rd degree

Mechanism of AV Blocks

1   Abnormal tissue around and in the AV node causes physiological blockage affecting the entry of the atrial impulse into the ventricles.

2   In 1st degree block—the impulses are merely slowed.

3   In 2nd degree block—only a portion of the atrial impulses penetrate to the ventricles.

4   In 3rd degree block—no atrial impulse enters the ventricles, so that the atria and ventricles beat independently.

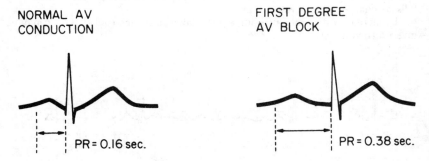

NORMAL AV
CONDUCTION

FIRST DEGREE
AV BLOCK

PR = 0.16 sec.

PR = 0.38 sec.

Figure 1.27. 1st degree AV block. Since the tissue around the AV node is abnormal, the impulse takes longer to traverse this area, which leads to a prolonged PR interval.

1st Degree AV Block (Fig. 1.27)

1   The PR interval is prolonged. (The PR interval represents the impulse going through the atrium and the area of the AV node.) It should not exceed 0.2 s (five small blocks on ECG paper when one block equals 0.04 s) at normal heart rates.
2   Since the atrial and AV nodal tissues are diseased, the electrical impulse takes a longer time to traverse its pathway (as reflected by the increased length of the PR interval).
3   All P waves penetrate the ventricles to form QRS complexes (in contrast to 2nd and 3rd degree block).

2nd Degree AV Block

1   Some P waves do not pass through the ventricles, but others do.
2   A ratio of 2:1, 3:1, 4:1 or any such combination appears on ECG. (Figure 1.28 represents a 2:1 ratio.)
3   2nd degree block is distinguished from 3rd degree block by the fact that some P waves conduct QRS complexes and others do not.

3rd Degree AV Block

1   Also called a complete AV block.
2   *No* P waves penetrate the AV node and enter the ventricles; therefore, the P waves and QRS complexes are beating *independently*.
3   P waves are seen before the QRS complexes, but the PR interval varies and there is no constant relationship of the P waves to the QRS complexes (Fig. 1.29).
4   The pulse rate is usually slow since the ventricles are beating at their own inherent rhythm, which is about 35 beats/min.

Treatment of AV Blocks

1   1st degree block:
    No treatment needed.
2   2nd degree block:
    a. When certain types of 2nd degree heart block occur in a myocardial infarction, many cardiologists insert a pacemaker which is activated when the cardiac rate falls to unacceptable levels.
    b. To increase rate while awaiting a pacemaker, atropine (0.5–1.0 mg) may be given intravenously.

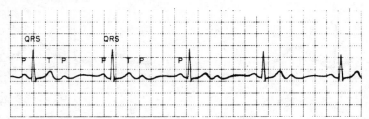

Figure 1.28.   2nd degree AV block. Some P waves pass through to the ventricles, but others do not.

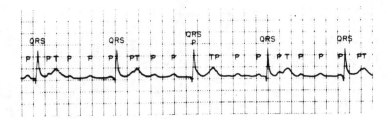

Figure 1.29.   3rd degree AV block. The P waves and QRS complexes are beating independently against each other.

    c. If the rate cannot be maintained with atropine, 1 mg of isoprenaline hydrochloride added to 250 ml of 5% glucose in water may be infused by the 'piggyback' technique to stimulate the heart to function at an acceptable rate.

3   3rd degree heart block:
    a. In myocardial infarction, 3rd degree block is frequently treated with a pacemaker.
    b. While awaiting insertion of the pacemaker, patient may be maintained on atropine or isoprenaline hydrochloride (Isuprel) as in 2nd degree block.

The Artificial Pacemaker

Normally Functioning Pacemaker (Fig. 1.30).

1   The ECG of a patient with a normally functioning artificial pacemaker shows a *vertical line* just at the beginning of the QRS complex. This represents the electrical stimulus of the artificial pacemaker.

Poorly Functioning Pacemakers

1   Due to lack of contact between pacing catheter and heart wall.
    a. May occur when patient performs a sudden movement.
    b. On the ECG the small vertical line denoting the pacemaker stimulus is *not* followed by a QRS complex (Fig. 1.31).

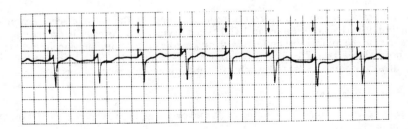

Figure 1.30.   Normal pacemaker function. In this ECG each QRS complex is preceded by a small vertical line (arrows) which represent the electrical stimulus of the artificial pacemaker.

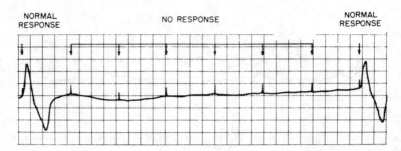

Figure 1.31. Poor pacemaker contact. Notice that the first and last pacemaker stimuli are followed by ventricular complexes and that the other pacemaker deflections failed to produce a cardiac impulse because of the lack of pacemaker contact with the heart wall.

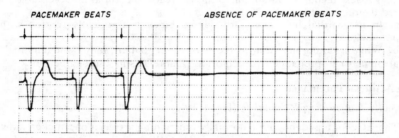

Figure 1.32. Malfunctioning pacemaker. Notice the eventual absence of pacemaker stimuli which in this case resulted in cardiac standstill. The patient had a faulty pacemaker.

2   Due to malfunctioning:
   a. Examples: wires break or disconnect from pacemaker; battery fails to function.
   b. Noted on ECG by the absence of vertical pacer lines (Fig. 1.32).

Premature Ventricular Contractions (PVCs)

Premature ventricular contractions represent one of the most easily recognized rhythm disturbances seen on an ECG. They occur in all forms of heart disease and are seen in the majority of patients with myocardial infarction. They occur frequently in normal hearts and can be secondary to smoking, coffee or alcohol. While not usually symptomatic, PVCs, when frequent, may cause palpitations.

Altered Physiology

1   Contractions come early in the cycle and originate in the ventricle *below* the AV node.
2   QRS configurations are wide and bizarre, since a PVC does not begin normally and therefore does not follow the true conduction path in the ventricle.

Mechanism of a PVC

Normal Pathway   PVC Pathway

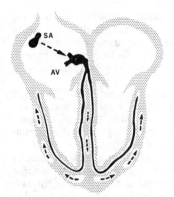   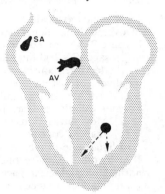

Since a PVC begins in the ventricle outside the AV node a bizarre ventricular QRS complex will be inscribed.

ECG of PVCs

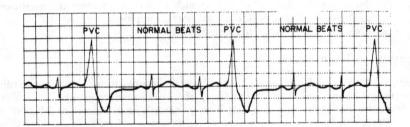

PVCs occur early in the cycle and are wider than the normal beat.

Danger of PVCs

PVC can be especially dangerous when they:

1 Occur more frequently than once in 10 beats.
2 Occur in groups of two or three.
3 Land near the T wave.
4 Take on multiple configurations—this indicates the PVCs come from different foci, which in turn means that the ventricle is more irritable.

Treatment

If a patient has an infarct, PVCs are treated vigorously since they *can precipitate ventricular fibrillation by hitting a T wave.*

1 Lignocaine (Xylocaine) can be given—PVCs are usually seen with a cardiac rate of over 60/min; lignocaine (a cardiac muscle suppressant) is drug of choice because PVCs are most likely to come from an irritable focus such as an infarct.
   a. Dosage: 75–100 mg intravenously as a bolus over a 2- to 3-minute period.
   b. If effective, a continuous intravenous drip of lignocaine should be started with a delivery of 1–4 mg/min.
     (1) Addition of a 50-ml bottle of 2% lignocaine to 1000 ml of 5% glucose in water will give a concentration of 1 mg of lignocaine per ml of fluid.
     (2) Most intravenous sets are calibrated to deliver 1 ml in 10 drops of fluid.
     (3) If above concentration results in too much fluid for the patient, the amount of lignocaine in the intravenous solution should be increased.
2 If heart rate is *slow* secondary to a myocardial infarction involving the heart's normal physiological pacemaker (SA node), PVCs (better termed 'ectopic ventricular beats' since in this circumstance the beats are not 'premature' but late in the cycle) may occur as a compensatory mechanism to maintain a reasonable rate so as to provide some type of cardiac contraction for pumping blood to the body tissues. (A PVC does not pump as much blood as a normal impulse from the SA node, but it does provide some circulation.)
   a. Xylocaine would be contraindicated since it would decrease circulation by extinguishing the PVCs which are pumping needed blood.
   b. Atropine is treatment of choice in this case (since a slow rate results in PVCs).
     (1) Increases the sinus node rate, which in turn terminates the inefficient ectopic beats by replacing them with normal impulses.
     (2) Dosage: 0.5–1.0 mg intravenously.

Ventricular Tachycardia

Ventricular tachycardia is one of the dreaded complications of a myocardial infarction and can be considered as multiple (three or more), consecutive, premature ventricular contractions that originate from an ectopic focus below the AV node in the ventricles and thus cause the complexes to be wide and bizarre in configuration.

Dangers of Ventricular Tachycardia

1 Leads to a reduced cardiac output (the ventricles are not being stimulated normally from the AV node, but from a focus farther down in the ventricle wall, which leads to an incomplete and inefficient contraction of the heart muscle).
2 Is a precursor of ventricular fibrillation, in which there is no cardiac output.

Mechanism of Ventricular Tachycardia

1 Pathway is the same as for PVC since ventricular tachycardia can be thought of as a series of PVCs.
2 Like the PVCs, the complexes of ventricular tachycardia show a bizarre configuration.

Normal Pathway

Ventricular Tachycardia Pathways

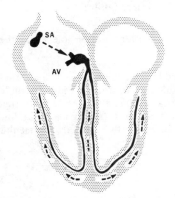 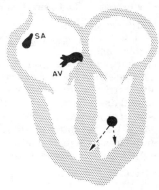

ECG of Ventricular Tachycardia

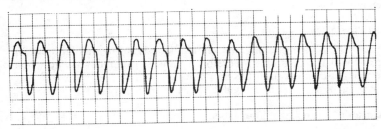

1 Since this arrhythmia begins below the AV node, the atria are beating independently.
2 On the ECGs of 20% of patients, when the ventricular rate is not too fast and the ventricular complexes are not too wide, P waves which are independent of the QRS complexes can be seen.
3 The rate is fast and the QRS complexes are wide. A width equivalent to 0.12 s (three small blocks) or more is considered abnormal for a QRS complex.

Treatment

1 If patient is tolerating the arrhythmia fairly well:
   a. Give lignocaine (Xylocaine):
   (1) 75–100 mg intravenously as a bolus over a 2-min period.
   (2) If effective, a continuous intravenous drip of lignocaine should be started (with delivery of 1–3 mg/min.)
   (3) If a 50-ml bottle of 2% lignocaine is added to 1000 ml of 5% glucose in water, 1 ml will contain 1 mg of lignocaine. Most intravenous sets are calibrated to deliver 1 ml in 10 drops of fluid. If concentration results in too much fluid for the patient, the amount of lignocaine should be increased in the intravenous solution.

Nursing Alert: Because the heart muscle is weakened, the cardiac patient should not receive excessive fluid since this may precipitate congestive failure.

2 Cardioversion.
   a. Used when lignocaine does not work or if patient is not tolerating the arrhythmia well.
   b. Start with about 200 W/s.
   Cardioversion is a *timed* electric shock delivered by a machine which is set so that its electrical output does not hit a T wave, which is considered the vulnerable period on the cardiac cycle. If an electrical shock, such as that from an external source or from an electrical impulse within the heart itself (such as a PVC), hits the T wave, ventricular fibrillation may ensue. If not terminated, ventricular fibrillation results in death.

Ventricular Fibrillation

Ventricular fibrillation is a lethal condition seen most commonly in the setting of a myocardial infarction. The patient will die within minutes if the arrhythmia is not terminated.

Altered Physiology

1 The heart is being stimulated simultaneously from numerous ectopic foci throughout the ventricles; therefore, there is no effective contraction of the cardiac musculature and thus no pulse.
2 Characterized by totally irregular appearance on ECG.

Mechanism of Ventricular Fibrillation

Normal Pathway   Ventricular Fibrillation Pathway

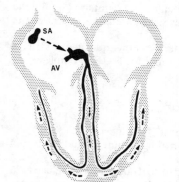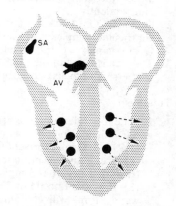

In ventricular fibrillation the presence of multiple ectopic foci in the ventricle prohibits an effective heart beat.

ECG of Ventricular Fibrillation

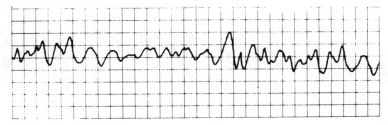

The complexes are completely distorted and irregular.

NOTE: It is extremely important to be sure that the chaotic undulations on the ECG do not represent artifacts since movement by the patient or of the monitor wires can give the same appearance. If the patient is alert or has a pulse, the rhythm does *not* represent ventricular fibrillation.

Treatment

Electrical defibrillation at 200–400 W/s. (In children, start with lower energies.)

1   If successful, the defibrillation shock stops the erratic uncoordinated electrical activity of the ventricle. After a moment the heart resumes its normal innate rhythm from the SA node.

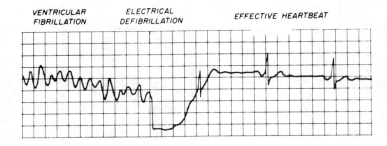

VENTRICULAR FIBRILLATION   ELECTRICAL DEFIBRILLATION   EFFECTIVE HEARTBEAT

2   Differs from cardioversion in that timing of the defibrillation shock is not necessary since there are no T waves in ventricular fibrillation.
3   Paddle placement (Fig. 1.33).
   a. The centre of one paddle is applied just to the right of the upper sternum in the second interspace.
   b. The rim of the other paddle is placed just below the left nipple.
   c. Paddles should be well lubricated and in firm contact with the skin.
4   See p. 29–31.

Summary

See Table 1.4.

Table 1.4. Emergency Diagnosis and Treatment of Arrythmias

Type of Arrythmia	Appearance of ECG	Treatment	Pathway
Normal rhythm		None	
Sinus tachycardia		Treat cause	
Sinus bradycardia		Atropine, Isoprenaline hydrochloride or pacemaker when condition is pathological	
Sinus arrhythmia		None	
PACs		Usually none. Quinidine may be used	
PAT		Carotid sinus pressure or metaraminol (Aramine)	
Atrial flutter		Digitalis if rate is above 100. Cardioversion* is very effective	
Atrial fibrillation		Digitalis if rate is above 100, and if fribrillation is not caused by too much digitalis. Cardioversion* may be effective	

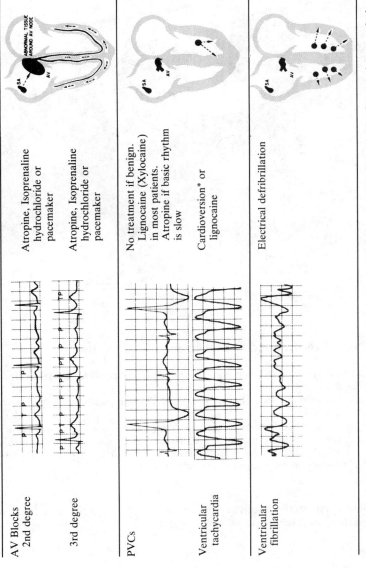

AV Blocks
2nd degree

3rd degree

Atropine, Isoprenaline hydrochloride or pacemaker

Atropine, Isoprenaline hydrochloride or pacemaker

PVCs

No treatment if benign. Lignocaine (Xylocaine) in most patients. Atropine if basic rhythm is slow

Ventricular tachycardia

Cardioversion* or lignocaine

Ventricular fibrillation

Electrical defibrillation

* Cardioversion can be very dangerous when a patient has a significant level of digitalis in his bloodstream since ventricular fibrillation or other lethal arrhythmias can be precipitated.

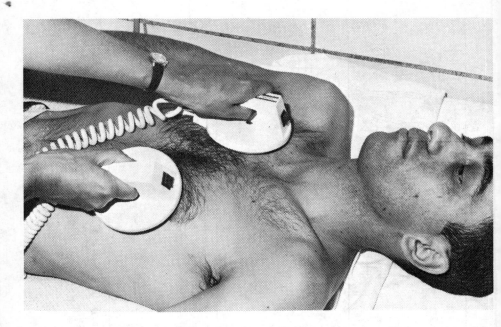

Figure 1.33.   Paddle placement in ventricular defibrillation.

GUIDELINES: Synchronized Cardioversion

Synchronized cardioversion is a *timed* electrical shock to the heart for the purpose of terminating certain arrhythmias.

Asynchronized cardioversion is the same as defibrillation and is used principally for ventricular fibrillation.

Both types of cardioversion use the same type of electricity, but timed shock is not needed in ventricular fibrillation because there are no T waves. (Synchronized cardioversion is timed *not* to hit the T wave, since an electrical discharge during this phase of the cardiac cycle may cause ventricular fibrillation.)

Purpose

To stop the abnormal electrical activity of the heart and allow the SA node (heart's natural pacemaker) to resume normal sinus rhythm.

Contraindications

Synchronized cardioversion is relatively *contraindicated* when a patient has been taking a significant amount of *digitalis*, since more lethal arrhythmias may ensue after electrical discharge.

Equipment

Cardioverter and ECG machine
Conduction jelly and cardiac medications
Resuscitative equipment including:

Endotracheal tubes	Manual breathing bag
Laryngoscopes	Pacing equipment
Suctioning equipment	

Procedure

1 If the procedure is elective it is advisable to fast the patient for 6–12 hours before the cardioversion.
   a. Reassure patient and see that the consent form has been signed.
   b. Make sure patient has not been taking digoxin and that the serum potassium is normal. Inform the doctor as necessary.

2 Make sure that the intravenous infusion is patent. (An intravenous line may be necessary for medications, such as lignocaine or atropine.)

3 As instructed by the doctor obtain a 12-lead ECG before and after cardioversion with the ECG machine. The ECG wires are left on the patient for use in the analysis of complicated arrhythmias. (An ECG is taken to ensure that the patient has not had a recent myocardial infarction, either just before or following the cardioversion).

4 **a.** Allow the patient to receive oxygen before and after cardioversion. (Oxygen will help prevent unwanted arrhythmias after cardioversion.)
   b. Do *not* give oxygen during the procedure. (An explosion could occur if a spark from the paddles should ignite the oxygen during the procedure).

5 Place the paddles in one of the following two positions:
   a. *Anterior-posterior position:*
   One paddle—left infrascapular area.
   Other paddle—upper sternum at third interspace.
   b. *Anterior position:*
   One paddle—just to right of sternum at second interspace.
   Other paddle—just under left nipple.

6 Determine if the machine's synchronization mechanism is working before applying the paddles.
   a. Discharge should hit near the peak of the R wave. (If the electrical discharge hits the T wave, ventricular fibrillation may occur.)
   b. The R wave usually has to be of substantial height; if it is not, turn up the gain or change the lead. On many machines, the R wave must be upright before there is synchronization. (Synchronization is not used for ventricular fibrillation. The machine will not work for *defibrillation* if the synchronization mode is on).

7 Apply electrode paste to the entire paddle surface, but make sure there is no excess around the edge of the paddles.
   a. The paste should be rubbed into the skin very thoroughly, since this allows more electricity to penetrate the body surface.
   b. Make sure paddles are clean because surface material will interfere with the flow of electricity.
   c. Apply firm pressure to the paddle. (If there is excess paste around the paddle

the discharge may run onto the skin, causing a burn. If there is not firm contact between the paddle and skin, a burn may occur, and also electricity is lost from the heart.)

8   Set dial for lowest level of electrical energy that can be expected to convert the arrhythmia as directed by doctor. Some arrhythmias (such as atrial flutter) can be converted with very low energies, e.g. 25 W/s (J). (Excessive energies cause myocardial infarction.)

9   Diazepam should be given if the patient is conscious.

10   Once the patient is in a light sleep from the intravenous diazepam, the doctor will discharge the cardioverter. Ensure that no one is touching the patient or the bed, or they will receive an electric shock. If cardioversion does not occur, higher energy levels will be used.

11   Monitor the ECG after conversion occurs. (The patient may revert to his previous arrhythmia after conversion.)

12   Blood pressure should be recorded at 15-min intervals until the precardio-version blood pressure has returned.

3. Vascular Disorders

Vascular disorders is a term that refers to conditions of the blood vessels.

   Peripheral vascular disease (PVD) refers to disease affecting the blood vessels that supply the extremities: veins, arteries and lymphatics.

Nature of the Disorder

1   Long-term. This is often discouraging to the patient: treatment may be painful and tedious; healing is slow.

2   Appears minor, but hospitalization or disability may last for months before healing takes place.
   Patient may have financial concerns and may worry about loss of job, separation from family and community responsibilities.

3   Older people are especially prone to peripheral vascular disease.

4   This condition is often compounded by other medical problems, such as diabetes.

5   If lesions heal, recurrence of the condition, with accompanying incapacity, is frequent.

Thrombus and Embolus Formation

1   *Thrombus*—a blood clot which partially or completely occludes a blood vessel.
   a. Thrombosed vessel—an occluded vessel.
   b. Thrombosis—the condition of having a thrombosed vessel.

2   Spontaneous clotting of the blood will not usually occur unless there is damage to the intimal surface of the vessel wall.
   a. Injury by trauma.
   b. Inflammation.
   c. Degenerative changes due to arteriosclerosis.

3   Injured intima—causes platelets to collect, fibrin to form and thrombus to develop.

4 *Embolus*—a fragment of a thrombus or a thrombus that has broken away from the point of formation.
   a. *Embolism*—occurs when an embolus moving through a blood vessel arrives at a narrowing of the vessel and thus occludes it.
   b. Air embolism—a bubble of air in the bloodstream.
   c. Fat embolism—multiple droplets of fat in the bloodstream.

Ischaemia

Ischaemia is lack of blood supply sufficient to meet tissue needs. This can develop as a result of:

1 Gradual occlusion of the lumen of the artery by encroachment of the thickened wall (atherosclerosis).
2 More rapid development of ischaemia due to formation of a blood clot (thrombus) at the atherosclerotic site.
3 Rapid occlusion of an artery when a free-flowing clot (embolus) lodges at a bifurcation or narrowing of the vessel.

PATHOPHYSIOLOGICAL MANIFESTATIONS OF VASCULAR DISORDERS

Coldness

1 Due to deficient blood supply to a part even though the environment is warm.
2 One extremity may be compared to another to note the difference.
3 The patient notices that the part feels uncomfortably cold.

Pallor (Paleness)

1 Normally the pink hue of the skin is due to adequate superficial circulation.
2 Diminished blood supply produces paleness, or lack of colour.
3 Blanching occurs when the part is elevated about the level of the heart and the arterial pressure in that part is lower than normal.

Rubor (Redness)

1 Instead of a normal rosy pink, the part may be red or reddish-blue. This is due to injury of superficial capillaries which causes them to remain dilated; it may also occur with chronic ischaemia.
2 Circulation is impaired.
3 Anoxia or coldness may be the cause of rubor.

Cyanosis (Blueness)

1 Indicates that less than normal amount of oxygen is in the blood.
2 When localized, it implies very slow circulation in that part.

Pain

1 Due to inadequate blood supply.

2   This is common, but varies with the condition.
      May be constant and severe, e.g. ulceration.
3   When it occurs only after a certain amount of exercise it is called *intermittent claudication*. (This disappears after rest, but returns with exercise.)
4   When it occurs at rest (rest pain), it indicates a more severe degree of ischaemia.

Diagnosis of Vascular Conditions (Fig. 1.34).

Oscillometry

1   Degree of arterial occlusion may be measured by an oscillometer, which measures pulse volume. One extremity may be compared with the other.
2   An inflatable cuff is wrapped around the extremity and the *oscillometric index* is determined by inflating the cuff and reading the dial.
3   Normal readings (points of pressure at which circulation ceases)
    a. Lower extremity:

Midthigh	4–16 mmHg
Upper third of leg	3–12 mmHg
Above ankle	1–18 mmHg
Foot	0.2–1.0 mmHg

   b. Upper extremity:

Upper arm	4–16 mmHg
Elbow	3–12 mmHg
Wrist	1–10 mmHg
Hand	0.2–2 mmHg

Phlebography

An x-ray picture of the vascular tree after the injection of a radiopaque dye (renografin).

1   Inform the patient that he may experience an intense burning sensation in the vessel where the solution is injected. This will last for only a few seconds.
2   Note any evidence of allergic reaction to the dye; this may occur as soon as the dye is injected or it may be delayed and occur when the patient reaches his room.
    a. Perspiring, dyspnoea, nausea, vomiting.
    b. Rapid heart rate, numbness of extremities.
    c. Hives.
    d. Treatment:
       (1) Notify doctor.
       (2) Have adrenaline available for injection, as well as antihistamine drugs and oxygen.
3   Nursing care:
    a. Observe injection site for the following:
       (1) Signs of redness, swelling, bleeding; signs of thrombosis (loss of distal pulses).

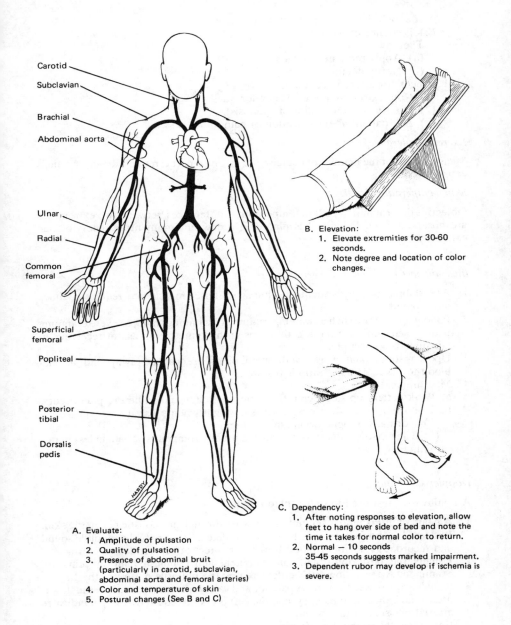

A. Evaluate:
1. Amplitude of pulsation
2. Quality of pulsation
3. Presence of abdominal bruit
   (particularly in carotid, subclavian,
   abdominal aorta and femoral arteries)
4. Color and temperature of skin
5. Postural changes (See B and C)

B. Elevation:
1. Elevate extremities for 30-60
   seconds.
2. Note degree and location of color
   changes.

C. Dependency:
1. After noting responses to elevation, allow
   feet to hang over side of bed and note the
   time it takes for normal color to return.
2. Normal — 10 seconds
   35-45 seconds suggests marked impairment.
3. Dependent rubor may develop if ischemia is
   severe.

Figure 1.34.   Salient points in evaluating peripheral arterial insufficiency.

> If above signs occur, notify doctor.
> (2) Evidence of bleeding.
> Therapy
> (a) Apply pressure dressing.
> (b) Notify doctor.
> **b.** Check for arterial occlusion.
> (1) Note extremity pulses; check for quality.
> (2) Observe colour (pallor or cyanosis).
> (3) Ask patient about sensation of pain, numbness.

Exercise Tolerance

Measurement of the amount of exercise the involved part can tolerate before pain is experienced.

Skin Temperature Studies

Objective determination of skin temperature—differences between two extremities are observed when individual is placed in a new environment: coolness of one extremity.

Intermittent Claudication Determination

1 At rest, blood supply is adequate—but an exercised muscle may require 10 times more blood.
2 Following exercise such as walking, running or climbing stairs, a severe cramping pain or sensation of tiredness develops in those muscle areas not receiving an adequate blood supply.
3 Upon resting, pain is relieved; metabolites are carried away and normal blood-to-tissue demand ratio is restored.
4 Measurement
   a. Walk patient up steps, counting number of steps taken before pain occurs.
   b. Use a foot-pedal device which lifts a weight when pressed.
   (1) Normally, fatigue occurs in 5–10 min.
   (2) The person with arterial occlusion usually complains of pain in less than a minute.

Doppler Ultrasound

A noninvasive test used to detect blood flow.

1 A beam of ultrasound is sent into the tissues through an acoustic gel on the skin. Reflected sound from moving blood cells is detected, amplified as audible sound and recorded; velocity of blood flow has a direct effect on the waveforms.
2 Usually the posterior tibial, calf, popliteal and common femoral veins are examined. Arterial flow can be detected by the pulsatile nature of the flow.
3 Signals are assessed for venous patency and valvular competence. Arterial flow is used as an indicator of patency, and the cuff pressure required to stop it indicates arterial pressure at that point.
4 Entire test takes about 5–10 min.

GENERAL MANAGEMENT OF PATIENTS WITH VASCULAR DISORDERS

Therapy Used to Increase Blood Supply to Tissues

Postural Therapy

Objective

To increase blood flow through use of gravity by intermittent filling and emptying of capillaries, veins and arteries.

Observation

Arterial blood supply to a section or part of the body can be increased by positioning it lower than the heart (gravity-assist).

Walking

A simple but very effective exercise.

1   A level surface is preferred.
2   Encourage patient to set realistic goals; each week these goals may be extended in keeping with his tolerance.
3   Use assistive devices as necessary—walker, cane, etc.
4   Evaluate patient's ability to climb stairs.

Jogging

A means of stimulating collateral blood flow not only to legs but also to the myocardium.
    May be practised as long as it is comfortable and pleasurable.

Buerger's Exercises

Prescribed according to condition of extremities and condition of patient.

1   Elevate extremity for a minute.
2   Place extremities in a dependent position until cyanosis or rubor becomes maximal.
3   Lie with extremities horizontal for a minute.
4   See Buerger-Allen exercises below.

Buerger-Allen Exercises

Exercises by which gravity alternately fills and empties the blood vessels (Fig. 1.35).

1   Procedure:
    a. Begin with patient lying flat in bed. Elevate legs to above level of heart—2 min or until blanching takes place.
    b. Allow legs to be dependent; exercise feet—3 min or until legs are pink.
    c. Instruct patient to lie flat—5 min.
    d. Repeat a, b and c five times; do entire set three times a day.
2   Tolerance and proper pacing:
    a. Advise patient to rest when he feels pain.

POSITION 1
Place legs on a pillow-cushioned chair
for one minute to drain blood.

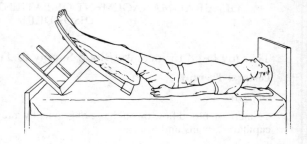

POSITION 2
Hold each of these
stretching positions
for 30 seconds
to enhance blood return.

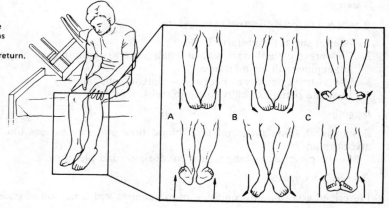

POSITION 3
Lie flat on back, with legs straight.
Hold position for one minute.

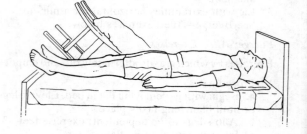

Figure 1.35.   Buerger–Allen exercises. Do exercise series six times four times a day. (From: Forshee, T and Minckley, B (1976) Lumbar sympathectomy, RN, July)

b. Avoid chilly environment since it causes vasoconstriction, which in turn further diminishes flow.

c. Maintain stability, particularly if postural hypotension is a problem.

3   Comfort:

a. Improvise equipment that will provide comfortable support for the patient in the leg-elevated position.

b. Well-padded straight-back chair can be placed on the bed so that the back of the chair supports the leg—top of chair is towards the top of the thigh.

c. Bed-table may be used with a pillow.

Oscillating Bed

Provides postural exercises using a passive method.

1   Aids indirectly in prevention of pressure areas—pressure sores.
2   Prescribed according to patient needs.
3   Explain to the patient that the bed will assist in relieving his circulatory difficulty.

a. Explain how the bed is turned on, regulated and stopped.

b. Advise him whether he can stop for meals, treatments, rest periods, etc.

4   Introduce motion of bed gradually to eliminate possibility of headache, dizziness or nausea.
5   Follow prescribed cycle for the individual patient.

Cycle: Degree of angle and the length of time to be elevated.

Degree of angle and the length of time to be lowered.

6   Prevent the patient from slipping downward by providing a padded footboard.

Thermotherapy

Nursing Alert: When heat is applied externally to an extremity—demand for circulation is increased. When applied to diseased tissues—sensations are impaired; may result in damaging burn and necrosis.

Dry Heat

1   Warm water bottles:

a. Check temperature of water before filling bottle—not to exceed 48.8°C (120°F).

b. Apply cover to bottle so that it does not come into direct contact with skin.

2   Heat cradle (thermostatically controlled or regulated with electric bulbs):

a. Pad metal edges of cradle to prevent injury to extremities.

b. Control temperature so that it will not exceed 32.2°C (90°F).

c. Ensure that bulbs are not likely to be touched by extremity (usually legs and feet).

d. Higher temperatures would stimulate metabolism (not desired).

e. Reduce temperature if patient complains of pain in extremity.

3   Ultrasound (acoustic vibration with frequencies beyond human ear perception):

a. Useful in small areas where deeper penetration of heat is desired and where circulation needs to be stimulated.

b. Application time is under 10 min.

c. Avoid areas where metal sutures may be present.

4   Paraffin bath.

Moist Heat

1   Hydrotherapy:
   a. Sitz baths—used for perineal therapy (see Rectal Surgery).
   b. Basin—for hands or feet with prescribed temperatures and for prescribed times.
2   Whirlpool bath:
   a. In addition to moist heat, the effect of agitated water provides hydromassage.
   b. May be used for one or two extremities or the whole body.
3   Warm compresses:
   a. Applied directly to the skin
   b. When hot, apply over towelling.

Pressure Gradient Therapy (Compression Devices and Garments)

Cuffs, Sleeves or Boots

1   Circulator—electrically produced air pressure alternately inflates and deflates a boot in which the extremity is encased.
   Rhythm of occlusion and release as well as pressure can be regulated to correspond to pulse.
2   Pressor sleeve or boot—a plastic tube filled with air.
   a. Can be maintained at low pressure for several hours.
   b. Can be regulated to function intermittently. (Useful in lymphoedema of arm following mastectomy).

Elastic Garments

1   Support for an extremity can be tailor-made: A unique measuring tape was devised by Jobst* so that exact 'fabric pressures' are produced with their custom-made venous pressure gradient supports (Fig. 1.36).
2   Method of applying supporting hose is demonstrated in Fig. 1.37.

Anticoagulant Therapy

Composite Physiological Action of Anticoagulants

1   Extrinsic prothromboplastin (tissue).
2   Intrinsic ingredients (blood)—plus:
3   Plasma Factors (V, VII and X)—acting in presence of:
4   Ionized calcium—assist in converting:
5   Prothrombin to thrombin→
6   Thrombin and fibrinogen form fibrin.

Clinical Indications

Authorities disagree about the justification of long-term use of anticoagulants in various disease entities.

* The Jobst Institute, Box 653, Toledo, Ihio 43694.

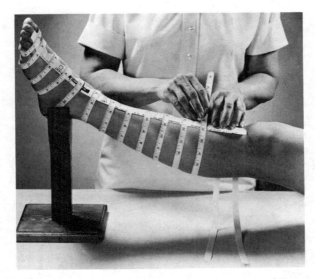

Figure 1.36.   By using a special measuring tape, exact measurements of the extremity can be obtained. Measurements are taken while the patient is lying down with the extremity slightly elevated. The foot is in a normal relaxed position. The horizontal spine of the measuring tape is placed anteriorly; key cross straps are fastened and then each succeeding strap is fastened. All straps are calibrated in centimetres. When properly and completely fastened, this measuring device can be cut according to directions and sent to the manufacturer for made-to-order support. (Courtesy: Jobst.)

1 *Venous thrombosis*—because of the danger of extension and the danger of emboli.
2 *Pulmonary embolism*—prophylactically, if patient is known to be suspect; also indicated during recovery phase to prevent further clot formation.
3 *Patient susceptible to embolism*—such as a surgical patient who has rheumatic heart disease, one who has had valve surgery.
4 *Coronary occlusion with myocardial infarction.*
5 *Cerebral vascular accident caused by emboli or cerebral thrombi*—to reduce sludging of blood: useful in prevention and treatment of strokes.

Contraindications

1 May cause spontaneous bleeding—therefore not used when there is likelihood of bleeding because of increased capillary fragility, aneurysm.
2 Individuals with peptic ulcer and chronic ulcerative diseases are considered poor risks, because of the possibility of bleeding.
3 Should not be given following neurosurgery because of danger of haemorrhage in brain or spinal cord.
4 Liver disease may present a problem because of interference with plasma protein clotting factors.

Put on supports early in the morning, before swelling occurs.

Always begin with supports "inside-out" ... as they are when you receive them.

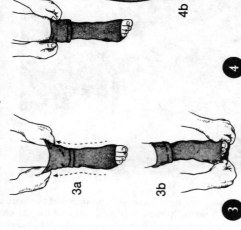

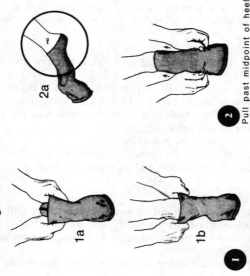

1

Sit with feet in easy reach. Support must be "inside out," with its foot inverted back to heel. Seam faces down (sketch 1a). Grasp each side firmly and pull onto foot (sketch 1b).

2

Pull past midpoint of heel (sketch 2a) so support will not slip back. Then, reach just beyond toes and grasp fabric between fingers and start pulling over foot. Pull from sides ... never by seams.

3

Pull all the way up past ankle (sketch 3a). Seat heel in place. Pull foot portion of support out toward tips of toes (sketch 3b) to set fabric evenly on foot. Allow to settle back normally.

4

Using short (2 inches at a time) snappy pulls (sketch 4a) pull support up to point it was measured to end (sketch 4b). Smooth evenly down leg. **Never allow top to roll or turn down.**

Figure 1.37. Method of applying supporting hose. (Courtesy: Jobst.)

5 Liver and kidney insufficiency diseases may preclude use of anticoagulants because of difficulty in metabolizing and eliminating them—resulting in toxicity and difficulty in responding to antidotal medication (not true of heparin).
6 Poor follow-up by patients; unless the patient co-operates by reporting for blood tests, etc., he should not be on anticoagulants.
7 Severe diabetes, infections or severe traumatic conditions are circumstances in which anticoagulant therapy may be contraindicated.

Heparin Sodium (parenteral anticoagulant)

Pharmacological Action

1 Affects coagulation time by its effect on the clotting mechanism.
2 Inactivates thromboplastin, which in turn interferes with changing of prothrombin to thrombin.
3 Inactivates any thrombin which manages to form.
4 May decrease adhesiveness of platelets.
5 May promote resolution of a newly-formed clot.
6 Does not dissolve fibrin of a well-established clot.

Advantages

1 Chief advantage is its rapid action which makes it the medication of choice in emergency situations and for short-term therapy.
2 When administered by vein, it acts within seconds and is both predictable and controllable (action time intramuscularly or subcutaneously is 30 min).
3 Its effect can be readily neutralized by injecting protamine sulphate or other heparin antagonists intravenously, and it is therefore the safest anticoagulant.
4 It has little cumulative effect and dissipates quickly (within 4 hours).
5 It is the most effective agent available in treatment of phlebitis.

Table 1.5. Anticoagulants

Type	Generic Name (BP)	Brand Name (UK)
Heparin sodium	Heparin sodium	Pularin Minihep Hepacort Plus Heparin Inj. Mucous, etc.
Heparin calcium	Heparin calcium	Calciparine Pularin Ca
Oral		
Coumarin derivatives	Warfarin sodium	Marevan Warfarin sodium
	Nicoumalone	Sinthrome
	Ethlbisoumacetate	Tromexan
Indanedione derivatives	Phenindione	Dindevan

Disadvantages

1   Chief disadvantage is that it must be given parenterally; it is unpleasant when used for long-term maintenance therapy.
2   For continued effectiveness, heparin must be given frequently.
3   Heparin is expensive—price varies greatly.

Side-Effects and Contraindications

1   Bleeding may occur; therefore, heparin should not be given to those patients listed under contraindications (p. 129), to those who have lost large areas of skin or to those with clotting-factor deficiencies.
2   Allergic reactions may appear in patients sensitive to substances of animal origin (redness, itchy skin, urticarial weals) but are uncommon.
3   Heparin sodium in full therapeutic doses is contraindicated when suitable blood coagulation tests, such as Lee–White whole-blood clotting time, activated partial thrombo-plastin time (APTT), etc., cannot be performed at the required intervals.

Nursing Alert: All anticoagulants should be used with extreme caution in disease states in which there is increased danger of haemorrhage.

Antidotes

1   Protamine sulphate—this should be available in the department where the patient is receiving heparin anticoagulant therapy.
2   Blood transfusion.

Coumarin Derivatives (oral anticoagulants)

Most Commonly Used

1   Warfarin sodium/Warfarin, Marevan

Pharmacological Action

1   Acts to reduce blood coagulability by its effect on prothrombin activity.
2   Interferes with vitamin K absorption—the latter being required in the synthesis of prothrombin.
3   Failure of Factor VII leads to prolonged clotting time.
4   Has no effect on clotting factors already in circulation—hence, the delayed action of these drugs is noted later and can be measured by prothrombin time tests.

Prothrombin Time Testing

1   Normal prothrombin time—11–13 s.
2   By lengthening prothrombin time to about 19–24 s, coagulability of blood is depressed sufficiently to lessen danger of thrombosis but not enough to cause spontaneous bleeding. This represents the *desired therapeutic range*.

Prothrombin Activity

Prothrombin range may also be reported in percents of normal—the activity of the plasma prothrombin.

1   Desired therapeutic range is 20–30% of normal.

2   Probability of haemorrhage exists when activity is less than 10% of normal. In other words, when prothrombin activity lessens, hypoprothrombinaemia increases.

Advantages

1   Is convenient since it is given by mouth; efficient absorption from gastrointestinal tract.
2   Unnecessary to keep the patient in the hospital.
3   Since it is synthetically produced, dosage and strength are uniform; it is also less expensive than parenteral heparin.

Disadvantages

1   Effects are unpredictable; dosage varies from one person to another and even from one time to another in the same patient, i.e., decreased liver or kidney function and fever enhance or prolong response. Many drugs enhance or antagonize effects of oral anticoagulants.
2   Because the prothrombin level must be tested frequently, laboratory facilities must be available. (This is often a problem.)
3   There is a cumulative effect:
     Dicumarol has a slow onset (2–3 days) and extended cumulative effect (up to 9 days after last dose).
     Coumadin onset occurs within 18–24 hours; cumulative effect lasts up to 7 days.
     Phenindione onset is within 10–12 hours; effects disappear after 24–48 hours; however, there are side-effects with which to reckon.
4   Cannot be quickly counteracted.

Antidotes to Coumarin Anticoagulants

1   Administer vitamin K (Phytomenadione) or Konakion intravenously or Konakion tablets by mouth.
     Usually brings prothrombin values back to safe levels within 8–24 hours.
2   Provide fresh whole blood if immediate antidote action is required, e.g. physical injury or other emergency.

Nursing Management

1   Since heparin may be given with longer lasting hypoprothrombinaemic agents, for the first few days of treatment each day's medication orders should be checked *after* reports of daily prothrombin time tests are know.
2   Have on hand the antidotes to anticoagulants being used:
     Heparin—protamine sulphate
     Coumarin—vitamin K (Phytomenadione, Konakion).
3   Note that the relatively long duration of action of oral anticoagulants makes it easier to maintain low prothrombin levels for long periods.
4   Observe carefully for any possible signs of bleeding and report immediately so that anticoagulant dosage may be reviewed and altered if necessary:
     a. Urine—note evidence of haematuria.

    b. Stool—check for tarry colour (occult blood).
    c. Vomit bowl following tooth brushing—note any pink or bloody return.
5 Later, when anticoagulant medication is stabilized, patient must be reminded to keep prothrombin test appointments as scheduled—once a week or however often they are required.
6 Tell patient the precautions to take and observations to make while on anticoagulant therapy after he leaves the hospital.
    Observe for any signs of bleeding.
    a. Skin discolouration or bruises on arms or legs.
    b. Undue oozing from small skin abrasions.
    c. Frequent nosebleeds.
    d. Blood in urine.

NOTE: Patients on phenindione produce orange or broth-coloured urine: when acidified, this colouration disappears. With true haematuria, acid does not affect colour.

    e. Red or tarry stools.
    f. Excessive menstrual flow.
    g. Faintness, dizziness or unusual weakness.
7 If prolonged diarrhoea occurs, anticoagulant requirements increase.
8 Drug interactions:
    a. Recognize that aspirin and salicylates interfere with the same clotting mechanisms that coumarin-type medications act on; hence avoid these drugs unless specifically approved by the doctor.
    b. Advise patient to avoid drinking alcoholic beverages to excess since this may affect absorption of vitamin K or anticoagulant from the intestines.
    c. Note that multivitamin supplements may contain vitamin K—patients on these will require a higher dose of anticoagulant.
    d. Report use of mineral oil—can cause vitamin K deficiency because it interferes with absorption of fat-soluble vitamins.
    e. Note that barbiturates increase metabolism of coumarin medications—therefore an increased dose of anticoagulants is in order.
    f. Be aware of the following with regard to sensitivity to coumarin derivatives:

May be intensified by	*May be decreased by*
antibiotics	antacids
mineral oil	barbiturates
quinidine	oral contraceptives
salicylates	adrenal corticosteroids
tolbutamide (Rastinon)	

Nursing Alert: Drug interactions can alter the effect of anticoagulants. Review with the doctor the effect of other medications the patient may be taking during anticoagulant therapy.

9 Remind patient to tell his dentist, chiropodist, or other doctors whom he may visit that he is taking anticoagulant medications.

GUIDELINES: Subcutaneous Injection of Heparin

Purpose

When prolonged therapy is indicated, heparin may be given subcutaneously into fatty tissues (Fig. 1.38).

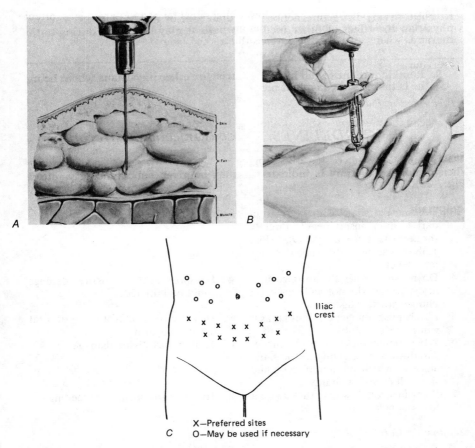

Figure 1.38 Subcutaneous injection indicating technique and sites for herapin therapin. a. When prolonged therapy is indicated, herapin is most conveniently given subcutaneously into the fatty tissue, which is a distinct layer beneath the skin. b. First stretch skin to empty vessels so they are less apt to be pierced by needle. Then insert the needle directly through the skin at a right angle (see a). c. Since the site of injection of herapin must be changed each time herapin is administered a suggested division of the abdomen into suitable areas is indicated. Do not inject into a bruised area or within 5 cm (2 in) of the umbilicus or any scar. (Courtesy: Wyeth Laboratories, Philadelphia, PA.)

Equipment

1- or 2-ml syringe or disposable tuberculin syringe
Fine sharp needle, No.25, 1.6 cm (0.625 in) long
Skin antiseptic

Considerations

1   Most convenient sites are along lower abdominal fat pad—to avoid inadvertent intramuscular injection and haematoma formation.
2   Areas where subcutaneous layer is thin should be avoided.

Procedure

Nursing Action	Reason
Performance Phase	
1 Clean the area *gently* with alcohol.	1 Rubbing or pinching skin might initiate damage to the tissue and heparin would aggravate any bleeding.
2 Attempt to stretch skin out, using palm of hand.	2 Try to empty vessels in local area to lessen likelihood of their being pierced by needle—with subsequent haematoma formation.
3 Holding the shaft of the syringe in dart fashion, insert needle directly through the skin at a right angle (Fig. 1.38a) just into the subcutaneous fatty layer.	
4 Do not move needle tip once it is inserted and do not pull back on plunger for testing.	4 Haemorrhage or tissue damage could be initiated.
5 Firmly push plunger down as far as it will go (Fig. 1.38b).	5 This ensures administration of total dose of heparin.
6 When injection has been made, withdraw needle gently at the same angle at which it entered, releasing skin roll as you withdraw.	6 To minimize tissue damage.
7 Press an alcohol swab to the site for a few seconds.	7 To minimize oozing or bleeding.

Follow-up Care

Nursing Action	Reason
1 Do not rub area. Tell the patient not to rub area.	1 Rubbing would increase the likelihood of bleeding.
2 Site of injection. **a.** Change site of injection each time herapin is administered.	

Nursing Action	Reason

b. Figure 1.38c shows a suggested division of abdomen into suitable areas.

c. A chart can be marked with time, date and measured dosage so that rotation of assured.

Nursing Management of the Patient with a Peripheral Vascular Problem

Nursing Objectives and Health Teaching

To Encourage Patient to Avoid Those Practices Which Cause Vasoconstriction in the Vessels of the Extremities

1 Impress upon the patient the *dangers of smoking*, especially inhaling.
2 Promote an atmosphere that is devoid of emotional tension; restrict those visitors who appear to upset the patient.
3 Maintain a warm and properly humidified environment.
4 Advise the patient against wearing constrictive garments, such as pantigirdles, garters, belts and tight pantihose.
5 Use analgesic and tranquillizing medications as required to keep the patient comfortable.

To Encourage the Following Measures and Activities to Increase the Blood Flow to the Patient's Extremities

Instruct the patient as follows:

1 Put on warm clothing before going out into cool air; protect hands and feet with sheepskin lining in gloves and boots to prevent vasoconstriction.
2 Take a warm bath to offset chilling; replace vigorous rubbing of the skin after a bath with gentle patting.
3 Avoid excessive heat to extremities (using hot water bottle, electric pad, etc.)—increases metabolism, so that more oxygenated blood is demanded.
4 Sleep with the head of the bed elevated about 20.3 cm (8 in); wear bedsocks to keep feet warm if necessary.
5 Walking is the best form of exercise; otherwise, active or passive exercise of the extremities is recommended.
6 Take prescribed vasodilating medications even though they may not appear to help; at times they maintain the status quo and keep the problem from worsening.
7 Take prescribed antilipaemic drugs to slow progress of accompanying sclerotic disease by reducing serum lipids.

To Recognize the Signs and Symptoms of Circulatory Disturbances Affecting Peripheral Tissues

1 Pain in the extremity—(note whether this occurs at rest, with limited activity or with more pronounced exercise).
2 Colour changes of the skin or nails—pallor, pinkness, rubor, cyanosis.

3   Impaired or peculiar growth of nails.
4   Shiny, taut skin.
5   Discrepancy in size of one extremity when compared to contralateral (opposite) extremity.
6   Enlarged veins or abnormal pulsations of veins.
7   Temperature variations—abnormally cold or abnormally warm.
8   Ulcerations, necrosis or gangrene.

To Keep Metabolic Demands on the Body to a Minimum

Instruct the patient as follows:

1   Take precautions to prevent injury and infection, particularly of the extremities.
2   Practise daily hygienic cleanliness and care of the feet: trim nails properly, avoid strong medications, use sheepskin for pressure areas, wear shoes and hosiery that fit correctly.
3   Avoid exposure to cold or excessive heat.
4   Exercise within recognized limits; set up a reasonable rest plan.
5   Remain in bed if there is evidence of necrosis, ulceration or gangrene.

Foot Care in the Patient with a Vascular Disorder

Patient Instruction

1   Keep the feet clean to prevent irritation and infection.
    a. Wash daily with a bland soap and warm water.
    b. Dry thoroughly, paying particular attention to areas between the toes; pat rather than rub dry.
    c. Apply lanolin to prevent drying and cracking of skin.
    d. Wear clean hose daily: woollen socks for winter, cotton for summer.
2   Avoid injury, excessive pressure or other irritants to the feet.
    a. Shoes:
       (1) Wear properly fitting shoes with a comfortable heel.
       (2) Check inside of shoe; avoid wearing shoes with protruding seams, torn lining, piercing nails or faulty lumps.
       (3) Wear shoes when out of bed; avoid going barefoot.
       (4) Break in new shoes gradually; alternate with an older pair.
       (5) Leather is preferred to rubber or synthetics because the latter interfere with proper circulation of air.
       (6) Allow wet or damp shoes to dry slowly on shoe trees to prevent misshaping.
    b. Hose:
       (1) Wear proper length and size—if too short; toes are compressed; if too long, wrinkles form and exert pressure on skin.
       (2) Avoid seams, holes or lumpy darned areas.
       (3) Use bedsocks rather than hot water bottle or heating pad if feet are cold in bed.
       (4) Use woollen or cotton hose; they absorb moisture; nylon is not absorbent.

(5) Avoid constricting garments—foundation garments, garters and even support hose unless they are specifically prescribed.

c. Pedicure:

(1) Trim toenails straight across after soaking the feet in warm water.

(2) Place wisps of cotton under corner of great toenail if there is a tendency toward ingrowing toenails.

(3) Visit a chiropodist to cut corns and calluses; do not use corn pads or strong medications.

d. Heat and cold

(1) Keep feet warm; avoid exposure to cold for long periods of time.

(2) Use heating devices only on advice of doctor; excessive heat can be as damaging as insufficient warmth.

(3) Rely on warm socks, fleece-lined boots or mittens, lightweight blankets, etc., rather than on heating extremities near a fire, oven or radiator.

e. General measures:

(1) Avoid areas where injury to feet is likely, e.g. crowded subways, building sites, sports shows, etc.

(2) Prevent sunburn in the summer and avoid wading in very cold water.

3   Prevent pressure on feet; rest and exercise in moderation.

a. Place a pillow under covers at end of bed to provide a footrest and prevent weight of top bedding from exerting pressure on toes.

b. Avoid remaining in one position for long periods of time.

c. Do not cross legs when sitting because of pressure on nerves and blood vessels.

d. Elevate feet on a chair or footstool with proper support of leg; do this for about 15 min every 2 hours.

4   If damage or injury occurs to any part of foot or leg, report to doctor.

a. Redness, swelling, irritation, blistering

b. Itching, burning—athlete's foot

c. Bruises, cuts, unusual appearance of skin.

PHLEBITIS OR THROMBOPHLEBITIS

Phlebothrombosis is the formation of a thrombus or thrombi in a vein; in general the clotting is related to (1) stasis, (2) abnormality of the walls of the vein(s) and (3) abnormality of clotting mechanism.

Phlebitis is an inflammation of the walls of a vein.

Thrombophlebitis is a condition in which a clot forms in a vein secondary to phlebitis or due to partial obstruction of the vein.

Aetiology

1   Venous stasis—following operations, childbirth or bed rest for any chronic illness.

2   Prolonged sitting or as a complication of varicose veins.

3   Injury (bruise) to a vein: may result from direct trauma to veins from intravenous injections, indwelling catheters.

4   Extension of an infection of tissues surrounding the vessel.

5   Continuous pressure of a tumour, aneurysm, heavy pregnancy.

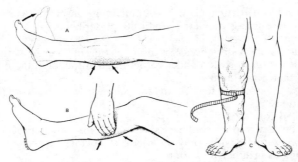

Figure 1.39   Assessment of signs and symptoms of phlebothrombosis. a. With the leg in extension, the patient may complain of pain in the calf on dorsiflexion (Homas' sign)—this was considered an unmistakable sign of early and subclinical thrombosis: it may or may not be present. b. Gentle compression reveals tenderness of the calf muscles (note arrow). c. The affected leg may swell, veins are more prominent and may be palpated easily.

6   Unusual activity in a person who has been sedentary.
7   Hypercoagulability associated with malignant disease, blood dyscrasias.

Basically, there are three causes: stasis, injury to a vessel wall and hypercoagulability (or a combination of these factors).

Clinical Manifestations

1   For phlebothrombosis there are no clinical signs since there is no inflammation.
2   Slight swelling around ankle; obvious prominence of leg veins in affected leg.
3   Calf pain may be aggravated when foot is dorsiflexed with the leg extended (Fig. 1.39a). Unfortunately, this is not a clear sign of early or positive thrombosis. In some patients with obvious thrombophlebitis, the sign is not present and in other kinds of involvement (irritation of sciatic nerve roots and myositis) the sign may be positive.
4   Muscle ache—may be falsely assumed to result from wearing flat bedroom slippers postoperatively (Fig. 1.39b)

Nursing Alert: Do not massage the leg; this may dislodge blood clot and cause pulmonary embolism.

Preventive Measures

1   Encourage early ambulation of surgical patients—encourage leg exercises for the bedridden patient, to prevent venous stasis.
2   Suggest deep breathing exercises that produce increased negative pressure in the thorax, which in turn assists in emptying large veins.
3   Recommend properly applied elastic stockings for the bedridden patient—to increase deep venous blood circulation. (Remove twice daily and check for skin changes or calf tenderness.)
4   Electrical stimulation of calf and pneumatic compression of leg
5   Use of oral anticoagulants preoperatively; not usually done because of fear of

increasing possibility of haemorrhage during operation. Mini-doses of heparin may be prescribed.

6   Prophylactic measures for bedridden patients who are prone to develop thrombosis.*

a. Lie in bed in the slightly reversed Trendelenburg position, because it is better for the veins to be full of blood than empty.

b. Place a footboard across the foot of the bed.

c. Instruct patient to press the ball of the feet against the footboard, just as if he were rising up on his toes.

d. Then instruct the patient to relax the foot.

e. Ask the patient to do this 1000 times a day.

Nursing Assessment

1   Inspect the lower extremities by removing top bedding from foot end up to patient's groin (remove any temperature-controlling devices such as heavy wool socks, ice bag, at least 10 min before clinical inspection.

2   Note symmetry or asymmetry.

Measure and record calf circumference daily (Fig. 1.39c)—mark on skin with felt tip pen where the measuring tape is used so that the same area is measured each time.

3   Observe for evidence of venous distension or oedema, puffiness, stretched skin, hardness to touch.

4   Hand test extremities for temperature variations.

a. The examiner's hands should be placed in cold water and then dried.

b. Hands are then placed simultaneously on each leg—first compare ankles, then move to the calf and up to the knee.

5   Examine for signs of obstruction due to occluding thrombus:

Swelling, particularly in loose connective tissue of popliteal space, ankle or suprapubic area

Treatment

Objective

To achieve early resolution of thrombi and prevention of sequelae.

1   Avoid massaging or rubbing calf because of the danger of breaking up the clot, which can then circulate as an embolus.

2   Check with doctor concerning proper position of the extremity since there may be differences of opinion.

a. Some recommend elevation—reduces venous congestion and oedema.

b. Others do not recommend elevation—because of possibility of releasing emboli.

3   If prescribed, apply heat in the form of hot wet dressings or a heat cradle to promote circulation and comfort.

4   Place the patient on anticoagulant therapy (see p. 128).

*Suggested by Linton, K (Discussion) (1974) Venous thromboembolic disease. Arch. Surg., 109: 668.

Health Teaching

Objectives

To increase venous return from lower extremities.
To avoid further injury to damaged vessel walls.

1 Prevent venous stasis by proper positioning in bed.
   a. Support full length of legs when they are to be elevated (Fig. 1.40).
   b. Prevent bony prominence of one leg from pressing on soft tissue of other leg (in side-lying position, place a soft pillow between legs).
   c. Avoid hyperflexion at knee as in jackknife position (head up, knees up, pelvis and legs down); this promotes stasis in pelvis and extremities.
2 Initiate active exercises, *unless contraindicated*, in which case use passive exercises.
   a. If patient is on bed rest
      (1) Simulate walking if lying on back—5 min every 2 hours.
      (2) Simulate bicycle pedalling if lying on side—5 min every 2 hours.
   b. If contraindicated resort to passive exercises—5 min every 2 hours.
   c. If permissible, ask patient to sit up and move to side of bed in sitting position.
      Provide a foot support (stool or chair)—dangling of feet is not desirable since pressure may be exerted against popliteal vessels and may cause obstruction to blood flow.
   d. If patient is permitted out of bed, encourage him to walk 10 min each hour; otherwise carry out passive exercises.
   e. Discourage crossing of legs because compression of vessels can restrict blood flow.
3 Promote circulation and prevent stasis by applying elastic hose.
      Apply elastic hose or elastic bandage from the toes up the leg; support must be consistent along entire leg.
4 Avoid straining or any manoeuvre that increases venous pressure in the leg.
      Eliminate the necessity to strain at stool by providing increased bulk in the diet and administer laxatives if necessary.
5 Also follow Nursing Objectives in Management of the Patient with Peripheral Vascular Disease (p. 137).

Chronic Venous Insufficiency (Postphlebitic Syndrome)

Postphlebitic syndrome is a form of chronic venous stasis; it may be a residual effect of phlebitis. It results from chronic occlusion of the veins or destruction of the valves.

Aetiology

1 Smaller vessels have dilated because main channel for returning blood from the leg to the heart was blocked by a thrombus.
2 Valves of diseased veins can no longer prevent backflow, thereby leading to →chronic venous stasis→swelling and oedema→superficial varicose veins.
3 Lower leg becomes discoloured due to venous stasis and pigmentation ulceration (postphlebitis).

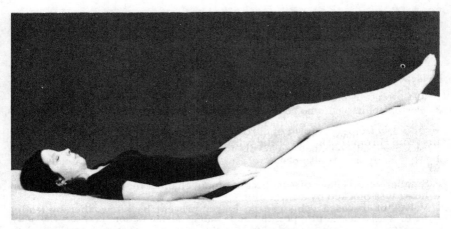

Figure 1.40.   This leg elevator is of foam construction with a removable cotton cover which can be machine washed. It is clamped to the lower end of the mattress. This position is anatomically correct and provides adequate support to all parts of the leg. Oedema and stasis of the lower extremities can be controlled. (Courtesy: Jobst.)

Altered Physiology

1   Pressure in veins at ankle is much greater than normal when leg is dependent—leads to transudation of fluid from intravascular to interstitial space.
2   Stasis, intractable induration, chronic oedema, discolouration, pain, venous congestion, ulceration, recurrent thrombosis→cellulitis.

Treatment

1   Best treatment is prevention of phlebitis and constant use of compression if phlebitis has occurred.
2   After this syndrome has developed, only palliative and symptomatic treatment is possible because the damage is irreparable.
3   Health Teaching.
    Instruct the patient as follows:
    a. Wear elastic stockings to prevent oedema.
    b. Avoid sitting or standing for long periods of time.
    c. Elevate legs on a chair for 5 min every 2 hours.
    d. Elevate legs above level of head by lying down (two to three times daily).
    e. Raise foot of bed 15–20 cm (6–8 in) at night to allow venous drainage by gravity.
    f. Apply bland oily lotions to prevent scaling and dryness of skin.
    g. Avoid constricting bandages.
    h. Prevent injury, bruising, scratching or other trauma to skin of leg and foot.

Stasis Ulcers

Stasis ulcer is a common and often disabling complication of chronic venous insufficiency.

Incidence

1 Occurrence is increasing, particularly in the older age group.
2 Postphlebitic syndrome and stasis account for most leg ulcers (Fig. 1.41).
3 Other causes include obstruction of one of the main veins by pregnancy or abdominal tumour, incompetency of valves of the ileofemoral vein, burns, sickle-cell anaemia, neurogenic disorders.
4 Hereditary factors also play a role in the predisposition of certain individuals.

Prevention

1 Prevent oedema:
   In stasis dermatitis, pruritus and scaling pigmentation may be the only manifestations; bed rest and a 30° elevation of the lower extremity may alleviate the oedema
2 Avoid trauma.

Diagnosis

Phlebography

1 A radiopaque dye is injected into a foot or ankle vein and forced into the deep system.
2 Films are taken before and after exercises.
3 Normal results show intact deep venous circulation and good valves.
4 Exercise clears dye from the deep veins after the test is completed. (See also Diagnosis of Vascular Conditions, p. 123)

Objectives of Treatment and Nursing Management

To Promote Rest and Reduce the Inflammation

1 Elevate the leg and maintain bed rest.
2 Initiate proper cleasing routine.
   a. Handle leg very gently.
   b. Use mild soap, warm water and cotton wool balls.
3 Remove devitalized tissue.
   a. Flush out necrotic materials with hydrogen peroxide.
   b. Apply enzymatic solutions, e.g. streptokinase, varidase, chymotrypsin.

To Stimulate Healing by Reducing the Infection and Providing Physiological and Nutritional Support

1 Again, elevation of the extremity is most important.
2 Participate in physiotherapy and maintain a regular exercise programme.
3 Control excess weight and provide proper vitamin and protein dietary supplements.

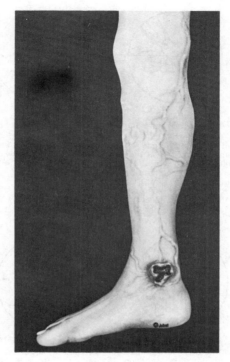

Figure 1.41.   Diagram showing leg ulcer resulting from concomitant postphlebitis and varicose veins. (Courtesy: Jobst.)

4   Check with individual doctor for specific therapy; treatment varies from clinic to clinic.

To Stimulate and Maintain Healthy Tissue in the Skin Surrounding the Ulcer

1   Use sterile saline compresses if area is inflamed or oozing.
2   Apply compression bandages to the leg (gelatin compression boot—Fig. 1.42).

To Encourage the Patient Who is Likely to get Discouraged During Prolonged Treatment

1   Stress the importance of following explicitly the recommendations of the doctor–nurse team.
2   Explain the hazards of trying other remedies on his own at home.
3   Indicate that the treatment may be long but that patience is an important aspect.
4   Maintain healthy tissue when the ulcer is healed by continuing with the safeguards practised before, because breakdown of healthy tissue unfortunately is frequent.

Patient Education (see objectives above)

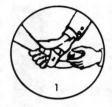

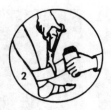

1. Apply right from can. Hold knee in slight flexion. Pad instep and ankle with cotton wad. Start at inner ankle. Make overlapping turns. Figure of eight turn around ankle joint. Use firm equal compression up to the knee.

2. If a turn does not fit snugly, nip edges with scissors or cut bandage off and start a new turn.

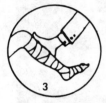

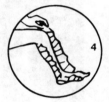

3. Mold cast during application with free hand until cast appears even and smooth. Make a cut 5 cm. (2″) long below knee to avoid constriction. Cover cast with loosely woven gauze bandage.

4. Patient can be fully ambulatory. Boot is usually changed once a week. Remove by cutting with scissors.

Figure 1.42.   Application of gelatin compression boot. (Manufactured by Graham-Field Surgical Co. Inc., New Hyde Park, NY.)

VARICOSE VEINS

Primary varicose veins—bilateral dilatation and elongation of saphenous veins; deeper veins are normal. As the condition progresses, because of hydrostatic pressure and vein weakness, the vein walls become distended with asymmetrical dilatation and some of the valves become incompetent. The process is irreversible.

Incidence

This is a common venous disorder of the lower extremity; 10% of the population are affected.

Aetiology

1   Dilatation of the vein prevents the valve cusps from meeting; this results in increased back-up pressure, which is passed into the next lower segment of the vein. The combination of vein dilatation and valve incompetence produces the varicosity (Fig. 1.43).
2   Varicosities may occur elsewhere in the body (oesophageal and haemorrhoidal veins) when flow or pressure is abnormally high.
4   Predisposing factors
   a. Hereditary weakness of vein wall or valves
   b. Long-standing distension of veins brought about by pregnancy, obesity or prolonged standing
   c. Old age—loss of tissue elasticity

Clinical Manifestations

1   Disfigurement due to large, discoloured, tortuous leg veins.
2   Easy leg fatigue, cramps in leg, heavy feeling, increased pain during menstruation, nocturnal muscle cramps.

Complications

1   Leg oedema, pain from superficial thrombosis.
2   Haemorrhage due to the weakening of the vein wall and pressure upon it.
3   Skin infection and breakdown, producing ulcers (rare in primary varices).

Diagnosis

Trendelenburg Test (for valvular competence)

1   Lie the patient down; elevate leg 65° to allow veins to empty.
2   Apply tourniquet high on upper thigh to constrict superficial veins (not deep veins).
3   Instruct patient to stand with tourniquet in place.

a. Veins fill slowly from below in 20–30s. Rate of filling not accelerated when tourniquet is removed.	**a.** Considered normal
b. Veins fill rapidly from below. Lower-leg 'blowouts' may be evident. Rate of filling not accelerated when tourniquet is removed.	**b.** Incompetence of communicating veins of lower leg.

4   Remove tourniquet.

a. Rapid flow of blood down saphenous vein from above.	**a.** Incompetence of values of saphe nofemoral and superficial veins.
b. Veins fill as in 3b; in addition, there is rapid flow of blood downward.	**b.** Incompetence of saphenofemoral veins, valves, superficial veins and valves of communicating veins.

Phlebography

Injection of radiopaque substance into veins, followed by observation of blood flow and valve action via x-ray.

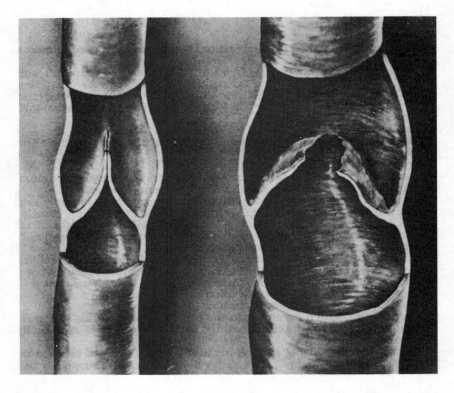

Figure 1.43.   Valve incompetence develops as dilatation of a vessel prevents effective approximation of the valve cusps. (Courtesy: Jobst.)

1   If dorsal vein of foot is used, dye usually remains in superficial veins unless tourniquet is used.
2   If dye injection is done directly into medial malleolus to the marrow cavity, regional or general anaesthesia is required (because of pain).

Treatment and Nursing Management

Objective

To decrease or eliminate blood flow in the affected vessels, forcing the blood to return through deep veins.

Medical Treatment (nonoperative) *and Patient Education*

Patient is instructed to:

1   Avoid activities that cause venous stasis by obstructing venous flow.

a. Wearing tight garters, tight girdle.
b. Sitting or standing for prolonged periods of time.
c. Crossing the legs at knees for prolonged periods while sitting (reduces circulation by 15%).
2 Control excess weight gain.
3 Wear firm elastic support as prescribed, from toe to thigh when in upright position. Put elastic stockings on in bed before getting up.
4 Elevate foot of bed 15–20 cm (6–8 in) for night sleeping.
5 Avoid injuring legs.

Surgical Treatment

Indications:
a. Progressively advancing varicosities.
b. Stasis ulceration
c. Cosmetic needs.
2 A single method or combination of methods is tailored to meet the needs of the individual:
a. *Sclerosing injection*—not used as frequently today; may be combined with ligation or limited to treatment of isolated varicosities. The affected vessel may be sclerosed by injecting sodium tetradecyl sulphate or similar sclerosing agent. Compression bandage is then applied without interruption for 6 weeks; inflamed endothelial surfaces adhere by direct contact.
b. *Multiple vein ligation.*
c. *Ligation and stripping* of the greater and/or lesser saphenous systems. This procedure is the most effective.
3 Preoperative patient care:
a. Prepare the skin each day beginning 3 or 4 days prior to surgery by thoroughly cleansing the lower abdomen and legs with a detergent-germicidal soap.
b. Prepare the patient on the day before surgery (and after his daily skin cleansing) for the surgeon to mark his skin with a felt tip pen (indelible). Usually the patient stands on a chair in proper light so that the incision sites, paths of veins, dilated tributaries, etc., can be marked to aid the surgeon during the operation.
4 Postoperative nursing care and patient support:
a. Elevate the legs about 30° and provide adequate support of the entire leg.
b. Observe the patient for complaints of pain in specific areas of the foot or ankle; if the elastic bandage is too tight, loosen the bandage—later, have it reapplied.
c. Observe circulation to detect constriction or haemorrhage.
d. Follow the individualized therapeutic plan for the following:
(1) Permit ambulation according to the preoperative condition of the skin and subcutaneous tissues; if skin is healthy, bathroom privileges are usually permitted the day after surgery.
(2) Discourage dangling of the legs because it causes stasis of blood in the lower leg.
(3) Encourage the patient to walk with a normal gait; offer support if necessary; this activity should be progressive, depending on tolerance.

e. At first the legs are encased in pressure bandages from the toes to the groin; this is followed by knee-level elastic stockings for 3–4 weeks after surgery.
f. If there are significant trophic changes in the leg, due to long-term varicosities (past history), then postoperative care requires more bed rest and slow ambulation; in this event, leg and foot exercises in bed are helpful.
g. Note that complaints of patchy numbness can be expected but should disappear in less than a year.
h. Recognize that varicosities may recur; therefore conservative measures, learned preoperatively, should be continued.

ARTERIAL EMBOLISM

Causes

1   Arterial emboli usually (about 85%) originate from thrombi in the heart chambers.
2   Arteriosclerosis may cause roughening or ulceration of atheromatous plaques which can lead to emboli.

Clinical Manifestations

1   May vary from the patient's being totally unaware of the event, to
2   Acute pain—severe,
3   Loss of function—motor and sensory:
   a. Paralysis of part ⎫ Due to embolic block of artery.
   b. Anaesthesia of part ⎬ Due to associated vasomotor reflex.
   c. Pallor and coldness ⎭

Treatment and Nursing Management

1   Heparin should be administered intravenously to reduce tendency of emboli to form or expand—useful in smaller arteries.
2   Protect the extremity by keeping it at or below the horizontal plane; protect leg from hard surfaces and tight or heavy overlying bed linens.
3   Administer analgesics as prescribed for relief of pain.
4   Prepare patient for surgery; surgical intervention (embolectomy) is essential when an embolus blocks a large artery, such as the iliac.

NOTE: This is an emergency and is life-threatening; it requires immediate operative intervention if the embolus has major effect.

5   Postoperative nursing management
   a. Encourage activity in the leg to prevent stasis—obtain specific recommendations from surgeon concerning type and duration of exercises.
   b. Administer anticoagulants with full knowledge of what to watch for.
      (1) Inspect for bleeding anywhere, including surgical wound; this may be indicative of overdose of heparin.
      (2) Monitor vital signs.

(3) Recognize cardiovascular history of this patient; hence be able to assess cardiac and circulatory manifestations.

Prognosis

1 Arterial embolism is a threat not only to the extremity (5–25% possibility of amputation) but also to the patient (15–40% mortality rate).
2 Mortality rate increases because of cardiac disease; development of gangrene also contributes to increase in number of deaths.
3 Other cardiovascular difficulties compound the problem.

ARTERIOSCLEROSIS AND ATHEROSCLEROSIS

Arteriosclerosis is an arterial disease manifested by a loss of elasticity and a hardening of the vessel wall.

Atherosclerosis is the most common type of arteriosclerosis, manifested by the formation of atheromas (patchy lipoidal degeneration of the intima).

Significance

1 Arteriosclerosis is one of the chief causes of death in the U.K. (see p. 43).
2 One of the major clinical manifestations of arteriosclerosis is coronary heart disease.
3 Studies indicate that arteriosclerotic heart disease is partially preventable if attention is paid to 'risk' factors.

Aetiology

A combination of many factors.

1 Predisposition to arteriosclerosis is thought by many authorities to be hereditary.
2 Other aetiological factors include metabolic disturbances, arterial hypertension.
3 Risk factors:
    a. Age.
    b. Sex—death rate (ages 35–44) is greater in males than in females.
    c. Emotional tension.
    d. Elevated serum lipids.
    e. Hypertension.
    f. Cigarette smoking.
    g. Obesity.
    h. Impaired glucose tolerance (diabetes mellitus).
    i. Physical inactivity—since substantial collateral circulation is not established.
    j. Gout—uric acid levels of 6.9 mg/100 ml and above.
    k. Softness of drinking water; some authorities report that the softer the water, the higher the mortality from cardiovascular conditions.

Altered Physiology

1   Arteriosclerosis→narrowing or arterial vessels→malnutrition of tissue cells→ischaemic necrosis→fibrosis→sclerosis.
2   Sclerosis→degeneration of major organs due to lack of blood supply (nutrition): brain, myocardium, kidney.
3   Calcium deposits in tunica media of arterial vessel cause loss of elasticity.
4   Atheromas (plaque-like deposits) of cholesterol, fatty acids and often calcium form on intima of arterial vessels (atherosclerosis).
5   Dislodging of plaque may occur or a thrombus may be formed near the plaque; subsequent embolus may cause arterial occlusion and infarction in distant body sites.
6   After menopause, women are no longer protected by oestrogen.

General Patient Assessment

1   Arteriosclerosis is a generalized vascular disease; however, it varies from patient to patient in that it may affect one area more than another.
2   Often it limits itself to a segment of the vascular tree.
3   Five areas which are the most dangerous and cause disturbing symptoms are:
    a. Brain—cerebroarteriosclerosis.
    b. Heart—coronary artery disease.
    c. Gastrointestinal tract.
    d. Kidneys.
    e. Extremities.
4   Prognosis depends on extent of pathology and area of involvement.

Treatment

1   Since arteriosclerosis and atherosclerosis affect many different parts of the body, treatment is described where the major condition occurs. For example: angina pectoris and myocardial infarction are brought about by atherosclerosis of coronary arteries; treatment is discussed under the disease entity (p. 44).
2   Attention is directed to reducing risk factors by avoiding tension, reducing excess weight, giving up cigarette smoking, controlling diabetes and adjusting diet to reduce cholesterol intake (Table 1.6).
3   Operative reconstruction of involved vessels.

Foods Useful in Low-Cholesterol Diets

Fruits—all are low in cholesterol

Vegetables—if prepared and served without butter, cream, lard or suet. Vegetable-oil margarine, vegetable oils and mayonnaise may be used for flavouring

Breads and cereals

Skim or non-fat milk, buttermilk and cottage cheese to replace whole milk and cheese

Lean meat and lean fish

Marmalade, jelly, jam, syrup and sugar may be used in place of butter and other fats unless calories are restricted

Table 1.6. Cholesterol in foods*

The following foods are listed in the order of their content of preformed cholesterol, from the highest to the lowest, based on 100-g portions:

Food	Cholesterol (mg/100 g)	Food	Cholesterol (mg/100 g)
Egg yolk, dried	2950	Veal	90
Brains, raw	2000	Cheese (25–30% fat)	85
Egg yolk, fresh	1500	Milk, dried, whole	85
Egg yolk, frozen	1280	Beef, raw	70
Egg, whole	550	Fish, steak	70
Kidney, raw	375	Fish, fillet	70
Caviar or fish roe	300	Lamb, raw	70
Liver, raw	300	Pork	70
Butter	250	Cheese spread	65
Sweetbreads (thymus)	250	Margarine ($^2/_8$ animal fat,	
Oysters	200	($^1/_3$ vegetable)	65
Lobster	200	Mutton	65
Heart, raw	150	Chicken, flesh only, raw	60
Crab meat	125	Ice cream	45
Shrimp	125	Cottage cheese, creamed	15
Cheese, cream	120	Milk, fluid, whole	11
Cheese, cheddar	100	Milk, fluid, skim	3
Lard and other animal fat	95	Egg white	0

Foods Useful in Low-cholesterol Diets

Fruits—all are low in cholesterol
Vegetables—if prepared and served without butter, cream, lard or suet. Vegetable-oil margarine, vegetable oils and mayonnaise may be used for flavouring
Breads and cereals

Skim or non-fat milk, buttermilk and cottage cheese to replace whole milk and cheese
Lean meat and lean fish
Marmalade, jelly, jam, syrup and sugar may be used in place of butter and other fats unless calories are restricted

* From Church, F C, and Church, H N (1975) Food Value of Portions Commonly Used, 12th edition, Philadelphia, J B Lippincott.

ARTERIOSCLEROSIS OBLITERANS

Arteriosclerosis obliterans is a form of arteriosclerosis in which the vascular system of the leg becomes blocked.

Incidence

Men affected more often than women
Parallels that of arteriosclerotic heart disease.

Clinical Manifestations

Symptoms appear gradually.

1   Intermittent claudication (see p. 124).
2   Coldness of extremity.
3   Colour change—pallor.
4   Decrease in size of leg.
5   Tingling, numbness of toes.
6   Later—pain, even when leg is at rest; occurs at night, requiring patient to get out of bed to walk to relieve pain.
7   Cramp-like excruciating pain in calf muscles.
8   Ulcers of toes and feet develop.

Diagnosis

1   Vascular physical examination.
2   Doppler ultrasound probe.
3   Angiography.

Treatment and Nursing Management

Objectives

To preserve the extremity.
To relieve the intermittent claudication.

See p. 137, General Management of the Patient with a Peripheral Vascular Problem.

1   Where conservative measures clearly are not enough, grafting is the treatment of choice.
2   If the arteriogram does not show a suitable situation for grafting, a sympathectomy may be done.

THROMBOANGIITIS OBLITERANS (BUERGER'S DISEASE)

Thromboangiitis obliterans is a disease characterized by inflammation in the arteries and veins, usually of the lower extremities. It is associated with venous and arterial thrombosis and frequently leads to gangrene.

Aetiology

1   It appears to be due to a hypersensitivity to use of tobacco.
2   Primarily affects males between the ages of 20 and 45; almost all are tobacco smokers.
3   Incidence has decreased in the last several years.

Altered Physiology

1   Structural changes in the walls of the arteries and veins produce a roughening of the intima; a thrombosis then results.
2   Arterial involvement predominates over venous involvement.

3   Coronary, abdominal visceral and cerebral vessels may be involved in the late stages of the disease.

Clinical Manifestations

1   Onset may be gradual or sudden.
2   Coldness, numbness, tingling or burning sensation in extremities.
3   Involvement of the upper extremities (particularly in the ulnar artery). Occurs in a high proportion of patients; fatigue with writing.
4   Intermittent claudication—cramps in the legs after exercise (relieved with rest).
5   Painful red lumps appear under the skin, heal and migrate to nearby areas as phlebitis shifts.
6   More persistent pain is noted in the pregangrenous stage; this becomes more severe when ulcers are present or gangrene has begun.
7   Symptoms are aggravated by smoking, chilling and emotional disturbances.
8   Dependent position of extremity—rubor
     Elevated above heart level—pallor } Indicative of arterial insufficiency.
9   Coldness of extremity is common.
10   Arterial pulses are diminished or absent as the disease advances.

Diagnosis

1   *Angiography*—useful in demonstrating focal, distal, occlusive arterial changes in otherwise smooth arteries.
2   *Allen test*—a test to demonstrate arterial occlusion of the radial or ulnar arteries.
     a. The patient is instructed to raise his hand and close his fist.
     b. Examiner grasps patient's wrist tightly, compressing radial and ulnar arteries.
     c. The patient opens and closes his hand until pallor is observed (Fig. 1.44).
     d. Patient is instructed to lower his hand and open his fist—meanwhile the examiner after 1 min releases pressure on ulnar artery, while maintaining pressure on radial artery.
     e. Observe hand; if ulnar artery is patent, the whole hand will be flushed. (Conversely, if there is ulnar artery obstruction, the hand will be partially or completely blanched.)

Objectives of Treatment and Nursing Management; Patient Education

To Improve Circulation in the Extremities and to Maintain Cleanliness to Prevent the Spread of Necrosis

Instruct patient as follows:

1   Wash feet with a bland soap and warm water.
2   Pat the washed areas dry with a soft towel; powder unbroken skin.
3   Massage the extremities gently with a bland lubricating oil.
4   Wear clean fresh socks or stockings each day.
5   Initiate Buerger–Allen exercises (see p. 125) if intermittent claudication is in evidence.

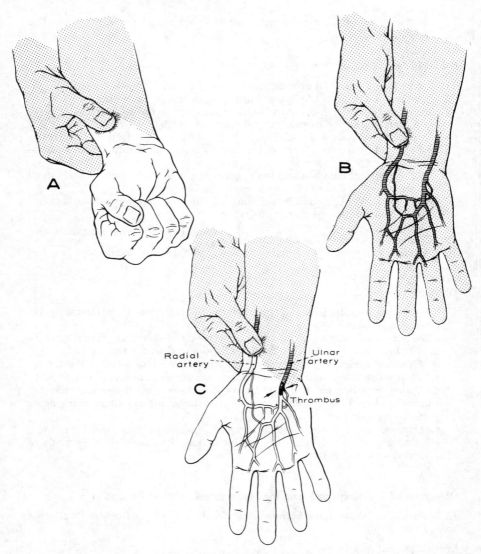

Figure 1.44.   Allen test. a. Diagrammatic representation of the procedure for determining patency or occlusion of the ulner artery distal to the wrist. b. The ulcer artery is patent as determined by the prompt return of the colour to the skin of the hand while the radial artery is still compressed. c. Occlusion of the ulnar artery is demonstrated by persistence of pallor as long as the radial arterial inflow is blocked by the examiner's finger. (Modified from: Juergens and Fairbairn, Arteriosclerosis obliterans, Heart Bulletin, 8: 22–24. By permission of the American Heart Association.)

To Urge Adoption of a Therapeutic Regimen to Block the Spread of the Disease

Instruct patient as follows:

1   *Avoid smoking in any form*, because it is the cause of the disease.
2   Obtain rest so as to minimize demands on the circulatory system.
3   Maintain adequate hydration to assist in avoiding stasis in the affected vessels.

To Protect the Extremities From Trauma and Infection

Instruct patient as follows:

1   Wear properly fitting shoes and hosiery.
2   Protect the feet from chilling and exposure to cold.
3   Avoid overheating leg by injudicious use of hot water bottles or heating pads.
4   Never use circular garters, constricting bands or garments which would impair circulation.
5   Seek medical attention for evidence of tissue disturbance, e.g., colour changes, blister development, abrasion, infection, changes in sensation such as tingling, numbness or pain.

To Perform a Temporary Sympathetic Block in Selected Patients

1   Inject lumbar sympathetic ganglia and trunk with procaine in order to abolish vaso-constricting influence of the sympathetic nervous system.
2   Evaluate effects of the temporary block; if definitely favourable, a lumbar sympathectomy may be done for more permanent effect.

To Initiate More Drastic Attempts to Treat the Effects of the Disease

1   Recognize that amputation of a part or parts, such as toes, may be necessary if necrosis develops.
2   Be prepared to repeat the process if gangrene develops in other toes or foot.

DISEASES OF THE AORTA

Aortitis

Aortitis is inflammation of the aorta—usually of the aortic arch.

Types of Aortitis

Arteriosclerotic Aortitis

1   Accompanies the generalized disease of arteriosclerosis.
2   Appears after the age of 60, usually—may occur earlier.
3   May cause pain, dilatation (aneurysm), aortic valve insufficiency.
4   Degeneration and sclerosis of entire surface of intima occur.

Syphilitic Aortitis

1   Appears before age 50.
2   Begins at root of aorta and spreads in patch-like areas over normal intima to involve aorta, aortic arch.

3   Symptoms are variable—may be severe or mild.
   a. Sensations of substernal oppression or weight (vicelike pains).
   b. Sudden attacks of dyspnoea may be agonizing and last 5–15 min. Accompanied by tachycardia, deep cyanosis, profuse perspiration.
   c. Symptoms lead to aortic insufficiency and aneuryms which may erode bone.

Diagnosis

Aortic insufficiency without associated mitral lesion, paroxysmal dyspnoea, anginal attacks or aneurysm suggest syphilitic aortitis.

Treatment and Prognosis

1   Antisyphilitic therapy for syphilitic aortitis (see Volume 1, Chapter 6).
2   Damage cannot be repaired completely—may require graft and prosthetic valve.

Aortic Aneurysm

Aneurysm is a distension of an artery.

Types of Aneurysms

Morphologically, they may be classified as follows:

1   Saccular—distension of a vessel projecting from one side.
2   Fusiform—distension of the whole artery, i.e. entire circumference is involved.

Aetiology

1   Local infection, pyogenic or fungal (mycotic aneurysm).
2   Congenital weakness of vessels.
3   Arteriosclerosis.
4   Syphilis.
5   Trauma.

Thoracic Aneurysm

Clinical Manifestations

1   Subjective Symptoms:
   a. At first no symptoms; later symptoms may come from congestive heart failure or a pulsating tumour mass in the chest.
   b. Pain and pressure symptoms:
      (1) Constant, boring pain because of pressure, or
      (2) Intermittent and neuralgic pain because of infringement on nerves.
   c. Dyspnoea causing pressure against trachea.
   d. Cough, often paroxysmal and brassy in sound.
   e. Hoarseness, voice weakness or complete aphonia resulting from pressure against recurrent laryngeal nerve.
   f. Dysphagia due to impingement on oesophagus.

g. With syphilitic aortic aneurysm there may be anginal and paroxysmal dyspnoea due to concomitant syphilitic aortitis.

2 Objective Signs:

a. Oedema of chest wall—infrequent.

b. Dilated superficial veins on chest.

c. Cyanosis because of vein compression of chest vessels.

d. Ipsilateral (on the same side) dilatation of pupils due to pressure against cervical sympathetic chain.

e. Pulse difference in two wrists if aneurysm interferes with circulation in left subclavian artery.

f. Abnormal pulsation may be apparent on chest wall—due to erosion of aneurysm through rib cage—in syphilis.

Treatment

1 The prognosis is poor for untreated patients.

2 Surgical—remove aneurysm and restore vascular continuity.
   Aortic arch aneurysms are the most difficult to treat.

Abdominal Aneurysm

Clinical Manifestations

1 About 40% of these patients display symptoms; the rest are asymptomatic.

2 Abdominal pain is most common; persistent or intermittent—often localized in middle or lower abdomen to the left of midline.

3 Low back pain.

4 Feeling of an abdominal pulsating mass.

5 Hypertension may be present.

Diagnosis

1 Normally the systolic blood pressure of the thigh exceeds that in the arm; in many of these patients the opposite is true.

2 A palpable pulsating abdominal mass; fluoroscopy will reveal pulsating tumour.

3 Angioaortogram allows visualization of vessels and aneurysm.

4 Ultrasound allows visualization of vessels and aneurysm.

5 Computerized tomography allows visualization of vessels and aneurysm.

Treatment and Nursing Management

1 If untreated, the prognosis is poor.

2 Abdominal aortic aneurysm.

a. Surgery to excise area affected.

b. Replacement of excised segment by a graft.

3 Dissecting aneurysm of aorta.

a. This is a type of aneurysm in which there is a tear in the intima of the aorta; as a result of pressure, blood splits the wall and may produce a large haematoma or may continue to rip the wall.

b. Symptoms may resemble coronary occlusion; diagnosis is confirmed by aortography.

    c. Prognosis is poor, but surgical removal of involved aneurysm and replacement of segment with a graft may be effective.

4 Peripheral vessel aneurysms.

    a. May involve renal artery, subclavian artery, popliteal artery (knee) or any major artery.

    b. These produce a pulsating mass and may cause pain or pressure on surrounding structures.

    c. Replacement grafts are used to repair these aneurysms.

RAYNAUD'S DISEASE

Raynaud's disease is a peripheral vascular disorder of the hands (occasionally the feet, less often the nose, ears, chin) in which there is paroxysmal contraction of the arteries.

NOTE: *Raynaud's phenomenon* is a symptom not only of Raynaud's disease but also of other conditions associated with paroxysmal vasoconstriction of the fingers.

1 Intermittent changes in colour of the skin of fingers and toes and, less commonly, of nose and ears.
2 Pallor phase—arteries and arterioles completely occluded.
3 Cyanotic phase—spasm causes partial occlusion of affected vessels.
4 Rubor phase—a period of hyperaemia.
5 The disease occurs chiefly but not exclusively in females between the ages of 20 and 40.

Cause

Cause is unknown; however, there appears to be a hereditary predisposition.

Altered Physiology

1 There is an abnormality of the peripheral sympathetic nervous system—sympathetic over-activity leading to toxic contraction of arterioles.
2 Intermittent vasospasm may completely interfere with the arterial blood flow to the fingers or toes, leading to ischaemia, pallor, coldness, prickling feeling, pain and numbness.
3 Responding, the capillaries become dilated because of an increase in metabolites; colour changes from pallor to cyanosis.
4 Following the spasm, circulation is re-established; colour changes from bluish to red to normal pink.
5 With repeated vasospasms, the artery wall thickens and thrombosis may develop, leading to occlusion, cyanosis, coldness, numbness, atrophy, gangrene.

Clinical Manifestations

1 Gradual onset: pallor of one or two fingers or toes when exposed to cold—then all digits may become involved; usually both hands are involved symmetrically in true Raynaud's disease.

2 Upon relaxation of vasospasm, tissue temperature change may move rapidly from cold to warm.
3 Nerve sensations may be apparent: tingling, numbness, dull ache.
4 Skin may appear white, smooth, taut, shiny; nail deformity may eventually occur.
5 Continued bouts of vasospasm may gradually progress to ulceration and gangrene.
6 Manifestations appear to be related to exposure to cold.

Treatment

Objective

To relieve and prevent vasospasm.

1 Exposure to cold, which causes vasoconstriction, should be avoided.
2 Patient should eliminate smoking, which has a tendency to constrict the peripheral vascular system.
3 Vasodilators are administered. Doses are gradually increased until therapeutic effect is noted or side-effects appear which suggest stopping drug increments.
4 Relief from emotionally stressful experiences may be in order since emotional stress appears to contribute to vasospasm.

Medication	Side-Effects
a. Phenoxybenzamine hydrochloride (Dibenyline)	Headache, tachycardia, nasal congestion, orthostatic hypotension.
b. Cyclandelate (Cyclospasmol)	Headache, nausea, heavier than usual perspiration, vertigo, flushing, tingling.
c. Tolazoline hydrochloride (Priscol)	Gastrointestinal upset, orthostatic hypotension, chilliness, tachycardia, palpitations.

5 Regional sympathectomy may be considered if condition worsens and does not respond to above measures; such surgery would remove vasoconstricting impulses.
   a. In most patients, this appears to have only transient benefit; a few patients have had significant improvement.
   b. If Raynaud's phenomenon is secondary to other underlying diseases, results of sympathectomy are usually poor since underlying condition is not affected.
6 Amputation may be necessary if gangrene affects digits (rare).

Health Teaching

1 Think through the possible causative factors which provoke a spasm; these should be avoided.
2 Use insulating clothing when it is necessary to go out into the cold: woollen gloves and socks, fleece-lined boots and footwear, etc.
3 Avoid exposing hands to cold objects, e.g. reaching into the freezer, handling a cold, ice-filled glass, etc.
4 Give up smoking; consider moving to a warmer climate, if possible.

HYPERTENSION

Hypertension is an abnormal condition of the small vessels of the arterial system in which the systolic or diastolic blood pressure is elevated. A rise in either systolic or diastolic pressure is associated with an increased mortality rate.

'Great as is the effect of hypertension on the incidence of myocardial infarction, it is even greater in relation to the incidence of stroke.'*

Normal Physiology

1 *Normal blood pressure* (normotension) is the pressure of the blood within the systemic arterial system. It ranges from 100/60 to 140/90.
2 *Systolic pressure* represents the greatest pressure of the blood against the wall of the vessel following ventricular contraction.
3 *Diastolic pressure* represents the least pressure of the blood against the wall of the vessel following closure of the aortic valve.
4 *Pulse pressure* represents the difference between the systolic and diastolic readings—the range of pressure in the arteries.
5 The *mean arterial pressure* is the average pressure attempting to push blood through the circulatory system.
   This can be determined electronically or mathematically as well as by using an intra-arterial catheter and mercury manometer.
   Mathematical determination. (Slightly less than average of systolic and diastolic).
   Mean arterial pressure = $\frac{1}{3}$ systolic pressure + $\frac{2}{3}$ diastolic pressure.
   Example: for blood pressure of 130/85
   Mean arterial pressure is 100 mmHg
   Kidney function requires a minimum of 70 mmHg (mean arterial pressure)
6 *Basal blood pressure* is the lowest blood pressure taken in supine position after several days of hospitalization without treatment.
   Basal sitting pressure and basal standing pressure are often taken for later comparison.

Factors Affecting Pressure of Blood

Blood volume, peripheral resistance, blood viscosity, cardiac output.

1 Blood pressure = cardiac output × total peripheral resistance.
   a. Pressure varies with exercise, emotional reaction, sleep, digestion, time of day.
   b. Such functions as renal, adrenal, vascular and neurogenic functions affect blood pressure.
2 Higher blood pressure = increased cardiac output × greater total peripheral resistance (circulatory overload).
3 Lower blood pressure = lessened cardiac output × lesser total peripheral resistance.
4 Increased diastolic pressure due to peripheral resistance indicates decrease in

* Tobian, L J Jr (1975) The clinical approach to essential hypertension, Hospital Practice, 10: 33.

diameter of arterioles. These are affected by sympathetic stimulation, hereditary factors, more vasopressor hormones in the blood.
5   Increased systolic pressure indicates increased cardiac output and systolic hypertension, which is always secondary.

Incidence

1   Hypertension is more common but better tolerated in women than in men.
2   Hypertensive women tend to be obese; hypertensive men do not appear to differ in size from other men.
3   There is a higher incidence in the black races.
4   It appears that a high sodium intake is related to the development of hypertension; when sodium intake is decreased, blood pressure often decreases.
5   Increase in incidence is associated with the following risk factors;
    a. Age: between 30 and 50.
    b. Race: black.
    c. Hyperlipidaemia.
    d. History of smoking.
    e. The higher the blood pressure, the greater the risk.

Aetiology and the Significance of Blood Pressure Elevation

1   Cause is unknown; however, there are several hypotheses:
    a. Hyperactivity of sympathetic vasoconstricting nerves.
    b. Presence of blood component which contains a vasoconstrictor that acts on smooth muscle, sensitizing it to constrictor substances.
    c. Increased cardiac output followed by arteriole constriction.
    d. Familial tendency.
2   Individual tolerance of increased blood pressure varies; however, there is a direct correlation between increase in blood pressure and the rate at which atherosclerosis and arteriosclerosis develop.
3   Onset of hypertension occurs in the early 30s; because it is asymptomatic, it is usually untreated for at least 20 years.
4   Rising blood pressure adversely affects the brain, the heart and the kidneys.
    a. Heart—myocardial infarction, congestive heart failure.
    b. Kidney—nephrosclerosis, kidney failure.
    c. Brain—headache, encephalopathy, cerebral haemorrhage, cerebrovascular accident.
    d. Eye—papilloedema, swelling of optic disc.
5   Emotional stress exacerbates the problem.
6   Obesity and diabetes mellitus are associated with hypertension.

Classification of Hypertension

Primary or Essential Hypertension (approximately 90% of patients with hypertension)

1   When the diastolic pressure is 90 mmHg or higher and other causes of hypertension are absent, the condition is said to be primary hypertension.
    More specifically, when the average of three or more blood pressures taken at

rest several days apart exceeds the upper limits of the following chart, an individual is considered hypertensive:

Infants	90/60 mmHg
3–6 years	110/70 mmHg
7–10 years	120/80 mmHg
11–17 years	130/80 mmHg
18–44 years	140/90 mmHg
45–64 years	150/90 mmHg
65 and older	160/95 mmHg

2   Genetic factors contribute to this condition; patterns of the patient indicate that he is hypersensitive to internal and external stimuli.
3   Benign—the presence of hypertension for years without any symptoms.
4   Labile—intermittently elevated blood pressure levels.
5   Malignant—a sudden and severe acceleration in arterial pressure producing many symptoms and vascular damage.

Secondary Hypertension

1   Occurs in approximately 5–10% of patients with hypertension.
2   More common in men and in black race.
3   Apparently follows other pathology.
   a. *Renal pathology* which may lead to hypertension.
      (1) Congenital anomalies, pyelonephritis, renal artery obstruction, acute and chronic glomerulonephritis.
      (2) Reduced blood flow to kidney (such as atherosclerotic plaque)—release of *renin*.
         (a) Renin reacts with serum protein in liver (alpha-2-globulin) → angiotensin I; this plus an enzyme → angiotensin II → leads to increased blood pressure.
         (b) Symptoms: proteinuria, polyuria, elevated blood pressure.
         (c) Therapy—endarterectomy, bypass graft, nephrectomy; blood pressure is reduced following correction of initial problem.
   b. *Coarctation of aorta* (stenosis of aorta).
      (1) Blood flow to upper extremities is greater than flow to lower extremities—hypertension of upper part of body
      (2) Correction—removal of stenosed section of vessel; anastomosis or graft to eliminate area.
   c. *Endocrine disturbance*—elevated blood pressure may be due to phaeochromocytoma.
      (1) Phaeochromocytoma—causes release of adrenaline and noradrenaline and a rise in blood pressure.
      (2) Adrenal cortex tumours lead to an increase in aldosterone secretion and an elevated blood pressure.
      (3) Cushing's syndrome leads to an increase in adrenocortical steroids and hypertension.
   d. *Retinal changes:*
      (1) Optic disc—blurring of disc margins and contour changes.
      (2) Papilloedema—choked disc.

(3) Arterial diameter lessened.
  e. *Arteriosclerosis*—renal pathology.

Phases of Hypertension

Prehypertensive Phase

1 Characteristics:
   a. Blood pressure elevation—no vascular change.
   b. Systole below 200 mmHG; Diastole below 100 mmHg.
   c. Pressure elevation may be the only sign for 10 or 15 years before other symptoms appear.
   d. Headache, giddiness, insomnia, forgetfulness, irritability, epistaxis.

Benign or Early Phase

1 Characteristics
   a. Systole below 200 mmHg.
   b. Diastole above 90 mmHg.
   c. Headache, giddiness, insomnia, forgetfulness, irritability, epistaxis, blurring of vision, shortness of breath, anginal pain.

Moderately Severe Phase

1 Characteristics:
   a. Systole above 200 mmHg.
   b. Diastole above 100 mmHg—no evidence of vascular damage.
2 Characteristics—with onset of arteriosclerosis, hypertension increases and diastolic blood pressure is persistently elevated:
   Therapy:
   a. If exceeding 130 mmHg (diastole), hospital rest is recommended.
   b. Immediate treatment if the following are present:
      (1) Convulsive movements.
      (2) Abnormal neurological signs.
      (3) Severe occipital headache.
      (4) Pulmonary oedema.
   c. Watch blood pressure; reduce gradually and avoid wide pressure variations—note that bringing pressure down to the usual normal may not be tolerated.
   d. Measure and record urinary output.

Malignant Phase

1 Blood pressure may elevate very rapidly with serious damage to vital organs.
   a. Hypertensive encephalopathy or cerebrovascular accident.
      Progressive headache—stupor—convulsion.
   b. Eye effect—visual impairment, haemorrhage, papilloedema, exudates.
   c. Kidney effect.
      (1) Blood flow decreased, vasconstriction.
      (2) BUN more than 100 mg/100 mm.
      (3) Plasma renin activity.
      (4) Specific gravity lowered.

(5) Proteinuria.
  d. Epigastric pain.
  e. Left ventricular failure.
  f. Morning headache, nausea and vomiting.
2   Onset of complications.
  a. Pathology:
    (1) Elevated diastolic pressure→strain on arterial wall→thickening and calcification of arterial media (sclerosis)→narrowed blood vessel lumen.
    (2) Sclerosis of vessels→increased wall permeability→deposits placed on intima and media of vessels→cerebral, myocardial or renal ischaemia.
  b. Cerebrovascular manifestations.
  Changes are determined by the type of onset symptoms.
    (1) *Rapid:*
      (a) Cerebral haemorrhage→headache, increase in cerebrospinal pressure→papilloedema→retinal haemorrhages→hemiplegia→coma.
      (b) Cerebral thrombosis→tingling sensations→numbness, limbparesis→aphasia.
      (c) Subarachnoid haemorrhage→stiffness of neck→pupil dilatation on side of haemorrhage→blood cells in cerebrospinal fluid→unconsciousness.
    (2) *Slow:*
    Gradual vascular insufficiency.
    (3) Neurological changes with recovery in a few hours→cerebrovascular spasms.

General Detection, Evaluation and Treatment of High Blood Pressure in Adults*

When there is group screening and measurement of blood pressure, resources for referral, confirmation and follow-up should be provided. Such screening is only available on a small scale in the UK.

1   Prior to blood pressure determination, ask the patient whether he has been or is currently under treatment for hypertension.
  a. Urge him to continue treatment even if blood pressure is normal.
  b. Urge him to report an elevated blood pressure to his doctor.
2   Take blood pressure with patient seated and resting comfortably.
3   Record both systolic and diastolic pressure (diastolic—*disapperance of sound*).
4   Use a mercury sphygmomanometer preferably.
5   Use a larger size cuff for persons with obese arms.
6   Inform the patient in writing of his blood pressure and whether further evaluation is necessary.
7   Refer promptly to a doctor all persons with diastolic pressure of 120 mmHg or higher.
8   See Fig. 1.45 for recheck schedule; this will separate those whose pressures have returned to normal (requiring only annual measurement) from those whose sustained pressure elevation warrants further study or treatment.

NOTE: Blood pressure should be taken on three different occasions before treatment is prescribed.

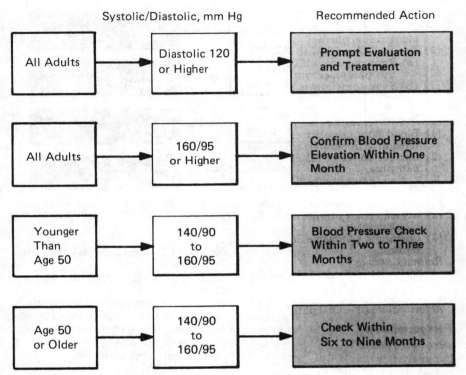

Systolic/Diastolic, mm Hg   Recommended Action

Figure 1.45. Recommended action after blood pressure measurement. (From: Moser, M et. al. (1977) High blood pressure, JAMA, 237: 256. Copyright 1977, American Medical Association.)

9 See Fig. 1.46 for recommended action following confirmed blood pressure measurements.
10 Be sure there are adequate systems for follow-up blood pressure measurement and for referral of patients with elevated blood pressures.
11 Make special efforts to detect high blood pressure in black communities since hypertension is more prevalent in this group.

Diagnostic Assessment of Patient

1 Careful medical history (including family history of hypertension); note any previous history of hypertension, excessive salt intake, use of birth control pills or other hormones, lipid abnormalities, cigarette smoking and history of headache, weakness, muscle cramp, palpitation, sweating
2 Physical examination.

* Based on the Report of the Joint National Committee on Detection, Evaluation, and Treatment of High Blood Pressure (JAMA, 237: 255–261, 17 Jan. 1977).

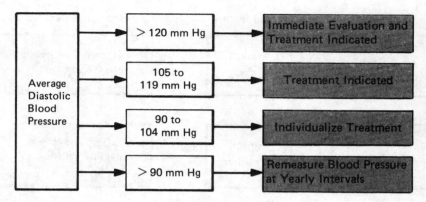

Figure 1.46   Recommended action after repeated or confirmation blood pressure measurements. (From: Moser, M et. al. (1977) High blood pressure, JAMA, 237: 256. Copyright 1977, American Medical Association.)

3   Blood pressure: supine and standing; also assess vital signs and evaluate function of vital organs.
4   Fundoscopic examination of the eye to detect vascular changes in the capillaries—note oedema, spasm, haemorrhage.
5   Careful examination of the heart; examination of peripheral pulse disparities.
6   Listen for bruits over all peripheral arteries to determine presence of atherosclerosis; also listen for bruits in abdomen to note signs of renal arterial stenosis.
7   Chest x-ray to determine cardiac size; auscultation of lungs.
8   Neurological tests to detect cerebral damage, neurological deficits.
9   Laboratory studies:
    a. Haematocrit (PCV) reading.
    b. BUN to determine renal excretory function.
    c. Serum potassium concentration to determine hyperaldosteronism.
    d. Electrocardiogram to establish a baseline.
    e. Urinalysis for blood, protein and glucose to determine renal parenchymal disease.

Guidelines for Treatment

Virtually all patients with a diastolic pressure of 105 mmHg or greater should be treated with antihypertensive drug therapy.

Objectives

To return blood pressure to normal or near normotensive levels.
To maintain a normal blood pressure with minimal side-effects.
To correct risk factors which directly affect the blood pressure.
To delay the progress of and to control the disease.
To slow the progression of atherosclerosis.
To recommend supportive psychotherapy in some form if it will lessen vasoconstriction.

Initial Conservative Therapy

1 Therapy is prescribed on an individual basis, depending on blood pressure, the extent of vascular damage and whether hypertension is primary or secondary.
2 Inform the patient of the significance of avoiding excessive fat and salt in the diet.
3 Initiate a programme of weight reduction if obesity is a problem.
4 Help the patient to understand the importance of giving up smoking.
5 Instruct the patient that he must learn to rest and must also become involved in a daily exercise programme to match his particular needs.
6 Emphasize the importance of avoiding or minimizing stressful situations.

Pharmacotherapy

'*Stepped Care*' is an approach (done on an individual basis) whereby initial therapy consists of a single medication; if this fails to meet the goal of lowering pressure, either the dose is increased or another drug is added; upon re-evaluation, perhaps another drug may be required. Increasing or decreasing dosages or adding or subtracting drugs is suggested following periodic re-evaluation.

NOTE: When there is a choice of two medications, the one with fewer side-effects, less patient inconvenience, less frequency of administration and less cost is preferred. No one combination of drugs works in all patients.

Step 1

Thiazides (diuretics)—See Fig. 1.47.

1 NOTE: The combination of a diuretic with digitalis requires attention because hypokalaemia induced by a diuretic potentiates the toxicity of digitalis.
2 Failure to achieve the therapeutic goal may be due to the following:
   a. Lack of patient compliance with medication schedule.
   b. Excessive salt intake.
   c. Use of other drugs which may interact with thiazides.

Step 2

1 If the therapeutic goal is not achieved with the diuretic alone, several alternative drugs may be tried. One or more may be effective in some patients and not in others.
   a. Reserpine (rauwolfia alkaloids) has the advantages of low cost and once-a-day administration (see Table 1.7).
   b. Usually, low doses are used initially and are increased gradually until therapeutic effect is achieved.
   c. The patient needs to be monitored for occurrence of fluid retention.
   d. Clonidine hydrochloride (Catapres) may be substituted for any Step 3 drug.
      (1) Clonidine side-effects—dry mouth, drowsiness.
      (2) Prazosin side-effects—weakness, postural dizziness, sudden collapse.

Step 3

Usually hydralazine hydrochloride is added.

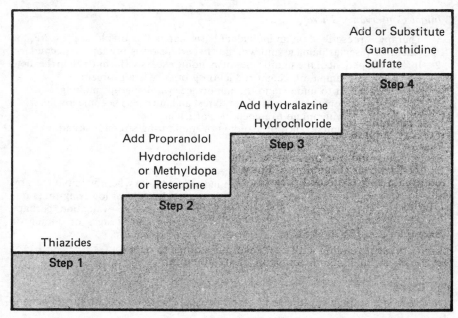

Figure 1.47.   Recommended antihypertensive regimes. (Experience with clonidine hydrochloride and prazosin hydrochloride, newly approved, moderately potent antihypertensive agents that may be added or substituted for step 2 or 3 drugs, is limited). (From: Moser, M., *et al.*, High blood pressure, JAMA 237: 260, 17 Jan. 1977. Copyright 1977, American Medical Association.)

1   This medication is an effective peripheral vasodilator.
2   It is used cautiously in patients with angina because its action increases cardiac output.
3   It is usually used with a sympathetic blocking agent (Step 2 medication) plus a diuretic.

Step 4

Followed when the first three steps are ineffective.

1   Guanethidine may be added or substituted for drugs used in previous steps.
2   Note the side-effects of this medication in Table 1.7.
3   This is a potent medication and is often effective in more resistant cases.

Blood Pressure Determination

Measure the blood pressure of the patient under the same conditions each time.

1   Place patient in the desired position (sitting, standing, etc.) according in preferences of the doctor.
2   Use the correct size of blood pressure cuff.

RULE: Width of an inflatable bladder should be 20% greater than the diameter of the extremity on which it is used. (Fig. 1.48a)

3   Record precisely the systolic and diastolic pressure:
a. Systolic—the pressure within the pressure cuff indicated by the level of the mercury column at the moment the Korotkoff sounds are first heard (Fig. 1.48b)
b. First diastolic—the pressure within the compression cuff indicated by the level of the mercury column at the moment the sound suddenly becomes muffled (beginning of Phase 4).
c. Second diastolic—the pressure within the compression cuff at the moment the sounds finally disappear (beginning of Phase 5).
4   If required, mark the blood pressure reading to indicate patient's position and the arm used:

        L (lying)   R.A. (Right Arm)
        St. (standing)   L.A. (Left Arm)

Example: L.A. 152/78/68 St.
5   Compare present reading with past several readings to note differences and detect trends.
6   Alert the doctor if significant changes are apparent.

Hypertensive Crisis

Hypertensive Crisis is a sudden rapid rise in blood pressure with effects on target organs that are life-threatening.

Aetiology

1   Malignant hypertension, hypertensive encephalopathy, acute congestive heart failure with hypertension, and eclampsia.
2   More rare is hypertensive crisis secondary to phaeochromocytoma or dissecting aneurysm.

Treatment

Objective

To first reduce diastolic pressure towards, but not below 90 mmHg and then to initiate oral therapy.

1   Use parenteral medications in hypertensive emergencies.
a. Diastolic blood pressure over 150 mmHg.
b. Pulmonary oedema, cerebral haemorrhage, encephalopathy in combination with diastolic pressure over 120 or 130.
2   Patient must be hospitalized and monitored constantly.
a. Record blood pressure frequently.
    Some drugs such as trimetaphan, sodium nitroprusside require blood pressure to be taken every 5 min.
b. Evaluate changes in cerebral state.
c. Measure urine output accurately.
d. Be prepared to administer vasopressors if severe hypotension develops.

Table 1.7. Side-effects of and Precautions to be Taken with Antihypertensive Drugs

Generic Name	Proprietary Name	Side-effects*	Precautions
Diuretics			
Thiazide and thiazide derivative diuretics (e.g. chlorthiazide)	(Saluric)	BUN↑, uric acid↑, calcium↑, serum K^+, glucose, gastrointestinal irritation, weakness, photosensitivity, blood dyscrasias, pancreatitis†	Hypokalaemia, gout, renal insufficiency
Loop diuretics (frusemide)		Calcium↓, BUN↑, uric acid↑, serum K^+, photosensitivity	Hypokalaemia, gout
Potassium-sparing diuretics			
Spironolactone	(Aldactone)	Hyperkalaemia, gynaecomastia, drowsiness, hirsutism, irregular menses	Hyperkalaemia, renal failure
Triamterene	(Dytac)	Hyperkalaemia, diarrhoea, nausea	
Non-diuretics			
Rauwolfia alkaloids	Reserpine (Serpasil)	Drowsiness, sedation, lassitude, nasal congestion, bradycardia, depression, gastric hyperacidity, nightmares	Mental depression
Methyldopa	(Aldomet)	Orthostatic hypotension, drowsiness, depression, abnormal liver function tests, positive direct Coombs test	Liver disease
Propranolol hydrochloride	(Inderal)	Insomnia, bradycardia, bronchospasm, heart failure, sedation	Asthma, heart failure, diabetes
Hydralazine hydrochloride	(Apresoline)	Headache, tachycardia, palpitations, exacerbation of angina or congestive heart failure, mesenchymal ('lupus like') reaction‡	Symptomatic coronary artery disease
Guanethidine sulphate	(Ismelin)	Orthostatic hypotension (especially in the AM), exertional weakness, bradycardia, diarrhoea, loss of ability to ejaculate	Symptomatic cardiovascular disease

* See also manufacturer's full prescribing information. Impotency may occur with any antihypertensive drug except hydralazine.
† Many side-effects, for example, blood dyscrasias and pancreatitis, are rare with diuretics.
‡ Rare with dosage under 300 mg/day.

Source: Table adapted from Moser, M et al. (1977) High blood pressure, JAMA, 237: 260. (Copyright 1977, American Medical Association.)

e. Administer diuretics such as frusemide and ethacrynic acid as adjuncts when prescribed.
They serve to maintain sodium diuresis when the arterial pressure falls.
f. Administer spironolactone when prescribed if hypokalaemia is a problem.
3 Pharmacotherapy.
a. Drugs which act in a few minutes but are not satisfactory for long-term management.
  (1) Diazoxide.
  (2) Sodium nitroprusside.
  (3) Trimetaphan.
b. Drugs which require 30 min or more to obtain full effects; they can later be used orally for long-term management of hypertension.
  (1) Methyldopa.
  (2) Hydralazine.
c. See Table 1.8.

Table 1.8. Drugs for Parenteral Treatment of Hypertension

Drug	Action	Side-effects and Pertinent Points
1. Diazoxide (Eudemine)	Orally—mildly antihypertensive Intravenously—strongly antihypertensive	Salt is restricted to prevent salt and water retention
2. Sodium nitroprusside (Nipride)	Has immediate antihypertensive effect Reduces total peripheral resistance (vasodilator) Produces a relaxation of arteriolar and venular smooth muscle	Useful in patients with hypertensive emergencies complicated by cardiac and aortic disease
3. Trimetaphan camsylate (Arfonad)	Has immediate antihypertensive effect—its effect disappears when infusion is discontinued (Ganglion-blocking agent)	Extremely potent hypotensive drug requiring adequate facilities, equipment and personnel for monitoring patient
4. Methyldopa (Aldomet)	Effective in lowering blood pressure in 4–6 hours—effect extends 10–16 hours after injection	Sedation sometimes occurs as a result of this medication but usually wears off in a few days when a maintenance dose is established Watch for kidney toxicity
5. Hydralazine (Apresoline)	Effective in treating hypertensive patients with acute glomerulonephritis Onset of action in 10–20 min Maximum response—1 hour Persists—12 hours	Monitor blood pressure every 15 min

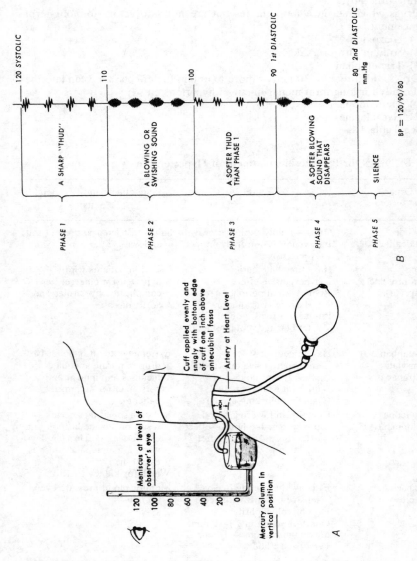

Figure 1.48. a. Important 'rules' for accurate recording of arterial blood pressure. b. The various phases of the Korotkoff sounds. Consult text for details (From: Burch, G E and DePasquale, N P Primer of Clinical Measurement of Blood Pressure, C V Mosby, St Louis).

Nursing Management of the Patient with Hypertension

1 Recognize the various effects of certain factors on symptoms of a patient with primary hypertension.
   a. Age, sex, occupation, race, environment, emotional response of the individual, etc.
   b. Understanding of his problem and his rapport with doctor, nurse, etc.
   c. Ability to adapt and adjust his activities in line with prescribed therapeutic regimen.
2 Gain the patient's co-operation in modifying his life-style in keeping with the guidelines of therapy.
   a. Give instructions to fit individual requirements.
   b. Reassure patient when encouragement is needed.
3 Make modifications meaningful and methodical.
   a. Be available when the doctor visits the patient so that his instructions can be explained.
   b. Tell the patient the meaning of the various diagnostic and therapeutic activities to minimize his anxiety and to obtain his co-operation.
   c. Seek the assistance of the patient's wife or husband—provide information regarding the total treatment plan.
   d. Be aware of the dietary plan developed for this particular patient.
4 Measure the blood pressure of the patient under the same conditions each day.
      Place patient in the desired position, sitting, standing, etc., according to the preferences of the doctor.
5 Observe patient for signs of cerebral nervous system complications.
   a. Note signs of confusion, irritability, lethargy, disorientation.
   b. Listen for complaints of headache, difficulty with vision; be alert for evidence of nausea or vomiting.
   c. Be prepared to offer protection to the patient if he exhibits convulsions—padded bed sides, nonrestrictive garments, anticonvulsive medications.
6 Prevent those reactions or activities which will increase arterial pressure.
   a. Avoid situations which might engender feelings of anxiety, anger or annoyance in the patient. Psychological stress has a direct effect on physiological function.
   b. Prevent alterations in the ordinary functions of eating, sleeping or elimination which might lead to discomfort or annoyance—physiological disturbance may increase stress reaction.
   c. Provide rest period and maintain a pleasant, comfortable environment.
      (1) Advise patient to rest for a short time before and after eating.
      (2) Remind him to rest during the waking hours for a full hour.
   d. Serve food in small quantities frequently rather than in three heavier meals.
      (1) Cardiac output increases with food intake.
      (2) Blood pressure is elevated with large intake of fluids.
      (3) Sodium intake may be restricted depending on severity of hypertension.
7 Practise supportive psychotherapy by observing the patient's reactions, appearance and personality as he relates to the professional staff, visitors, ancillary personnnel, etc.
   a. Permit him to express his feelings; promote positive reactions; analyse negative reactions in an attempt to avoid their recurrence.

   b. Note side-reactions which can be easily missed; investigate these.
   (1) Failure to make eye contact in conversation.
   (2) Suggestions of uneasiness, nervousness, restlessness.
   (3) Side remarks or 'under-the-breath' comments.

Plans for Discharge and Patient Education

1 Explain the meaning of hypertension, risk factors and their influences on the cardio-vascular system; hypertension is a lifetime problem
2 Usually there can never be total cure, only control of essential hypertension; emphasize the consequences of uncontrolled hypertension.
3 Stress the fact that there may be no correlation between high blood pressure and symptoms; the patient cannot tell by the way he feels whether his blood pressure is normal or elevated.
4 Help the patient to recognize that hypertension is chronic and requires persistent therapy and periodic evaluation; effective treatment improves life expectancy, therefore follow-up visits to the doctor are mandatory.
5 If elevated blood pressure can be brought down to normal range, there is very clear evidence that congestive heart failure, strokes and renal failure can be almost completely prevented; therefore treatment should continue in spite of medication cost or inconvenience.
6 Develop a plan of instruction which will be practised when the patient goes home.
   a. Teach him the proper method of taking his blood pressure at home and at work if his doctor so desires. (Some authorities recommend this practice.) Tell him which readings should be reported to the doctor.
   b. Plan his medication schedule so that the many medications are given at proper and convenient times; set up a daily checklist on which he can record the medication he has taken.
   c. Determine recommended dietary plans, e.g. extent of salt restriction, exchange foods, etc.
7 Assist the patient to manage the side-effects of the therapeutic medications.
   a. Recognize that the drugs used to control effectively the elevated blood pressure will very likely produce side-effects.
   b. Warn the patient of the possibility that hypotension may occur following the intake of certain drugs.
   (1) Instruct him to get up slowly to offset the feeling of dizziness.
   (2) Encourage him to lie down immediately if he feels faint.
   c. Alert patient to expect such effects as nasal congestion, asthenia (loss of strength), anorexia (loss of appetite), orthostatic hypotension (dizziness on changing position).
   d. Inform the patient that the goal of treatment is to control his blood pressure, reduce the possibility of complications, and use the minimum number of drugs with lowest dosage necessary to do the task.
8 Educate the patient to be aware of toxic manifestations and report them so that adjustments can be made in his individual pharmacotherapy.
   a. Note that dosages are individualized; therefore, they may need to be adjusted since it is often impossible to predict reactions.

b. Remember that certain circumstances produce vasodilatation—a hot bath, hot weather, febrile illness, consumption of alcohol.

c. Be aware that blood pressure is increased when circulating blood volume is reduced—dehydration, diarrhoea, haemorrhage.

d. Suspect the presence of oedema as a reportable symptom particularly when guanethidine is taken; these medications are less effective in the presence of oedema.

THE LYMPHATIC SYSTEM

The *lymphatic system* is a network of vessels and nodes that are interrelated with the circulatory system. It removes tissue fluid from intercellular spaces and protects the body from bacterial invasion. Lymph nodes are located along the course of the lymphatic vessels and filter lymph before it is returned to the bloodstream.

Significance of Lymphangiography

Radiological visualization of the lymphatic system is possible when a dye in injected into a lymphatic vessel of the hands or feet;

It is a means of detecting lymph node involvement due to metastatic carcinoma, lymphoma or infection in otherwise inaccessible sites (except by surgery) such as the pelvis, retroperitoneum, deep axilla.

Lymphangitis

Lymphangitis is an acute inflammation of lymphatic channels.

Aetiology

Arises most commonly from a focus of infection in an extremity.

Clinical Manifestations

1 Displays characteristic red streaks that extend up an arm or leg from an infection that is not localized and that can lead to septicaemia.
2 Produces general symptoms: high fever, chills.
   Produces local symptoms: local pain, tenderness, swelling along involved lymphatics.
   Produces local lymph node symptoms: enlarged, red, tender (acute lymphadenitis).
   Produces an abscess: necrotic, pus-producing (suppurative lymphadenitis).

Treatment and Nursing Management

1 Administer antibiotic agents since causative organisms are usually streptococci and staphylococci.
2 Treat affected part by rest, elevation and the application of hot, moist dressings.
3 Incise and drain if necrosis and abscess formation take place.

Acute Cervical Adenitis

Acute cervical adenitis is an acute infection of the lymphatic glands of the neck.

Aetiology

1 Usually cervical adenitis is secondary to an infection of the mouth, pharynx or scalp.
2 Occurs more frequently in children.
   a. Inspect teeth, tonsils, etc., since they are often foci of infection.
   b. Examine scalp for evidence of pediculosis.

Clinical Manifestations

1 Swelling on one side of neck: markedly tender and oedematous.
2 Systemic signs indicative of an infection: temperature elevation, malaise, increased pulse, etc.
3 Process may continue, leading to abscess formation and spontaneous rupture if not treated.

Treatment

1 Determine the source of infection and treat it.
2 Administer antibiotics.
3 Apply warm, moist compresses to localize infection.
4 Incise and drain; continue with moist, warm compresses until drainage ceases and infection is cleared.

Lymphoedema

Lymphoedema is a swelling of the tissues (particularly in the dependent position) produced by an obstruction to the lymph flow in an extremity.

Clinical Manifestations

1 Oedema may be massive and is often firm.
2 Obstruction may be in lymph nodes as well as in the lymphatic vessels.
   Observed in arm following radical mastectomy.

Treatment and Nursing Management

1 Apply elastic bandages of stocking.
2 Keep patient at rest with affected part elevated, each joint higher than the preceding one.
3 Administer diuretics to control excess fluid.
4 Give antibiotics as prescribed.
5 Recommend isometric exercises with extremity elevated.
6 Suggest moderate sodium restriction in diet.
7 Advise patient to avoid infection and trauma and to practise good hygiene to avoid superimposed infections.

FURTHER READING

Books

Andreoli, K G et al. (1975) Comprehensive Cardiac Care, C V Mosby
Ashworth, P and Rose, H (1973) Cardiovascular Disorders, Ballière Tindall
Bain, W H and Kennedy Watt, J (1970) Cardiovascular Surgery, Churchill Livingstone
Belcher, J R and Sturridge, M F (1972) Thoracic Surgical Management, 4th edition, Ballière Tindall
Brainbridge, M V (1972) Postoperative Cardiac Intensive Care, 2nd edition, Blackwell Scientific Publications
Brainbridge, M V and Fleming, J S (1974) Lecture Notes in Cardiology, 2nd edition, Blackwell Scientific Publications
Conway, N (1977) An Atlas of Cardiology, Wolfe Medical Publications
Davies, I J T (1977) Postgraduate Medicine, 3rd edition, Lloyd Luke
Ellis, H and Calne, R Y (1976) Lecture Notes on General Surgery, revised 4th edition, Blackwell Scientific Publications
Fleming, J S (1979) Interpreting the Electrocardiogram, Update Books
Fontaine, Y and Welti, J J (1976) The Essential of Cardiac Pacing, Collection Tardieu, William Heinemann, Cedig-Editeur-France
Goodland, N L (1978) Coronary Care, 3rd edition, Wright
Jordan, S C and Scott, O (1973) Heart Disease in Paediatrics, Apley, J (Ed) Butterworth
Julian, D G (973) Cardiology, 2nd edition, Concise Medical Textbooks
Kocham, M S and Daniels, L M (1978) Hypertension control for Nurses and other Health Professions, C V Mosby
Laurence, D R (1973) Clinical Pharmacology, 4th edition, Churchill Livingstone
Owen, S G, Stretton, T B and Vallance-Owen, J (1968) Essential of Cardiology, 2nd edition, Lloyd Luke
Partridge, J et al. (1975) The Acute Coronary Attack, Pitman Medical
Phibbs, B (1975) The Human Heart, 3rd edition, C V Mosby
Schamroth, L (1976/1978) An Introduction to Electrocardiotherapy, 5th edition, Blackwell Scientific Publications
Stoddart, J C (1975) Intensive Therapy, Blackwell Scientific Publications
Update Postgraduate Centre Series (1973) Hypertension, Update Books
Walker, W F (1980) A Colour Atlas of Peripheral Vascular Diseases, Wolfe Medical Publications
Zoob, M (1970) Cardiology for Students, Churchill Livingstone

Pamphlets

The Chest and Heart Association (1970) The Human Side of Heart Illness.
Breton Smith, C (1971) My Husband had a Coronary

Articles

Atherosclerotic Heart Disease

Adams, N R (1976) Reducing the perils of intercardiac monitoring, Nursing, 6: 66–74

Allendorf, E E et al. (1975) Teaching patients with nitroglycerin, American Journal of Nursing, 75: 1168–1170

Rute, D (1976) The road back begins in the CCU, Nursing, 6: 48–51

Cardiac Pacing

Westfall, W E (1976) Electrical and mechanical events in the cardiac cycle, American Journal of Nursing, 76: 231–235

Cardiogenic Shock: Counterpulsation

Dorr, K S (1975) The intra-aortic balloon pump, American Journal of Nursing, 75: 52–54

Central Venous Pressure

Drake, J J (1974) Locating the external reference point for central venous pressure determination, Nursing Research, 23: 475–482

Chapter 2

BLOOD DISORDERS

CELLULAR COMPONENTS OF NORMAL BLOOD

Erythrocytes (Red Blood Cells)

1   Comprise the vast majority of all blood cells; chiefly responsible for the colour of blood.
2   Approximately 5 million erythrocytes mm^3 of blood.
3   Normal red cell is a biconcave disc; red cell in normal blood has no nucleus.
4   Principal function is to transport oxygen—accomplished through the loose valence of an iron-containing pigment, haemoglobin, which accounts for 34% of mass of cells.
    Total normal concentration of haemoglobin—15 g/100 ml of blood.
5   Red blood cells are produced in red bone marrow, which also provides most of the blood's leucocytes and all of its platelets.
    Red cells of normal adults found in short and flat bones—ribs, sternum, skull, vertebrae, bones of the hands and feet, pelvis.
6   Bone marrow requires a number of nutrients, including iron, vitamin B$_{12}$, folic acid and pyridoxine for normal erythropoiesis (formation of red cells).
7   Normal life expectancy of a red cell is between 115 and 130 days—then eliminated by phagocytosis in the reticuloendothelial system, predominantly in spleen and liver.

Leucocytes (White Blood Cells)

1   Normally are present in a concentration of between 5000 and 10 000 cells in each cubic millimetre of blood (1 white cell for every 500–1000 red cells).
2   Leucocytes have a nucleus and are capable of active movement.
3   Major categories of leucocytes include the granulocytic series, lymphocytes, monocytes, and plasma cells.
4   Leucocytosis—white cell count over 10 000.
5   Leucopaenia—white cell count below 5000.
6   *Granulocyte*—leucocytes produced in the marrow.
    a. Comprise 70% of all white cells.
    b. Called *granulocytes* because of the abundant granules contained in their cytoplasm or *polymorphonuclear leucocytes* since their nuclei, when mature, are of a highly irregular, multilobed configuration.
7   *Lymphocytes*—most numerous of the *mononuclear cells*; comprise about 25% of the circulating white cells.
    a. Produced in lymph nodes throughout the body and to a lesser extent in the bone marrow.
    b. Responsible for the immunological competence of an individual.
8   *Monocytes*—derived from components of the reticuloendothelial system (particularly spleen, liver, lymph nodes and bone marrow).
    a. Constitute a ready source of mobile phagocytes, congregating and performing their scavenging function at sites of inflammation and tissue necrosis.
    b. Account for about 5% of the white cell count.
9   *Plasmocytes*—formed in the lymph nodes and bone marrow.
    a. Are the main and probably sole source of the circulating immune globulins (antibodies).
    b. Represent approximately 1% of the blood leucocytes.

Table 2.1. Common Problems of Patients with Blood Disorders

The Problem	Nursing Management
Fatigue and weakness	Plan nursing care to conserve the patient's strength Give frequent rest periods Encourage ambulation activities as tolerated Avoid disturbing activities and noise Encourage optimal nutrition
Haemorrhagic tendencies	Encourage patient to protect himself from injury Keep the patient at rest during the bleeding episodes Apply gentle pressure to the bleeding sites Apply cold compresses to the bleeding sites when indicated Avoid disturbing clots Use topical haemostatic agents as directed Use small gauge needles when administering medications by injection Observe for symptoms of internal bleeding Give ice-chips to the patient who is bleeding orally—induces vasoconstriction Carry out serial haematocrit evaluations to determine if there is continued bleeding Have a tracheostomy set available for the patient who is bleeding from the mouth or throat; observe for signs of asphyxiation Transfuse the patient with appropriate agents
Ulcerative lesions of the tongue, gums or mucous membranes	Avoid irritating foods and beverages Give frequent oral hygiene with mild, cool mouthwash solutions Use cotton-tipped applicators or soft-bristled toothbrush Keep the lips lubricated Give mouth care both before and after meals
Dyspnoea	Elevate the head of the bed Use pillows to support the patient in the orthopnoeic (sitting upright) position Administer oxygen when indicated Prevent unnecessary exertion
Bone and joint pains	Relieve pressure of bedclothes by using a bed cradle Administer either hot of cold compresses as directed Provide for joint immobilization when ordered
Fever	Administer tepid sponging Give antipyretic drugs as ordered Give free fluids unless contraindicated Maintain a cool room temperature
Pruritus or skin eruptions	Keep the patient's fingernails short Use soap sparingly Apply oil-based lotions in skin care

(continued)

Table 2.1 (*cont.*)

The Problem	Nursing Management
Anxiety of patient and his family	Explain the nature, the discomforts and the limitations of activity associated with the diagnostic procedures and treatments Encourage the patient to verbalize his *feelings*, and listen carefully Show an empathetic and accepting attitude Promote the patient's relaxation and comfort Remember the patient's individual preferences Promote a sense of independence and self-care within the patient's limitations Encourage the family to participate in the patient's care (as desired) Create a comfortable atmosphere for the family's visits with the patient

Platelets (Thrombocytes)

1 Are the smallest and most fragile of the formed elements; are small particles (devoid of nuclei) that arise as a result of budding from giant cells called *megakaryocytes* in the bone marrow.
2 Number approximately 250 000–500 000 platelets per cubic millimetre of blood.
3 Prime function to halt bleeding—accomplished by congregating and clumping at all sites of vascular injury and by plugging with their own substance the lumen of the bleeding vessel. As they disintegrate they release a constituent (platelet factor 3) which initiates clot formation in their immediate vicinity, thereby checking the flow of blood through and the leakage of blood from a lacerated vessel.

COMMON PROBLEMS OF PATIENTS WITH BLOOD DISORDERS
See Table 2.1.

BLOOD AND BONE MARROW SPECIMENS
Blood may be obtained by (1) skin puncture (finger, toe, heel or ear-lobe) and (2) venepuncture.

A *skin puncture* is performed when only a small amount of blood is needed (for red and white cell counts, haemoglobin and haematocrit (packed cell volume; PCV) determinations, reticulocyte counts, blood films for differential smear). However, the values for the red blood cells, haematocrit, haemoglobin and platelets are lower in capillary blood than in venous blood.

A *venepuncture* is a puncture of a vein to obtain blood and is used when larger amounts of blood are needed (preferred method).

NOTE: A venepuncture is performed by the doctor in the majority of cases. Nurses working in special units, e.g. intensive care, cardiac care, are trained to perform venepuncture.

GUIDELINES: Obtaining Blood by Skin Puncture

Equipment

Disposable lancet   Slides
Pipette and tubing   Alcohol swabs and dry sterile swabs

Procedure

1   Cleanse site (preferably tip of finger) with alcohol swab and dry with sterile swab.
    (If the skin is wet with alcohol the blood will haemolyse and also it will not collect
    in a compact drop but will run down the patient's finger.)
2   Create stasis by pressing on the distal joint of the finger to produce redness at the
    end of the finger.
3   Use a sterile disposable lancet (Fig. 2.1). (This avoids the possibility of the
    transfer of the hepatitis virus.)
4   Prick the skin sharply and quickly with the lancet. (Pricking the skin sharply and
    quickly lessens pain and produces a free-flowing sample.)
5   Release pressure of the finger. Wipe off the first drop of blood (Fig. 2.2).
    (Epithelial or endothelial cells may be found in the first drop of blood and render
    the count inaccurate. Also platelets will begin to clump immediately in the blood
    at the puncture site.)
6   Obtain the blood sample (Fig. 2.3).
    a. Fill the pipette (Fig. 2.4).
    b. Make blood slides according to the study ordered. This procedure is
    performed by the doctor or laboratory staff (Figs. 2.5 and 2.6).
7   Apply pressure over the wound with a dry gauze swab until bleeding stops.

GUIDELINES: Obtaining Blood by the Syringe Method

Veins Used

Median basilar vein in antecubital area   Dorsum (back) of hand
Wrist   Top of foot

Equipment

70% alcohol and tincture of iodine   5- and 10-ml syringe
Dry sterile swab   20 gauge needle(s)

Procedure

1   Reassure the patient. Explain that relatively little blood will be taken.
2   Tell the patient to extend his arm. The arm should be held straight at the elbow.
3   Apply the tourniquet directly above the elbow with just sufficient pressure to
    prevent venous return. (A tourniquet increases venous pressure and makes the
    vein more prominent and easier to enter.)
4   Inspect the area to visualize the vein. Palpate the vein. (Select a vein that is
    visible, palpable and well fixed to surrounding tissue.)
5   Cleanse the skin with alcohol and dry thoroughly.

6   Fix chosen vein with the thumb and draw the skin taut immediately below the site before inserting needle. (The vein may roll beneath the skin when the needle approaches its outer surface especially in elderly and extremely thin patients.)
7   Insert the needle, bevel up, at a 30° angle so that it enters the skin first and then the vein.
8   Release the tourniquet.
9   Obtain blood sample by gently pulling back the plunger. (Use minimal suction to prevent haemolysis of blood and collapse of the vein.)
10 Withdraw the needle slowly. (Slow withdrawal of the needle is less painful.)
11 Apply gauze over the puncture site firmly for 2–4 min. (Firm pressure over the puncture site prevents leakage of blood into surrounding tissues with subsequent haematoma development. Merely flexing the arm may not prevent a haematoma as the vein can slip to the side of the area where pressure is applied.)
12 Assist the doctor to make blood smears as required.
13 Remove the needle from the hub of the syringe. Gently eject the blood sample into a specimen bottle containing anticoagulant.
14 Place stopper on the specimen bottle and invert gently several times to mix blood with anticoagulant.
15 Label specimens correctly and send to laboratory immediately. (Specimens should go to the laboratory with a minimum delay for optimum reliability.)

GUIDELINES: Bone Marrow Aspiration and Biopsy

Bone marrow aspiration or biopsy is done so that specimens of bone marrow can be obtained. It is performed for the following reasons:

1   To diagnose haematological disease—enables the precursors of cells in peripheral blood to be examined and their relative number determined. Also to estimate the iron content.

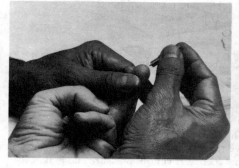

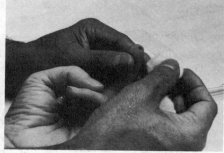

Figure 2.1.   To abtain blood sample, hold finger so that finger tip becomes red. The lancet has a flange (or guard) to prevent it from being inserted to deeply.

Figure 2.2.   The first drop of blood is wiped away with dry cotton so that the ensuing blood will form a round drop.

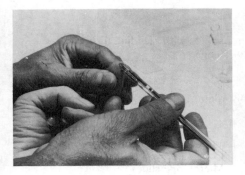

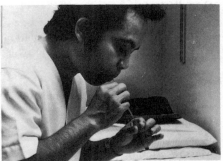

Figure 2.3.   The blood is drawn up into the capillary tube. The nurse is bracing the finger of the patient's right hand from the side to stabilize the patient's finger and keep the tip of the capillary tube in the drop of blood.

Figure 2.4.   The blood is dispensed into Drabkins solution for haemoglobin determination.

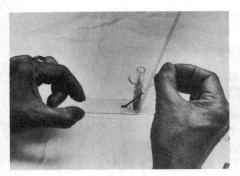

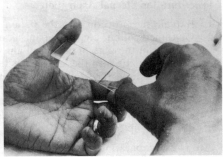

Figure 2.5.   A drop of blood is placed on the slide.

Figure 2.6.   The blood is smeared over the slide.

2   To follow the course of disease and the patient's response to treatment.
3   To diagnose diseases other than pure haematological disorders, such as primary and metastatic tumours, infectious diseases, certain granulomas and parasitic infections.
4   To isolate bacteria and other pathogenic agents by culture or animal inoculation.

Complications

1   Osteomyelitis (rare).
2   Bleeding and haematoma formation in patients with bleeding disorders.
3   Puncture of vital organs if biopsy is too deep.

Contraindications

Haemophilia and related haemorrhagic disorders.

Equipment

Bone marrow aspiration tray
Marrow aspiration needles with
   guards
Sterile towels
25 and 22 guage neddles
Two 20-ml syringes
Three 5-ml syringes
Local anaesthetic (1% lignocaine
Steril gloves
Skin antiseptic, e.g. chlorhexidine
   0.5% in spirit

Laboratory equipment
   Coverslips
   Microscope slides
   Specimen bottles (plain and
   with heparin)
Scalpel blade and handle
Gauze swabs
Elastoplast dressing
Nobecutane spray

Procedure for Sternal Aspiration

1   Explain the procedure to the patient.
2   Give medication, e.g. diazepam as ordered. Often not necessary. (Diazepam helps calm the patient and has light sedative effect.)
3   Place the patient in the supine position.
4   Shave the area. The following sites may be used:
   a. Sternum
   b. Iliac crest (anterior and posterior spines).
   c. Spinous processes of vertebrae (usually second or third lumbar vertebrae).
   d. Tibia—up to the age of 2 years.

After the preparation of the patient the procedure is performed by the doctor as follows:

1   The skin is cleaned with antiseptic and the site infiltrated with local anaesthetic.
2   The site selected is usually the midsternal line at the level of the second interspace. (The sternum is thinner and marrow more plentiful between the sternal interspaces.)
3   A small stab incision may be made before bone marrow needle insertion. (This technique avoids pushing the skin into the bone marrow.)
4   The marrow needle with guard in place is inserted through the cortex of the bone with a slight twisting motion. The doctor usually feels a 'give' in the marrow needle when the marrow cavity has been penetrated. (A sternal puncture is considered more dangerous than other sites because of its proximity to vital structures in the mediastinum.)
5   The guard is removed and a syringe attached to the hub of the needle. The

plunger is withdrawn slowly until marrow appears in the syringe. 0.2 ml of fluid is aspirated. (The marrow will appear as whitish granular particles through the bloody aspirate.)

6 Warn the patient that he will feel a brief episode of sharp pain. (The pain is caused by suction of the syringe and lasts only a few seconds.)

7 The syringe and needle are removed and smears are prepared by the doctor. (If repeated aspirations result in no marrow it indicates that the sternal marrow is not suitable for aspiration.)

8 Pressure is applied over the puncture site until bleeding (if any) ceases. (If the patient has thrombocytopaenia, pressure should be applied for 5–10 min.)

9 As indicated, Elastoplast dressing or Nobecutane spray may be used to cover the puncture site.

Procedure for Iliac Crest Aspiration/Biopsy

Anterior approach

1 Position the patient prone or on his side. (The anterior or posterior iliac crest has the advantage of having no vital organs near the puncture site.)

2 The needle is passed into the cavity of the ilium 2 cm behind and 2 cm below the anterior iliac spine and perpendicular to the flat surface of the bone. (Pain is an indicator that the needle is within the marrow cavity.)

3 A small hammer may be used to tap the needle gently in place, but this is rarely necessary. (The bone of the iliac crest is harder than that of the sternum.)

Posterior Approach

1 Position the patient on his side.

2 The needle is passed along an anesthetized tract that runs behind the prominence of the posterior iliac spine and at right angles with the anterior abdominal wall.

3 Tell the patient to lie on his affected side after the procedure. (Lying on the affected side promotes haemostasis.)

Follow-up Care

1 Give mild analgesic if needed, e.g. paracetamol tablets.

2 Observe patient for discomfort, continued bleeding and any untoward symptoms.

TRANSFUSION THERAPY

Blood

A unit of blood (drawn from a donor) consists of approximately 450 ml of whole blood and 60–70 ml of acid-citrate-dextrose (ACD) and citrate-phosphate-dextrose (CPD), both of which are one of the anticoagulant preservative solutions.

1 Whole blood is used for acute blood loss.

2 See p.191 for technique of administration.

Blood Components

Packed Red Cells

Erythrocytes separated from a unit of whole blood by centrifugation or sedimentation; about 80% of the plasma is removed, leaving a haematocrit of 60–70%.

1   The plasma is used for the preparation of various plasma fractions such as albumin, cryoprecipitate or gamma globulin.
2   Indicated for:
   a. Patients who need only red blood cells.
   b. Patients with severe anaemia who have relatively normal blood volume.
   c. Patients with risk of heart failure.
3   Packed cells are administered through a large bore needle at a flow rate slower than that of whole blood.

Platelet Transfusions

Given to patients with dangerous degrees of thrombocytopaenia (decrease of platelets in circulating blood) to control or prevent bleeding.

1   Viable platelets, may be supplied in form of:
   a. Fresh blood—replaces red cells and platelets.
   b. Platelet-rich plasma (PRP)—contains 80–90% of original platelets.
   c. Platelet concentrates (PC)—retain nearly all original platelets in a viable state, but reduced in volume.
      Eliminate risk of circulatory overloading.
2   The use of matched platelets is more advantageous and lessens the risk of antibody formation.
3   Platelet transfusions are given in the treatment of leukaemia, aplastic anaemia and thrombocytopaenia induced by chemotherapy or drugs.

Granulocyte Infusions

Given to patients with severe and temporary bone marrow depression.

1   Granulocytes are harvested from a donor by continuous flow centrifugation or are trapped in nylon wool filters. (Machine used is called a cell separator.)
2   The process is complex and costly; available only at a few centres at this time.

Whole Plasma

Fluid portion of the blood in which corpuscles are suspended.

1   Clinical usefulness (used with decreasing frequency):
   a. Treatment of clotting defects—all of the plasma factors can be supplied rapidly without overexpanding the patient's blood volume.
   b. Correction of hypovolaemia due to selective loss of plasma—mainly in burned patients.
   c. Correction of hypovolaemia in acute blood loss when whole blood is not immediately available.
2   As a plasma expander for hypovolaemia or as an exogenous source of plasma albumin for hypoalbuminaemia, whole plasma has largely been replaced by pure preparations of serum albumin and other plasma fractions that are comprised largely of albumin.

3 *Freshly frozen plasma*—plasma which has been separated immediately from freshly donated blood and then promptly frozen.

Factor V (one of the accelerators of prothrombin conversion) and factor VIII (the antihaemophiliac factor; A.H.F) are retained by this process.

4 *Factor VIII concentrates:* (There are numerous named and numbered clotting factors.)

Cryoprecipitate—effective in treatment of haemophilia A (factor VIII deficiency) and fibrinogen deficiency.

5 *Human serum albumin and other albumin preparations:*
Clinical usefulness:
   a. To combat plasma leakage and prevent haemoconcentration in burn patients.
   b. To expand blood volume in patients in hypovolaemic shock.
   c. To elevate the circulating albumin in patients with hypoalbuminaemia.

6 *Human fibrinogen*
Used for congenital and acquired hypofibrinogenaemia complicated by active bleeding.

GUIDELINES: Administering Blood Transfusions

Blood transfusion is the introduction of blood into the body circulation.

Purposes

1 To restore circulating blood volume.
2 To replace clotting factors.
3 To improve oxygen-carrying capacity of the blood.

Equipment

Blood administration set (disposable)   Blood as ordered
Needles no. 18–19 gauge   Skin antiseptic
Tourniquet

Procedure

1 Make sure that the blood has been grouped and cross matched. (Grouping is done to establish the blood group A, AB, B or O and Rh factor. A cross match is done to establish the compatibility between the patient's blood and the donor's.)
2 Give the blood within 20 min after taking it from the blood bank. (Storage at 1–6°C (33.8–42.8°F) should be maintained until just before administration. Rapid deterioration of the red blood cells can occur with uncooled blood.)
3 Inspect the blood for gas bubbles and any abnormal colour or cloudiness. (Gas bubbles may indicate bacterial growth, abnormal colour or clouding may warn of haemolysis.)
4 Explain the procedure to the patient.
5 Check the labels identifying the donor and recipient blood (number and group) and confirm the identity of the patient who is to receive it. Call the patient by his full name. Check his identification wrist band with the container identification, check his chart to make sure of his number and group. (Meticulous attention to

detail is essential to avoid giving the wrong blood to the wrong patient which may cause a fatal reaction.)

6   Infuse the blood at the rate prescribed by the doctor.
7   Maintain regular ($\frac{1}{2}$-hourly) temperature, pulse, respiration and blood pressure recordings.
8   Observe the patient for signs of adverse transfusion reaction, e.g. sweating, tachycardia, restlessness, loin pain.
9   Record carefully the amount of blood that the patient receives.

Complications

Nursing Alert: Transfusion therapy (whether of whole blood or blood components) entails a number of calculated risks. Some of these potential complications cannot be prevented with absolute certainty. There is a significant incidence of morbidity and mortality associated with blood transfusion.

Circulatory Overloading

Due to administration of excessive volume or at a rate faster than the heart can accept. Observe for rise in venous pressure, distended neck veins, dyspnoea and cough. Râles can be heard in base of lungs.

Prevention

1   Prevent by using packed cells, proper spacing of transfusions and give at a rate which can be managed by the circulatory reserve of the patient.
2   Monitor central venous pressure of patients with heart disease.

Treatment

1   Stop transfusion immediately and call the doctor.
2   Reassure the patient and sit him upright.
3   Administer diuretics, e.g. mannitol, as directed.

Transmission of Disease

Hepatitis A or B, malaria, cytomegalovirus and bacterial diseases may be transmitted from donor to recipient via infected blood.

Prevention

1   Screen donor carefully.
2   Reject donors with history of hepatitis or jaundice or if laboratory test is positive for hepatitis B antigen.

Pyrogenic Reactions (febrile reaction)

Usually due to presence of leucoagglutinins or platelet agglutinins in patient or to antigens in transfused blood.

Symptoms

May occur after transfusion is discontinued.

1   Sudden chilling and fever.

2   Headache.
3   Flushing; tachycardia.

Prevention

Keep blood recipients comfortably covered during transfusion.

Treatment

1   Stop transfusion and notify the doctor and the blood bank (for examination of blood).
2   Take temperature, pulse, respiration and blood pressure ½-hourly.
3   Give aspirin to reduce fever, as directed by doctor.

Bacterial Contamination

Due to transfusion of bacteria or their toxins in the blood.

Symptoms

1   High fever (over 38.4°C (101°F).
2   Intense flushing.
3   Severe headache or substernal pain.
4   Vomiting, diarrhoea.
5   Hypotension; shock-like state with dry flushed skin.
6   Pain in abdomen and extremities.

Prevention

1   Do not allow the blood to stand unnecessarily at room temperature—accelerates growth of any contaminating organisms.
2   Do not warm containers of blood before transfusion.
3   Inspect blood for gas bubbles and change in colour before starting transfusion.

Treatment

1   Stop transfusion and call the doctor.
2   Assist the doctor in obtaining cultures of donor's blood (and recipient's blood) and send the remainder of the blood to the laboratory.
3   Treat septicaemia as directed—antibiotics, intravenous fluids, fresh transfusion, steroids.

Allergic Reactions

Blood of allergic patient may contain antibodies capable of reacting with allergens in the donor's blood.

Symptoms

1   Flushing.
2   Itching and rash.
3   Urticaria (hives).
4   Asthmatic wheezing.
5   Laryngeal oedema.

Prevention

1   Screen and reject all donors with known allergies.
2   Ask patient whether he has a history of allergy.
3   Give prophylactic antihistamine as directed *before* blood is started to patients known to have allergies.

Treatment

1   Stop the blood and call the doctor.
2   Prepare adrenaline for administration if respiratory distress is severe.

Haemolytic Reaction and Incompatibility (most severe reaction)

Haemolysis occurs when incompatible red cells are injected into the patient's circulating blood. It may cause oliguric renal failure and death.

Signs and Symptoms

1   Chilliness; fever.
2   Back pain.
3   Flushing; feeling of head fullness.
4   Oppressive feeling in chest.
5   Distension of neck veins.
6   Tachycardia; tachypnoea.
7   Fall in blood pressure.

Prevention

1   Positively identify patient and blood before transfusion is started.
2   Stay with the patient during the first 15–30 min that he is receiving the transfusion—if the transfusion is stopped early, untoward (and possibly fatal) reactions may be averted.
3   Administer blood very slowly during this period.

Treatment

1   Stop the transfusion immediately—consequences are in proportion to the amount of incompatible blood given.
2   Call the doctor.
3   Assist with infusion of mannitol. Mannitol maintains urine flow, glomerular filtration and renal blood flow.
4   Maintain volume with intravenous infusions as directed if diuresis follows after the administration of mannitol.
5   Prepare patient for renal dialysis as directed.
6   Insert indwelling urinary catheter as directed and observe urine output hourly.
7   Send sample of patient's blood and urine to the laboratory for the presence of haemoglobin (indicative of intravascular haemolysis) and for tests for disseminated intravascular coagulation.

Hyperkalaemia (potassium excess)

Symptoms

1   Nausea, colic, diarrhoea.
2   Muscular weakness.
3   Paraesthesia of hands, feet, tongue, face.
4   Flaccid paralysis.
5   Apprehension.
6   Slow pulse rate.
7   Cardiac arrest.

Prevention

Avoid using old blood—stored blood causes potassium levels to increase.

Hypocalcaemia (calcium deficit)

Calcium deficit can occur with administration of a large volume of citrated blood.

Signs and Symptoms

1   Tingling of fingers and around the mouth.
2   Muscular cramps.
3   Hyperactive reflexes.
4   Convulsions.
5   Carpopedal spasms.
6   Laryngeal spasms.

Treatment

Clamp the tubing and notify the doctor.

Air Embolism

May occur if blood is transfused under pressure.

Signs and Symptoms

1   Chest pain.
2   Cough.
3   Dyspnoea.

Prevention

Prevent air from entering intravenous lines, especially when changing infusion sets.

Treatment

1   Clamp tubing and notify doctor.
2   Position patient on his left side in a slight Trendelenberg position—to trap air in the right side of the heart.

Nursing Responsibilities in Transfusion Reaction

1   Notify doctor and blood bank immediately when a suspected transfusion reaction has occurred.
2   Disconnect the transfusion set, but keep the intravenous line open with a dextrose or saline solution in case intravenous medication should be needed rapidly.
3   Save the blood bag and tubing; send to blood bank for repeat grouping and culture.
4   Take blood for plasma haemoglobin, culture and regrouping.
5   Collect urine sample and send to laboratory for a haemoglobin determination. Save subsequent specimens of urine.

ANAEMIA

Anaemia is a laboratory definition which implies a low red cell count and a below-normal haemoglobin or haematocrit (PCV) level.

Altered Physiology

1   The appearance of anaemia reflects (1) marrow failure, (2) excessive red cell loss, (3) a combination of (1) and (2) or (4) congenital defects in haemoglobin synthesis.
2   Marrow failure may occur as a result of nutritional deficiency, toxic exposure, tumour invasion or from unknown causes.
3   Red cells may be lost through haemorrhage or haemolysis (increased destruction).
    a. This problem may be rooted in some red-cell defect that is incompatible with normal red-cell survival or is explicable on the basis of some factor extrinsic to the red cell that promotes red-cell destruction.
    b. Red-cell lysis occurs mainly within the phagocytic cells of the reticulo-endothelial system, notably within the liver and spleen.
    c. As a by-product of this process, bilirubin, formed from haemoglobin within the phagocyte, enters the bloodstream, and an increase in haemolysis is promptly reflected by an increase in total plasma bilirubin.

Clinical Manifestations

1   The more rapidly the anaemia develops, the more severe its symptoms:
    a. Pallor.
    b. Susceptibility to fatigue.
    c. Shortness of breath.
    d. Headache; loss of concentration; dizziness.
    e. Predisposition to angina pectoris or congestive heart failure in susceptible individuals.
2   Severity of symptoms dependent upon:
    a. The speed and degree with which the anaemia has developed.
    b. Its prior duration, i.e. its chronicity.
    c. The metabolic requirements of the particular patient.

d. Any other disorders currently afflicting the patient, particularly cardiac conditions, etc.

e. Special complications or concomitant features of the condition producing the anaemia.

Iron Deficiency Anaemia

Iron deficiency anaemias are conditions in which the total body iron content is decreased below a normal level.

Aetiology

Iron deficiency develops when the body's need for iron exceeds the supply.

1   Chronic blood loss—bleeding via the gastrointestinal tract, excessive bleeding from menorrhagia, multiple pregnancies.
2   Impaired gastrointestinal absorption of iron—small bowel disease, certain gastric resections.
3   Inadequate dietary sources of iron
4   Increased iron requirements—during pregnancy, periods of rapid growth, menstruation (average of 20 mg of iron lost per menstrual cycle).

Dietary Implications

1   Average person ingests 10–15 mg of iron daily in food iron and inorganic iron salts; less than 10% of all iron ingested (including food and iron supplements) is absorbed.
2   Approximately 6 mg of iron is ingested per 1000 calories.
3   A nutritious diet should maintain normal iron balance, unless there is abnormal drain of iron (bleeding, pregnancy).
4   Food sources of iron:
       Red meat (particularly liver), green leafy vegetables, dried fruit (apricots, prunes).
5   Ascorbic acid has been shown to enhance iron absorption.

Clinical Manifestations

Reduction in haemoglobin concentration decreases the capacity of the blood to transport and deliver oxygen to the tissues.

1   Fatigue.
2   Headache, dizziness, tinnitus.
3   Palpitations and dyspnoea.
4   Paraesthesias.
5   Pallor of mucous membranes.
6   Glossitis.
7   Pagophagia (excessive ice eating).
8   Spooning of fingernails (koilonychia).

Treatment

1   Recognize and correct the underlying cause.
   a. Assist in the search for the site of chronic blood loss.
   (1) Question the patient concerning haematemesis, melaena, epistaxis, haematuria, menometrorrhagia, multiple diagnostic procedures.
   (2) Send urine and stool specimens to lab for occult blood examination.
   (3) Prepare patient for sigmoidoscopy, colonoscopy, barium enema, upper gastrointestinal studies.
2   Correct the haemoglobin and tissue iron deficiency with the administration of the prescribed iron preparation.

Oral Iron Therapy

1   Allows patient to regenerate haemoglobin. (Haematologic values should return to normal in 4–8 weeks). Therapy is continued for approximately 6 months following the return to normal of blood values to restore iron stores.
2   Choice of iron depends on (1) patient tolerance, (2) gastrointestinal absorption and (3) dosage according to estimate of haemoglobin deficiency.
3   Oral iron preparations:
   a. Ferrous sulphates (preferred).
   b. Ferrous gluconate.
   c. Ferrous fumarate.
4   Delayed-release forms of iron are not usually given. In this type of preparation the iron is released beyond the duodenum, which is the major site for iron absorption.
5   *Nursing Emphasis and Health Teaching.*
   a. Iron preparations are absorbed at all levels of the gastrointestinal tract below the stomach; maximal absorption occurs in the duodenum and upper jejunum.
   b. Give iron immediately after meals to minimize gastric irritation; then shift to a between-meal schedule for maximum drug absorption.
   c. Educate patient to anticipate a certain amount of dyspepsia from time to time.
   d. Iron salts alter the colour of the stools; tell the patient to expect colour changes (dark green to black).
   e. Ferrous sulphate is apt to deposit on the teeth and the gums; advise patient to use frequent oral hygiene measures.
   f. The dosage of iron may be gradually increased over a few days.
   g. If gastrointestinal side-effects are troublesome, the dosage may have to be halved.
   h. Iron administration should be continued for approximately 6 months after haemoglobin levels return to normal—to replenish iron stores.
   i. Emphasize that the patient should take the iron faithfully.

Parenteral Iron Therapy

1   Parenteral iron therapy is given (1) when the patient is unable to tolerate iron preparations orally, (2) when the patient has severe gastrointestinal disorders or (3) when there is continuing negative iron balance while patient is taking maximum oral dose tolerated.

Nursing Alert: Extravasation of iron medication results in painful local induration. Systemic reactions (flushing, nausea, vomiting, myalgia and fever) may occur.

2   Parenteral iron preparations:
   a. Iron dextran (Imferon).
   b. Iron sorbitol complex (Jectofer)—may cause patient's urine to turn black on standing, as about 50% of iron is excreted in the urine within 24 hours.

3   Technique of parenteral iron administration:
   a. Discard needle that is used to draw medication into syringe; use a fresh needle for injection.
   b. Use a needle 5 cm (2 in) long—medication is injected deep into muscle.
   c. Retract the skin over the muscle *laterally* before inserting needle—to prevent leakage along injection tract and staining of skin.

Health Teaching

1   Encourage the selection of a well-balanced diet.
   Adolescent girls should receive nutritional counselling.
2   Iron supplements should be given during pregnancy.

Pernicious Anaemia

Pernicious anaemia is a megaloblastic anaemia* due to vitamin B_{12} deficiency caused by lack of the intrinsic factor in the gastric juice. (B_{12} deficiency is also seen in diseases of the small intestine, i.e. malabsorption, blind loop syndrome, etc.)

Altered Physiology

1   Pernicious anaemia is produced by a defect in the gastric mucosa; the stomach wall becomes atrophic and fails to secrete the intrinsic factor.
2   This substance normally binds with the dietary vitamin B_{12} and travels with it to the ileum, where the vitamin is absorbed. Without intrinsic factor, no orally administered B_{12} can enter the body.
3   Therefore, after the body's stores of B_{12} are used up, the patient begins to show signs of the anaemia.
4   Vitamin B_{12} is the extrinsic factor necessary for the maturation of red blood cells.

Clinical Manifestations

1   Symptoms due to anaemia:
   a. Pallor.
   b. Dyspnoea or orthopnoea.
   c. Angina pectoris.
   d. Oedema of legs.

* Megaloblastic anaemias:
   1   A megaloblast is a nucleated red cell with delayed and abnormal nuclear maturation.
   2   The most common megaloblastic anaemias are B_{12} deficiency anaemia and folic acid deficiency.
   3   Anaemias due to deficiencies of the vitamins B_{12} and folic acid show identical bone marrow and peripheral blood changes. This is because both vitamins are essential for normal DNA synthesis.

2   Symptoms due to physiological changes in gastrointestinal tract:
   a. Sore mouth with smooth red, 'beefy' tongue.
   b. Loss of appetite.
   c. Indigestion and epigastric discomfort.
   d. Recurring diarrhoea or constipation.
   e. Weight loss.
3   Symptoms due to neurological changes (occur in high percentage of untreated patients):
   a. Tingling and numbness or burning pain (paraesthesia) involving hands and feet.
   b. Loss of position sense, leading to disturbances of gait.
   c. Disturbances of bladder and bowel function.
   d. Irritability; depression.
   e. Paranoia and delirium.

Diagnosis

1   Blood smear—reveals marked variation in size and shape of cells and a variable number of unusually large cells containing a normal concentration of haemoglobin.
2   Gastric analysis—the gastric juice lacks free hydrochloric acid (achlorhydria).
3   *Schilling test*—a test for vitamin B_{12} absorption.
   Purpose: to prove that the patient cannot absorb oral vitamin B_{12} unless intrinsic factor is added.
   a. The patient is given a small dose of radioactive B_{12} in water to drink followed by a large nonradioactive intramuscular dose.
   b. When the oral vitamin is absorbed, it will be excreted in the urine; the intramuscular dose helps to flush it into the urine.
   c. A 24-hour urine specimen is collected and measured for radioactivity.
   d. If very little has been excreted, the test is repeated several days later (the 'second stage') with a capsule of oral intrinsic factor added to the oral B_{12}.
   e. If the patient has pernicious anaemia, this time much more radioactivity will be found in the 24-hour urine specimen.
4   Bone marrow aspiration—reveals megaloblastic marrow.
5   Gastroscopy—gastric mucosa appears thin and grey.
6   Low B_{12} level in the serum.

Treatment

Objectives

To support the patient during the acute phase of his illness.
To give enough antianaemic factor (vitamin B_{12}) to produce a remission.
To help the patient accept that he must be on vitamin B_{12} maintenance for his lifetime.

Treatment During Acute Stage

1   Give cyanocobalamin (vitamin B_{12}) as directed.
   a. Reticulocytes begin to increase on 4th day after therapy is started; normal haemoglobin values are obtained in approximately 6 weeks.

b. Patient begins to improve in general well-being and mental status in a few days.

c. *Recent* neurological changes will usually be reversed.

2 Give transfusion of packed cells very slowly (if prescribed).

a. Transfusions are only given to patients whose anaemia is life-threatening (symptoms of hypoxia to heart or brain).

b. Place the patient in a sitting position in bed.

Too rapid administration of transfusion to patient with anaemia may produce acute pulmonary or cerebral oedema.

3 Support the patient with neurological involvement (see Management of Patient with Neurogenic Bladder, Volume 3, Chapter 1).

Maintenance Therapy

1 Impress upon the patient that vitamin B_{12} must be continued for his lifetime.

a. Maintenance dose schedule—vitamin B_{12} intramuscularly every 4 weeks.

b. Teach patient and family to give maintenance therapy. The health visitor is also involved with the therapy.

c. Untreated pernicious anaemia is fatal.

2 Instruct the patient to report for follow-up examinations every 6 months—for haematocrit and physical examination.

a. Patient may develop haematological or neurological relapse if therapy is inadequate.

b. Patients with pernicious anaemia have a higher incidence of gastric cancer and thyroid problems; therefore, periodic stool examinations for occult blood and gastric cytology, along with thyroid function tests, should be made.

3 Following total gastrectomy (and occasionally subtotal gastrectomy) patient should receive maintenance dose of vitamin B_{12} as often as indicated—removal of gastric fundus deprives the patient of all intrinsic factor; may take as long as 10 years for clinical symptoms to appear, due to small amount of daily vitamin B_{12} required and the large body stores available for use.

4 Parenteral vitamin B_{12} therapy is preferred—greater reliability, better patient supervision, less expensive.

Aplastic Anaemia

Aplastic anaemia is a condition of bone marrow failure which results in near absence of all blood cells (erythrocytes, leucocytes and platelets [pancytopaenia]).

Causes

1 Idiopathic—approximately 50% of aplastic anaemia cases are of unknown aetiology.

2 Chemical compounds—benzol (dry-cleaning agents) may induce permanent bone marrow damage.

3 Drugs—antibiotics (chloramphenicol), antitumour agents, antidiabetic agents, phenothiazines, antihistamines, insecticides, antidepressants, thyroid medication, heavy metals. (Almost any drug has potential).

4 Ionizing radiation—therapeutic, industrial or laboratory accidents.

5 Viral infections—viral hepatitis, mononucleosis, etc.
6 Congenital (Fanconi's anaemia)—congenitally constituted defect in the bone marrow.

Clinical Manifestations

1 Anaemia—resulting from depression of haemoglobin and rapidity of blood cell change
   a. Pallor; weakness
   b. Exertional dyspnoea, palpitation.
2 Infections with high fever—resulting from granulocytopaenia:
   a. Pharyngitis.
   b. Sepsis via gastrointestinal tract or genitourinary tract.
3 Abnormal bleeding—resulting from thrombocytopaenia:
   a. Purpura; petechiae; ecchymoses.
   b. Bleeding from gums, nose, gastrointestinal and urinary tracts.

Diagnosis

1 Peripheral blood smear shows pancytopaenia (deficiency in all the cellular elements of the blood).
2 Bone marrow aspiration—bone marrow is hypoplastic or aplastic; reduction of its cellular elements occurs, and there is an almost complete absence of haemopoietic activity.

Progress of Disease

1 The progress of the disease is variable: patients with severe pancytopaenia with totally aplastic marrow have a poor prognosis.
2 Approximately half of the patients with aplastic anaemia die of the disease, usually from *infection, haemorrhage* and *complications of chronic anaemia*.

Treatment

The appropriate treatment remains controversial.

Objectives

To bring the patient to remission.
To prolong his survival time with supportive therapy.

1 Attempt to identify and eliminate the underlying toxic agent(s)—gives marrow opportunity to recover before being damaged too severely. However, permanent damage often occurs.
   a. Question patient regarding all agents (chemicals, drugs) to which he has been exposed.
   b. Instruct patient to eliminate exposure to toxins and discontinue all unnecessary medications.
2 Support the patient undergoing bone marrow transplantation (replacement of affected bone marrow with marrow from healthy donor—preferably matched sibling). This treatment is performed at specialized centres, with variable results.

Treatment for Patient when Bone Marrow Transplantation is not Feasible

1   Give blood transfusions.
    a. Give packed red cell transfusions carefully—to maintain haemoglobin level compatible with patient's activities and to relieve symptoms of dyspnoea, palpitation and weakness.
    b. Give transfusion of whole blood for haemorrhagic emergencies.
    c. Give platelet transfusions from histocompatible donors if possible—to arrest bleeding in patient with thrombocytopoenia (Haemorrhagic complications occur with platelet counts below 20 000/mm³).
    d. Keep patient who receives multiple transfusions over a period of time under careful nursing observation—transfusion complications usually develop with these patients.
    (1) Eventually, patient may develop antibodies to minor red cell antigens and to platelet antigens so that transfusions no longer raise the counts sufficiently.
    (2) Multiple transfusions decrease chance for successful bone marrow transplantation.
2   Give agents (anabolic steroids, e.g. Prednisone) to attempt to stimulate marrow regeneration and bring about a remission.
3   Prepare patient for splenectomy (p. 228) if indicated—the spleen destroys large numbers of white cells and platelets; splenectomy may cause slight elevation of haemoglobin levels and decrease the transfusion requirements.
4   Watch for evidence of infection—patients with aplastic anaemia are susceptible to infections, due to low leucocyte count.
    a. Utilize careful aseptic techniques for patients with pronounced leucopaenia.
    b. Treat infections with appropriate agent.
    (1) Long-term antibiotic therapy may cause enteritis and diarrhoea from changes in intestinal flora.
    (2) Generalized moniliasis may also occur in weakened patients taking antibiotics for prolonged periods.

Discharge Planning and Health Teaching

Instruct patient as follows:

1   Be aware of drugs that may damage the bone marrow cell.
2   When taking drugs that can produce blood dyscrasias (chloramphenicol, phenylbutazone, sulphonamides), have regular blood counts; however, aplastic anaemia may develop after drug has ben discontinued.
3   During bleeding episodes use mouthwashes instead of brushing teeth with brush.
4   Prevent minor infections. Any abrasion or wound of mucous membranes or skin is a potential site of infection.

POLYCYTHAEMIA VERA

Polycythaemia vera (erythnaemia) is a disease of unknown cause characterized by an increase in the number of red blood cells and in the total blood volume. The bone marrow is dark red and intensely cellular. It is characterized by leucocytosis, thrombocytosis and splenomegaly.

Secondary polycythaemia is commonly associated with hypoxia (cardiovascular and pulmonary disease), with excessive production of erythropoietin, adrenocortical steroids or androgens, or to chronic chemical exposure.

Altered Physiology

1   Altered physiology due to increased blood volume because of increase in red cell mass.
2   Increased supply of precursor cells (to the erythroid, myeloid and megakarocytic line).
3   Striking increase in total blood volume; gradually increasing blood viscosity.
4   Decreased marrow iron.
5   Engorgement of all organs with blood.
6   Hyperplasia of all bone marrow elements.
7   Enlargement of spleen (sometimes).

Progress of Disease

1   Insidious and gradual onset—probably measured in years.
2   Clinical course of long duration—up to 20 years.
3   More frequent in males; most common during middle and later years of life.
4   Peptic ulcers are common in these patients; cerebral, gastrointestinal and nasal haemorrhages may occur at any time during the course of the disease.

Clinical Manifestations

This is a multiple organ system disease.

1   Weakness and fatigue.
2   Headache, dizziness, impaired mental ability, visual disturbances.
3   Pruritus.
4   Plethoric appearance.
5   Reddish-purple hue of the face, lips, hands, feet and buccal cavity; aggravated by cold.
6   Peripheral vascular complaints.
7   Paraesthesia.
8   Splenomegaly, producing abdominal discomfort.
9   Elevated systolic blood pressure.
10   Hepatomegaly (late in course of disease).

Diagnosis

1   Increased red cell mass—measured by an isotopic technique.
2   Thrombocytosis; often abnormal platelet aggregation.
3   Leucocytosis.
4   Elevated granulocyte alkaline phosphatase activity.
5   Increased cellular activity of bone marrow; decreased marrow iron.

Treatment

Objective

To reduce the red cell mass (e.g., to bring the haematocrit to within normal limits).

1 Assist with phlebotomy (venesection) to correct blood viscosity and circulating abnormalities and to lower the haematocrit.
  a. 500 ml of blood removed every 2–3 days until haematocrit reaches desired level.
  b. Repeated phlebotomies may be performed to lower haemoglobin, haematocrit and red cell mass to normal ranges.
2 Give chemotherapy:
  a. Melphalan (Alkeran).
  b. Chlorambucil (Leukeran).
  c. Busulphan (Myleran).
  d. Cytosine arabinoside.
  e. See Nursing Support of Patient Receiving Chemotherapy (Volume 1, Chapter 7).
3 Or prepare patient for radioactive phosphorus ^{32}P, either orally or intravenously—reduces myelopoiesis (formation of bone marrow).
4 Keep patient mobile—likelihood of thrombosis increases when patient is on bed rest.
5 Evaluate and treat for complications—the clinical course of polycythaemia is determined by the development of complications.
  a. Thrombotic complications—due to hypervolaemia and hyperactivity of the haematopoietic tissues.
     Includes deep vein thrombophlebitis, myocardial and cerebral infarction and thrombotic occlusion of the splenic, hepatic, portal and mesenteric veins.
  b. Haemorrhage—bleeding occurs spontaneously from engorgement of capillary beds.
  c. Gout—from overproduction of uric acid (secondary to nucleoprotein turnover of marrow cells).
  d. Congestive failure—from increased blood volume and hypertension.
  e. Acute leukaemia—may be a terminal complication.

AGRANULOCYTOSIS (Granulocytopaenia)

Agranulocytosis (granulocytopaenia) is an acute disease in which the white blood cell count drops to extremely low levels and neutropaenia becomes pronounced.

Aetiology

1 Hypersensitivity to certain drugs or chemicals—may suppress bone marrow activity and decrease production of white blood cells. Some agents occasionally associated with agranulocytosis include:
  a. Phenothiazines.
  b. Antihistamines.
  c. Analgesics (Butazolidin).
  d. Diuretics.

e. Dibenzazepine compounds.
f. Tranquillizers.
g. Antithyroid drugs.
h. Sulphonamides and their derivatives (including hypoglycaemic agents).
i. Certain antibiotics (chloramphenicol).
j. Anticonvulsants.
k. Agents that regularly depress leucopoiesis (alkylating agents, antimetabolites).
2   In some patients the cause cannot be identified.

Clinical Manifestations

1   Sore throat, ulcerations of mucosa of mouth and pharynx (agranulocytic angina); throat becomes increasingly sore and eventually necrotic.
2   Fever/chills.
3   Extreme prostration.
4   Vaginal and rectal ulceration—may occur as a result of local infection.
5   Pneumonia, urinary tract infection, sepsis.

Progress of Disease

Spontaneous restoration of marrow function (except in patients with neoplastic disease) may occur in 1–3 weeks if death from infection can be averted.

Diagnosis

Blood shows marked reduction in number of circulating neutrophils.
Bone marrow examination.

Treatment

Objectives

To eliminate the factor responsible for the bone marrow suppression.
To prevent and treat infection until the bone marrow has returned to normal.

1   Question the patient concerning any drugs he has been taking, including those taken without medical prescription.
2   Take the patient off the offending drug. Warn the patient to avoid re-exposure to offending drug.
3   Prevent and treat infection.

Nursing Alert: Granulocytes are the first barrier to infection. In patients with agranulocytosis, infection develops rapidly and may soon become overwhelming.

a. Watch for the occurrence of fever.
b. Patient may be placed in protective isolation; however, infection usually arises from patient's endogenous flora (in gastrointestinal tract, urinary tract) or from organisms in hospital environment.
c. Opportunistic fungal infections (which in normal host are not pathogenic) may be life-threatening to this patient.
d. The therapy of suspected sepsis is started as soon as cultures are taken—blood

cultures, throat, urine, sputum, etc. It is undertaken with a combination of antibiotics, since at this time no single agent provides an antibacterial spectrum broad enough to control all common pathogenic organisms usually involved.

(1) Patient is usually given aminoglycoside antibiotics (gentamicin plus a penicillin-type drug) if there is evidence of infection. These drugs have a broad spectrum of activity in vitro against most Gram-negative bacilli which are likely to be pathogenic for compromised host.

(2) If patient is severely neutropaenic, carbenicillin is added to this regimen because of the problem of *Pseudomonas*.

3 Administer anabolic steroids (testosterone, fluoxymesterone) as directed— stimulates the marrow stem cell.

4 Utilize measures to support the patient and increase comfort.

a. Using nursing and therapeutic measures to relieve throat pain—gargles, ice-packs, analgesics, anaesthetic lozenges.

b. Encourage patient to remain on bed rest.

c. Give high vitamin, high calorie, soft or liquid diet.

Complications

1 Sepsis.
2 Bronchial pneumonia.
3 Haemorrhagic necrosis of mucous membrane lesions.

LEUKAEMIA

The *leukaemias* are neoplastic disorders of the blood-forming tissues (spleen, lymphatic system and bone marrow). They are characterized by widespread proliferation within the bone marrow and other blood-forming tissues of immature precursors of one of the types of leucocytes. The leukaemic process drastically reduces the production of the principle constituents of normal blood, resulting in anaemia and increased susceptibility to infection and haemorrhage.

Classification

Classified according to:

1 The cell line involved (lymphocytic, granulocytic or monocytic).
2 The maturity of malignant cells:
   a. Acute (immature cells).
   b. Chronic (diffentiated cells).

Predisposing Factors

Aetiology unknown: several factors are associated with increase in incidence:

1 Exposure to radiation.
2 Chemical agents—benzene.
3 Infectious agents—viruses (currently being investigated).
4 Genetic abnormalities—increased risk of leukaemia in patients with Down's syndrome.

5   Chemotherapy treatment—particularly, melphalan (Alkeran).
6   Myeloproliferative disorders—polycythaemia vera, myelofibrosis (fibrosis of bone marrow).
7   Heredity—some families with incidence of leukaemia.

Acute Leukaemia

Acute leukaemia is a rapidly progressive disease involving primitive cells or blasts. It may be lymphocytic, granulocytic, monocytic, myelomonocytic or undifferentiated (stem cell).

Clinical Manifestations

Produced by proliferation and infiltration of bone marrow and other organs by immature white blood cells of the lymphocytic, granulocytic or monocytic group

1   General malaise; person tires easily; pallor from anaemia caused by depressed erythropoiesis, haemorrhage and haemolysis.
2   Persistent fever of unknown cause.
3   Enlarged lymph nodes and spleen; abdominal discomfort—from local tissue invasion.
4   Bone pain, arthralgia—from expanding marrow in bone and gout of hyperuricaemia.
5   Bleeding of gums, epistaxis, petechiae, prolonged bleeding following a surgical procedure—from thrombocytopaenia (lowered platelet count).
6   Tachycardia, weight loss, dyspnoea on exertion, intolerance to heat—from increased metabolism.
7   Leukaemia infiltration of the skin—tendency for leukaemic tissue to infiltrate other organs and tissues.
8   Cerebral haemorrhage, cranial nerve paralysis, increased intracranial pressure—from neurological complications (leukaemia cells frequently invade the central nervous system—usually in patients in long remission).
9   Pain—from infarction, particularly the spleen.

Diagnosis

1   Examination of the blood—total peripheral white count varies widely (10 000–100 000/mm³).
2   Bone marrow biopsy—characteristically large percentage of bone marrow's nucleated cells are immature leucocyte forms called 'blasts'.
3   Lymph node biopsy.
4   Chest x-ray—to detect mediastinal node and lung involvement.
5   Skeletal x-ray—to detect skeletal lesions.

Treatment

Objectives

To restore normal marrow function as quickly as possible.
To achieve complete remission.

To provide the patient with as long and as normal a life as possible.

Initial treatment in a specially equipped medical unit that treats patients with leukaemia with a team approach gives the best promise for prolonged remission.

Chemotherapy

1   The drugs are classified on the basis of their effects on cell chemistry.
2   Objective of chemotherapy—to induce remission (disappearance of all abnormal cell forms in the bone marrow and peripheral blood).

Underlying Principles of Chemotherapy

1   Chemotherapy inhibits growth of leukaemic cells by destroying or inactivating nucleic acids or by interfering with their synthesis; causes bone marrow depression and depresses the patient's immunological defence mechanism.
2   Drugs are usually given in combination (exert different biological effects) at high dose levels to produce greater leukaemia cell damage.
3   The treatment regimen is designed to affect cells in different phases of miotic cycle.
4   Usually there is intensive treatment with multiple agents at the beginning of therapy to induce a remission, followed by long-term 'maintenance' therapy.
5   The nursing management of the patient with acute leukaemia includes constant assessment of the patient for effects of drug toxicity.

Some Drugs Used in Acute Leukaemia

A large number of drugs have an antileukaemia effect. The drug protocol changes as research developments are received.

1   Antimetabolites—compete with the natural metabolite, thus blocking the pathway for the synthesis of DNA or another cellular constituent (thereby blocking cell growth).
      Methotrexate; antipurines (6-mercaptopurine); cytosine arabinoside (Ara–C).
2   Alkylating agents—may exert their anticancer effects by direct chemical interaction with the DNA of the cell.
      Cyclophosphamide (Cytoxan); melphalan (Alkeran); busulphan (Myleran).
3   Antibiotics—inhibit synthesis of cell proteins.
      Doxorubicin (Adriamycin); daunorubicin.
4   Plant alkaloids.
      Vincristine (Oncovin)—blocks process of cell division. Vinblastine (Velban).
      ban).
5   Hormones—suppress the growth of lymphocytes.
      Adrenal cortical steroid (prednisone).
6   Other drugs:
      L-asparaginase—an enzyme that breaks down asparagine, an amino acid frequently required by leukaemic cells for cell growth.

Nursing Management

Constant Nursing Observation of Patient Receiving Chemotherapy

1   Obtain baseline information before chemotherapy is started.
  a. Know the patient's 'normal' TPR and BP.
  b. Follow up the white blood cell count, differential count, haemoglobin measurements, platelet counts—to be aware of the drug's effect on the body.
  c. Follow up blood chemistry studies, electrolytes, urea nitrogen, creatinine, liver enzymes, bilirubin.
  d. Weigh the patient once or twice weekly.
  e. Assist with bone marrow aspirations as directed (see p. 186).
2   *Watch for toxic manifestations during chemotherapy.*
  a. Modifications of patient's chemotherapy regimen are based on laboratory and physical examinations before each course of treatment.
  b. Monitor intravenous infusion of drugs—may cause local irritation in the veins; patient may complain of burning sensations during infusions of methotrexate and prednisone.
    (1) Adjust infusion flow to a slower rate.
    (2) Change position of extremity to prevent muscular cramping.
    (3) Patient may complain of nausea, vomiting and burning sensation along the gastrointestinal tract during or immediately after drug infusion.
  c. Watch for mouth ulcers—frequently occur when patient is taking methotrexate. Offer medicated mouth rinses frequently to relieve oral discomfort.
  d. Be prepared for the patient to experience loss of hair during antileukaemic treatment—alopecia occurs in high percentage of patients receiving vincristine. Encourage the patient to experiment with wigs, hair pieces, head scarfs.
  e. Observe patient for footdrop, weakening hand grasp, ptosis of eyelids—vincristine may cause neuropathy.
  f. Assess for constipation and abdominal pain—vincristine may produce paralytic ileus.
  g. Watch for personality changes, fluid retention, hypertension, gastric ulcers and diabetes mellitus—occur with prednisone therapy.
  h. Watch for other drug side-effects—diarrhoea, maculopapular rash, stomatitis, phlebitis, bone marrow depression, evidence of cardiac toxicity (tachycardia, arrhythmias, tachypnoea, dyspnoea).
  i. Take ECG readings as prescribed—cardiac toxicity is associated with certain chemotherapeutic agents.

Supportive Measures for Patient with Leukaemia or Lymphoma

Underlying consideration: Failure to improve is usually due to complications—infection and haemorrhage.

Objective

To control complications so that chemotherapeutic agents can demonstrate their effectiveness.

1   To eliminate the morbidity and mortality resulting from haemorrhage.
  a. Major cause of haemorrhage is thrombocytopaenia (decrease in platelets).

b. Risk of haemorrhage is high at platelet levels below 15 000–20 000 (normal 250 000–500 000 platelets/mm³).

c. Prepare the patient for a transfusion of compatible platelets or pooled platelets when haemorrhage occurs.

Platelet transfusion may need to be repeated two to three times weekly—average platelet half-life is 3–5 days.

2   To prevent and treat infection—the major morbidity and mortality associated with leukaemia; bone marrow invasion of the leukaemic cell line prevents normal production and maturation of granulocytes. Also the pathogenic organism is usually part of the patient's own flora.

a. Monitor the concentration of circulating granulocytes. Concentrations below 1000/mm³—serious danger of infection.

b. Recognize infection promptly.

(1) Monitor temperature at regular intervals—fever is major symptom of infection.

(2) Usual manifestations of infection are altered in patient with leukaemia.

c. Obtain cultures (for both aerobes and anaerobes) of blood, urine, sputum, spinal fluid.

d. Obtain chest x-ray.

e. Broad spectrum antibiotics are usually given until organism is identified.

f. Watch for development of fungal infection (especially *Candida* and *Aspergillus*)—from indwelling catheters, antibiotics, immunosuppressive effects of chemotherapy and decreased resistance of patient.

3   To prevent infectious complications by control of environmental contamination.

a. Laminar air-flow room—a unidirectional air flow 'barrier' that establishes an air environment in which the infection-prone patient is free from contact with exogenous micro-organisms.

b. Utilize all appropriate measures to reduce environmental contamination when special units are not available (protective isolation).

4   On an experimental basis, the patient may be given leucocyte transfusions—used as a supporting therapy in bone marrow aplasia (not readily available at this time).

a. Chemotherapy gives rise to aplasia of bone marrow and produces a fall in the number of immunocompetent cells (lymphocytes and macrophages), which in turn results in acute exacerbation of infection.

b. Transfusions of leucocytes (from normal donors) can help patient with severe neutropaenia through the dangerous phase of his illness until bone marrow has sufficiently regenerated.

Other Measures

1   Assist the patient to accept and participate in his therapeutic regimen.

a. Give expert physical care and support—this encourages the patient to endure much discomfort associated with treatment.

b. Help the patient to adapt to an incurable illness.

(1) Patient may react with shock and anger when disease is first recognized; anger may be directed at health care personnel.

(2) Anger is a defence mechanism; patient realizes that death is inevitable; anger is also a defence against anxiety.

      (3) Develop ability to accept and deal with this anger—important for establishing a therapeutic patient–nurse relationship.

      (4) Allow patient and family to express their emotions.

      (5) Patient may use mechanism of denial, which may need to be supported or worked through.

2   Control the pain and discomfort.

    a. Use milder analgesics when possible; change to a stronger narcotic as the patient's condition requires.

    b. Give tranquillizers as directed to enhance the effects of narcotics.

    c. Give antiemetic medication before meals—to help relieve the patient's nausea; sedatives may also be helpful.

3   Maintain oral intake between 3–4 l daily—to prevent precipitation of uric acid crystals in the urine; overproduction of uric acid is due to the tremendous proliferation of blood cells and the destruction of these cells by antileukaemic agents.

4   Control fever—tepid sponging, increased fluid intake, antipyretic drugs.

5   Give frequent and special mouth care—to remove dried blood, combat odour and soothe oral ulcerations.

    a. Alternate solutions of mouth wash, dilute hydrogen peroxide solution and glycerine and lemon solutions.

    b. Use cotton applicators instead of a toothbrush when there is oral bleeding.

    c. Cleanse and lubricate the lips and nostrils—to prevent drying and cracking.

    d. Offer a soft diet if indicated—to reduce mechanical irritation to the gums.

6   Demonstrate continuing concern for the welfare of the patient.

Chronic Lymphocytic Leukaemia

Chronic lymphocytic leukaemia is a type of leukaemia characterized by a great increase in mature lymphocytes in the circulation and in the lymphoid organs of the body.

Clinical Features

1   Occurs most frequently between ages 45 and 60.

2   Insidious onset; symptoms closely resemble those of chronic myelogenous type (p. 213).

3   The course is variable.

Clinical Manifestations

1   Gradual appearance of generalized lymph node enlargement—cervical region, axillae, groin; splenomegaly.

2   Anaemia, fever, weight loss and haemorrhagic features.

3   Possible leukaemic infiltrations in retinae of eyes and in skin. (Skin may become pruritic and bronzed.)

4   Ascites; pleural effusion.

5   White blood cells may be in excess of 100 000/mm³ of blood; lymphocytes may comprise 90–99% of cells.

6   Abnormalities of erythrocytes, granulocytes and platelets are common.

Treatment

Objective

To achieve a remission of symptoms.

Asymptomatic Patient with Chronic Lymphocytic Leukaemia

1   May not require treatment for a period of years.
2   Support the patient with optimum nutrition, rest, exercise, recreation and mental activity.

Symptomatic Patient

Patient with massive adenopathy, severe anaemia, thrombocytopaenia, skin involvement, recurring infections.

1   *Chemotherapy*—brings symptomatic relief; decreases size of lymph nodes and spleen:
    a. Chlorambucil (Leukeran).
    b. Combination drug therapy (three or four drug regimen) may be given to patients with poorly differentiated lymphocytes who are unresponsive to a single chemotherapeutic agent)—reduces white blood cell count, improves constitutional symptoms.
2   For anaemia—from blood loss; from replacement of bone marrow by leukaemia cells:
    a. Radiation therapy for local disease.
    b. Corticosteroids (prednisone).
    c. Chemotherapy.
    d. Transfusions: whole blood for haemorrhage; packed red cells when haemolysis or bone marrow failure exists.
3   For adenopathy:
    Deep x-ray therapy for localized nodes, masses, or splenomegaly.
4   For haemorrhage—may occur when severe thrombocytopaenia and purpura are present or when bleeding, secondary to peptic ulcer, occurs as a complication of corticosteroid therapy.
    Transfusion to replace blood loss.

Nursing Management

See p. 210 for nursing support of patient receiving chemotherapy and page 211 for other aspects of management of a patient with leukaemia.

Chronic Granulocytic Leukaemia

Chronic granulocytic (myelocytic, myelogenous) leukaemia is a condition characterized by an increase in all phases of white blood cell development. It affects the granulocytes which are produced by the myeloid, or bone marrow. The condition is often associated with great enlargement of the spleen and liver. It may also occur in the acute form.

Clinical Features

1   Appears most often between ages 35–50 and 60–70.
2   Gradual, insidious onset. The disease runs a progressive course over several years.

Clinical Manifestations

1   Pallor, palpitations, dyspnoea—from anaemia.
2   Dragging sensation or enlargement of left side of abdomen—from splenic enlargement.
3   Haematological features: elevated platelet count, elevated granulocyte count; blood smear shows predominance of granulocytes at all stages of maturation.
4   Weakness, loss of weight, loss of appetite—from increased metabolic rate due to progress of disease.
5   Tenderness and pain in long bones (particularly tibia, ribs, sternum)—due to invasion by abnormal marrow.

Treatment

Objective

To achieve a remission of symptoms.

Chemotherapy.

1   Busulphan (Myleran)—will induce a complete or partial remission in majority of patients.
   a. Following initial treatment patient may be placed on long-term, low-dose maintenance therapy or high-dose therapy when evidence of disease recurs.
   b. Eventually patient will no longer respond; the acute exacerbation phase is termed myeloblastic or 'blast' crisis. The patient is then treated as for acute leukaemia. (See p. 208).
2   Other chemotherapeutic agents (second line drugs) may be used.

Nursing Management

1   See page 210 for nursing support of patient receiving chemotherapy.
2   See page 211 for other aspects of management of a patient with leukaemia.

MALIGNANT LYMPHOMAS

The *lymphomas* are a group of neoplastic diseases of the lymphoreticular system and include Hodgkin's disease and the non-Hodgkin's lymphomas.

1   Lymphomas are classified, according to the predominant malignant cell, as lymphocytic lymphoma (previously called lymphosarcoma), histiocytic lymphoma (previously reticulum cell sarcoma) or Hodgkin's disease.
2   These tumours usually start in lymph nodes, but can involve any lymphoid tissue in the spleen, gastrointestinal tract (tonsils, walls of stomach), liver or bone marrow.

3   They may spread to all these areas and to extralymphatic tissues (lung, kidneys, skin).
4   The aetiology of these diseases is unknown.

Hodgkin's Disease

Hodgkin's disease is a malignant disease of unknown aetiology that originates in the lymphoid system and involves predominantly the lymph nodes. It may occur in almost any lymphoid mass of tissues: spleen, bone marrow.

Altered Physiology

1   The malignant cell of Hodgkin's disease is the 'Reed–Sternberg' cell, which is a gigantic, atypical tumour cell, morphologically unique and of uncertain lineage.
2   The different histopathological types of Hodgkin's disease are associated with varying prognoses.
3   Hodgkin's disease shows a highly predictable pattern of spread—usually via the lymphatic channels from one chain of lymph nodes to another, often to the spleen, and ultimately to extralymphatic sites.
4   Hodgkin's disease may have a haematogenic spread as extra node sites involved include the gastrointestinal tract, bone marrow, skin, upper air passages and other organs.

Clinical Manifestations

1   Painless enlargement of lymph nodes on one side of neck.
2   Generalized pruritus (itching), sweating, weight loss.
3   Progressive anaemia.
4   Slight to high fever.
5   Enlargement of lymph nodes in other regions of the body.
6   Enlargement of mediastinal and retroperitoneal lymph nodes produces pressure symptoms.
    a. Dyspnoea from pressure against the trachea.
    b. Dysphagia from pressure against the oesophagus.
    c. Laryngeal paralysis due to pressure against the recurrent laryngeal nerve.
    d. Brachial, lumbar or sacral neuralgias due to pressure on the nerve.
    e. Oedema of the extremities due to pressure on the veins.
    f. Enlargement of spleen and liver.
7   Effusions into the pleura or peritoneum.
8   Obstructive jaundice.

Diagnosis

The extent of the disease is determined before treatment.

1   Biopsy of lymph node(s) to identify characteristic histological features.
2   Complete blood count.
3   Chest x-ray and tomography.
4   Skeletal survey.
5   Technetium bone scan.

6 Bone marrow biopsy.
7 Liver function tests and scan.
8 Lymphangiogram:
   a. Reveals size of lymph nodes.
   b. Detects abdominal lymph node enlargements which may not be seen or felt by ordinary means.
9 Laparotomy ('staging operation')—to determine extent of disease; splenectomy (may improve blood tolerance to extensive radiotherapy and chemotherapy); open liver biopsy; biopsy of para-aortic lymph nodes. These procedures are important in determining prognosis and treatment.

Staging of Hodgkin's Disease*

Staging is done to provide guidance in prognosis and to assist in therapeutic decisions.

Stage I: Involvement of a single lymph node region (I) or of a single extralymphatic organ or site (I_E).

Stage II: Involvement of two or more lymph node regions on the same side of the diaphragm (II) or localized involvement of extralymphatic organ or site and of one or more lymph node regions on the same side of the diaphragm (II_E).

Stage III: Involvement of lymph node regions on both sides of the diaphragm (III) which may also be accompanied by localized involvement of extralymphatic organ or site (III_E) by involvement of the spleen (III_S) or both (III_{ES}).

Stage IV: Diffuse or disseminated involvement of one or more extralymphatic organs or tissues with or without associated lymph node enlargement.

Treatment

Depends upon stage, symptoms and cell type.

Concepts

1 Radiotherapy to local field, to an extended field or to all node-bearing areas (total nodal irradiation) is the first choice of treatment in early Hodgkin's disease (without any symptoms).
   An important factor in treatment is the radiation dose administered.
2 Hodgkin's disease may be eradicated from any site that has received 4000–4500 rad within the space of 4 weeks. Megavoltage radiation techniques permit the delivery of such a dose to one or more entire lymph node chains.
3 Areas of the body in which the lymph node chains are located can tolerate doses of this magnitude without serious damage (as can the area of the spleen and the oronasopharynx); vital structures such as the lungs, liver and kidneys are protected by lead shields.
4 Radiotherapy usually given daily over a period of weeks.

---

* Committee on Hodgkin's Disease Staging Classification (1971) Cancer Research, 31: 1860–1861.

5 *Complications of intensive radiotherapy:*
a. Pneumonitis, myocardial and pericardial fibrosis, hepatitis, artificial menopause, impotence, development of second malignancy (leukaemia)—depending on site of irradiation and dose-related circumstances.
b. Acute reactions to irradiation—dryness of mouth; loss of taste; dysphagia; nausea and vomiting; apathy and lassitude; skin redness, dry peeling in treatment fields; loss of hair at back of neck and under areas treated; reduction of white blood cells.

Treatment in Advanced Hodgkin's Disease

Objectives

To produce tumour regression and remission.
To relieve pressure on a vital organ (brain, bronchi, kidney).

1 Radiation alone may be used as a palliative measure, or a combination of radiotherapy and chemotherapy may be used.
2 Chemotherapy is used since Hodgkin's disease is considered a drug-responsive tumour.
a. Multiple drug chemotherapy used (nitrogen mustard, vincristine, procarbazine and prednisone).
b. Other combinations have also been effective.
c. Dosage depends on patient's status and his response to treatment.
d. Intermittent maintenance therapy may be required to keep disease under control.
e. Toxic effects of these drugs often overlap, especially bone marrow depression.
f. See page 210 for discussion of patient undergoing chemotherapy.

Nursing Management

1 Support the patient having toxic effects from chemotherapy. (See p. 210).
2 Encourage the patient by saying that the therapy will end in 'a period of time'—serves as an incentive for the patient to continue with therapy.
3 Give laxatives to control constipation that accompanies chemotherapy.
4 Anticipate that patients on chemotherapy will develop leukopaenia, thrombocytopaenia, and anaemia.
5 Help patient cope with unpleasant side-effects of radiation.
a. Oesophagitis—bland soft foods at mild temperatures, aspirin gum (use moderately), anaesthetic lozenges, pain medication before eating if patient unable to eat.
b. Loss of taste—serve palatable meals.
c. Anorexia—encourage patient to make the effort to eat.
d. Nausea—antiemetics given to cover peak time of nausea.
e. Vomiting—reduction of radiation dose may be necessary.
f. Diarrhoea—antidiarrhoeal medication.
g. Skin reaction (sunburned/tanned appearance of treatment area)—avoid rubbing, heat, cold, application of lotions.
h. Lethargy—rest/sleep to keep energy level up; diversional activities to prevent boredom.

6   Prepare patient for surgical excision of localized lymph nodes if indicated (may be followed by radiation therapy).
   Surgery may also be used to alleviate complications caused by pressure or obstruction due to tumour masses.

Lymphocytic Lymphoma

Lymphocytic lymphoma is a malignant growth of lymphocytes in lymphoid tissue characterized by progressive generalized lymphadenopathy and splenomegaly, often progressing to involvement of one or more nonlymphoid organ systems. Marrow damage, manifested by anaemia and thrombocytopaenia, and immune dysfunction, with heightened susceptibility to bacterial and fungal infections, are also evident in these patients.

Clinical Manifestations

1   Prominent generalized lymphadenopathy.
2   Fatigue—attributable primarily to anaemia from impaired erythropoiesis and haemolysis.
3   Malaise, anorexia, weight loss.
4   Fever and sweating.
5   Abdominal distension—due to enlargement of spleen.

Clinical Evaluation

1   Bone scan.
2   Reticuloendothelial (liver, spleen) scan.
3   Intravenous pyelogram.
4   Retroperitoneal lymphography.
5   Bone marrow biopsy.
6   Liver biopsy
7   Laparotomy.

Treatment and Nursing Management

Objective

To induce a remission.

1   Give chemotherapy as directed.
   a. Combination drug therapy used (cyclophosphamide, vincristine, prednisone)—in different dosages and schedules.
   b. See p. 210 for nursing management of the patient having chemotherapy.
2   Prepare the patient for radiation—may be helpful in palliation.
3   Be on the alert for complications.
   a. Infection—by bacteria, viruses, fungi; due to deficiencies of cellular immunity.
   b. Anaemia—from bone marrow invasion, haemorrhage, chemotherapy, hypersplenism, failure of bone marrow, haemolysis.
   c. Spinal cord compression—from lymphomatous infiltration.
   d. Hyperuricaemia.
4   See also discussion of the care of patients with Hodgkin's disease (see above).

Mycosis Fungoides

Mycosis fungoides is a cutaneous lymphoma that may progress to involve the lymph nodes and other internal organs. The late stage of the disease closely resembles malignant lymphoma.

Clinical Manifestations

1 Generalized severe itching—may last for several years.
2 Erythematous, urticarial, eczematous or psoriasis-like lesions—there are exacerbations and remissions of these eruptions.
3 Ulcerating and necrotic tumours of the skin—lesions become indurated and more fungoidal until they are mushroom-like growth (scarlet or purplish in colour), varying in size from 1–15 cm; the body may be covered with these lesions.
4 Patient usually dies from systemic lymphoma.

Diagnosis

Biopsy of skin lesion—gives distinctive diagnostic pattern of mycosis fungoides.

Treatment and Nursing Management

Objective

To bring about a remission.

1 Radiation is applied by electron beam—gives very little skin penetration and permits total body irradiation without visceral damage; used primarily when there is no evidence of systemic involvement.
2 Chemotherapy—to arrest the disease.
  a. *Topical therapy* (for cutaneous manifestations):
    (1) Nitrogen mustard used as topical therapy—effective in certain stages of the disease.
    (2) Allergic contact hypersensitivity to the mustard may develop.
    (3) Other agents used include topical fluocinolone acetonide (under plastic occlusive dressings).
  b. Intralesional injections of triamcinolone or nitrogen mustard may be tried.
  c. Systemic chemotherapy is carried out when internal organs are involved to prevent progressive growth and dissemination of disease.
    (1) Single agent chemotherapy protocol may be used.
    (2) Antimetabolites, cytotoxic antibiotics and corticosteroids may be used.
    (3) See p. 210 for management of patient receiving chemotherapy.
3 Radiotherapy (electron beam therapy)—for patients with widespread mycosis fungoides.
4 Watch for evidence of infection (major cause of death, particularly septicaemia, bacterial pneumonia).
5 Support the patient who has painful ulcerative lesions.
  a. Place bed cradle over patient when he is unable to tolerate the weight of the bed clothing on his skin lesions.

b. Apply bacteriostatic ointment (as prescribed) to lesions as a prophylaxis against infection and to promote comfort by excluding air from open nerve endings.
c. Give analgesics for pain.
d. See p. 217 for discussion of the nursing management of patients with Hodgkin's disease.

Multiple Myeloma

Multiple myeloma (plasma cell myeloma; plasmocytoma; myelomatosis) is a malignant disease of the plasma cell that infiltrates bone and soft tissues. The cause is not known. It is a disease of older people and is not classified as a lymphoma.

Altered Physiology

1 The malignant cell is the plasma cell; neoplastic proliferation takes place mainly in the bone marrow. (The plasma cell is derived from lymphocytes and produces immunoglobulin [antibodies]).
2 The bones most commonly affected are the vertebrae, skull, ribs, sternum, pelvis, upper ends of humerus.
3 The malignant plasma cells usually produce abnormal amounts of an immuno-globulin or parts of an immunoglobulin protein (Bence Jones protein) that can usually be detected in urine by immunoelectrophoresis.
4 There is a constant threat of hypercalcaemia, hypercalciuria and hyperuricaemia due to skeletal destruction, because myeloma cells stimulate osteoclasts.
5 Increased loss of bone substance leads to collapse of vertebral bodies, rib fractures, etc.

Clinical Manifestations

1 Constant severe bone pain, especially on movement—marrow is infiltrated with plasma cells and there are destructive bone lesions.
   a. Low back pain—the most characteristic symptom.
   b. Skeletal lesions—producing swelling, tenderness, pain and *pathological fractures.*
2 Anaemia—due to malignancy and/or replacement of marrow with neoplastic plasma cells. May be associated with thrombocytopaenia and granulo-paenia—causes increased susceptibility to infection and abnormal bleeding.
3 Marked weight loss.
4 Symptoms of renal failure—may be due to precipitation of the immunoglobulin in the tubules or to pyelonephritis, hypercalcaemia, increased uric acid, infiltration of the kidney with plasma cells (myeloma kidney), renal vein thrombosis.
5 Bleeding tendencies.
6 Nausea, vomiting, constipation, lethargy (late stage).

Diagnosis

1 Abnormalities present in basic haemogram—anaemia, elevated sedimentation rate, leukopaenia with diminished granulocytes; decreased platelets.

2 Malignant plasma cells produce abnormal globulins which appear in serum electrophoresis as a paraprotein 'spike'—fragments of these globulins are excreted in urine as Bence Jones proteins.
3 Bone marrow biopsy—may show evidence of increased number of abnormal plasma cells in the marrow.
4 Bony lesions may appear on x-ray; numerous areas of localized bone destruction may be visible; demineralization of skeleton (osteoporosis) may occur.
5 Radioactive technetium bone scans—involved areas show increased uptake of technetium.

Treatment and Nursing Management

Objectives

To decrease the tumour mass.
To control pain.

Decrease the Tumour Mass and Relieve Bone Pain

1 Give the appropriate chemotherapy (foundation of treatment):
   a. Combination drug therapy appears more effective than single dose therapy in most patients.
   b. Melphalan, prednisone, cyclophosphamide—some of the agents currently being given.
   c. See p. 210 for supportive care of patient receiving chemotherapy.
2 Support patient receiving radiotherapy—given for relief of pain from large lesions (especially from nerve compression and fracture) and for reducing size of extraskeletal plasma cell tumours.

Give Attentive and Supportive Care

1 Keep the patient mobile unless lesion in spine produces danger of cord compression—prevents further bone resorption and hypercalcaemia.
   a. Avoid total immobilization.
   b. *Watch for pathological fractures*—may occur when patient turns, is placed on bedpan, transferred to a stretcher.
   c. Avoid excessive lifting and straining. Handle patient with smooth, unhurried movements.
   d. Use analgesics, supportive splints and back brace for patient with pathology of spine.
   e. Local irradiation may be employed to achieve mobilization.
   f. Assist patient to *walk* as much as possible.
2 Evaluate for spinal cord compression—from invasion of canal by neoplastic tissue. Watch for bladder distension (spinal cord compression).
   a. Radiation therapy—to prevent paraplegia.
   b. Laminectomy for decompression—for cord compression or vertebral fractures.
3 Watch for recurrent infections—patient has impaired capacity for antibody production.
   a. Record temperature frequently—patients on steroids may not have overt symptoms of infection. Observe for apathy, lethargy.

    b. Observe for symptoms of urinary tract infection and bronchopneumonia.

    c. Take cultures from skin lesions, blood, sputum and urine as indicated.

4 Observe the patient for signs and symptoms of renal insufficiency—from precipitation of Bence Jones protein in renal tubules, leading to tubular obstruction and dilatation and uraemia; or from pyelonephritis, hypercalcaemia (which may result from bony destruction and immobilization), amyloidosis, hyperuricaemia, myeloma kidney.

    a. Encourage free fluids—to prevent protein precipitation and to minimize hypercalcaemia.

    b. Give allopurinol as ordered—to control hyperuricaemia.

    c. Watch for symptoms of haemorrhagic cystitis in patient taking Cytoxan; maintain on free fluids.

    d. Give prednisone as prescribed by doctor—may be used in management of hypercalcaemia.

    e. Avoid dehydration—can precipitate acute renal failure; intravenous fluids may be necessary.

Nursing Alert: Patients with multiple myeloma should not be put on fasting regimens for diagnostic tests, since dehydrating procedures can precipitate acute renal failure.

5 Treat concomitant anaemia—occurs in most patients.

    a. Give packed red cell transfusions for patients with severe anaemia.

    b. Administer chemotherapy, steroid hormones and androgens—to stimulate erythropoiesis; may improve anaemia.

    c. Determine methods to conserve patient's energy; note this on nursing care plan.

6 Be aware of the complications.

    a. Infection—from decrease in normal circulating antibodies due to proliferation of abnormal plasma cells which produce ineffective globulins; extensive bone marrow involvement causes leucopaenia; chemotherapy and radiotherapy also cause marrow depression; steroid hormones increase susceptibility to opportunistic infection.

    b. *Neurological complications:*

      (1) Paraplegia—from collapse of supporting structures, from infiltration of nerve roots or from cord compression of plasma cell tumours.

    c. Bone complications—pathological fractures.

    d. Haematological complications:

      (1) Renal failure—from plugging of renal tubules by proteinaceous casts.

      (2) Renal stones from hypercalcaemia—due to bone destruction and increased bone resorption.

      (3) Infiltration of kidney from plasma cells, etc.

      (4) Hypercalciuria—excessive bone destruction creates increased excretion of calcium in urine.

      (5) Hyperuricaemia—may produce renal failure.

    e. Multiple primary neoplasms may occur—disordered immune surveillance may make patient susceptible to multiple tumour development.

BLEEDING DISORDERS

Vascular Purpuras

The term *purpura* refers to extravasation (escape) of blood into the skin and mucous membranes. Purpuric lesions may occur spontaneously as an isolated phenomenon or as an accompaniment of obvious disease.

Types of Purpura

1   *Petechiae*—small pinpoint haemorrhages under the skin.
2   *Ecchymoses*—escape of blood into tissues, producing a large bruise.
3   Petechiae and ecchymoses may occur as the result of vascular rupture, permitting the leakage of blood into the subcutaneous tissue of the mucous membranes.
4   *Symptomatic or secondary purpura*—certain types of bloodstream infections (e.g., meningococcaemia and infective endocarditis) exhibit this phenomenon due to damage to the vascular walls by the infectious agent.
5   Severe arterial hypertension—may cause the patient to bruise easily; Valsalva manoeuvre may cause petechiae.
6   *Anaphylactoid purpura*—generally regarded as an allergic disorder in which there are various skin lesions (purpuric and otherwise) and episodes of arthritis, abdominal pain, haematuria, gastrointestinal haemorrhages and fever.
    a. Attacks last several weeks and recur for years.
    b. Steroid therapy is often effective.
7   *Familial haemorrhagic telangiectasia*—a hereditary disorder manifested by an abnormal tendency to bleed and bruise.
    a. Precise nature of defect is obscure.
    b. Condition does not respond to any proved method of treatment.
8   *Toxic purpura*—a condition observed after exposure to certain drugs and poisons.
9   *Vitamin C deficiency*—a vascular purpura.
10   Senile purpura.
11   Collagen and vascular disease.
12   Steroid purpura.

Idiopathic Thrombocytopaenic Purpura

Thrombocytopaenic purpura refers to purpura (extravasation of blood into skin) which is accompanied by reduction in the number of circulating platelets. The cause is unknown.

Clinical Manifestations

1   Onset is usually sudden.
2   Bleeding—mild to severe (thrombocytopaenia not usually accompanied by bleeding unless the platelet count falls below 20 000/mm³).

   a. Skin lesions—small red haemorrhages; do not blanch on pressure.
   b. Purpuric lesions may occur in vital organ (brain).
   c. Bleeding may occur from nose, mouth, genitourinary tract.

Laboratory Manifestations

1 Platelets may be absent or only slightly decreased in number; abnormalities may be seen in platelet size or morphological appearance.
2 Anaemia—usually normocytic.
3 Proteinuria and microscopic and gross haematuria present in majority of patients.

Treatment and Nursing Management

Objectives

To search for possible causes of bleeding.
To treat patient during spontaneous bleeding episodes.

1 Give adrenal corticosteroids (prednisone)—may produce improvement by reducing bleeding (by affecting blood vessels, resulting in decreased capillary fragility; by elevating the level of circulating platelets; or by suppression of phagocytic cells of reticuloendothelial system). This form of therapy is controversial.
2 Prepare the patient for a splenectomy (p. 228).
   Splenectomy may bring about improvement by elevating the platelet levels and by removing major site of platelet breakdown.
3 Give immunosuppressive therapy—used for patients who do not respond to corticosteroids or splenectomy.
   Azathioprine, cyclophosphamide, vincristine, etc.
4 Support the patient receiving transfusions.
   a. Transfusions of fresh whole blood (blood collected within 24 hours)—fresh blood is a source of platelets as well as plasma-clotting factors.
   Given to enhance haemostasis during bleeding episodes, to restore circulating blood volume and to correct anaemia.
   b. Transfusions of platelets (in form of platelet concentrates, platelet-rich plasma, fresh whole blood).
   Used in treating patients with thromboytopaenia secondary to bone marrow suppression caused by drugs (chemotherapy) or an idiopathic thrombocytopaenic purpura.
5 Utilize other measures to help the patient.
   a. Avoid unnecessary trauma (intramuscular injections, etc.).
   b. Keep patient on bed rest during periods of active bleeding.
   c. Administer iron salts for iron deficiency anaemia from chronic blood loss.
   d. Suppress menstrual flow (by oral progestational-oestrogenic agents) if patient has recurrent menorrhagia.
   e. Avoid aspirin—interferes with the haemostatic function of platelets.

CLOTTING DEFECTS

Disseminated Intravascular Coagulation (DIC)

Disseminated intravascular coagulation (consumption coagulopathy) is the formation of microthrombi in the capillaries and small vessels with consequent consumption of coagulation factors, especially fibrinogen and platelets, causing bleeding tendency.

Clinical Features

1   Disseminated intravascular coagulation is a complication of many illnesses; often fatal.
   a. Infections.
   b. Obstetrical complications.
   c. Malignancies.
   d. Massive tissue injuries (burns)
   e. Vascular and circulatory complications
   f. Anaphylaxis.
   g. Haemolytic transfusion reactions.
2   Haemorrhagic tendency is the consequence of the acute activation of the clotting mechanism of the blood—results in intravascular consumption of the plasma clotting factors.
3   Clotting factors are consumed more quickly than they can be replenished by the liver.

Clinical Manifestations

1   Diffuse bleeding—skin and mucous membranes.
2   Ecchymoses; petechiae.
3   Bleeding from gastrointestinal and urinary tracts.
4   Prolonged bleeding from venepuncture.
5   Signs and symptoms of acute renal failure.

Diagnosis

1   Coagulation screening tests—prolonged.
2   Thrombocytopaenia.
3   Hypofibrinogenaemia.
4   Deficiences in prothrombin factors V and VIII and elevated levels of fibrin degradation products.

Treatment

Difficult to generalize about the treatment

1   Treat the cause of the syndrome since DIC seems secondary to some primary disease.
   a. Correct any condition that exaggerates coagulopathy (shock, acidosis, sepsis).
   b. Give antisepsis treatment for coagulation changes produced by bacteraemia.
2   Give heparin in initial stages (intravenously)—to stop the clotting (*controversial*).

  a. May be contradindicated in certain conditions (acute hepatic failure, intracranial haemorrhage).

  b. Follow heparin therapy with laboratory tests.

3 Administer blood component replacement and other types of treatment as indicated by individual patient's condition.

Haemophilia

Haemophilia is a hereditary coagulation disorder.

Acquired Defects in Coagulation

Acquired defects in coagulation may be associated with many conditions, including:

1 Vitamin K deficiency.
2 Administration of coumarin–indanedione anticoagulant drugs.
3 Heparin therapy.
4 Diseases of the liver.
5 Disseminated intravascular coagulation.
6 Uraemia.
7 Transfusion-induced clotting factor deficiency.
8 Chronic renal failure.
9 Certain antibiotics—inhibit coagulation factors.

Vitamin K Deficiency

Vitamin K deficiency produces a characteristic abnormality of blood clotting mechanisms.

General Considerations

1 Vitamin K is obtained partly from diet and partly from bacterial action in the intestinal tract.

  a. Foods high in vitamin K—leafy vegetables (spinach, cauliflower, cabbage, kale, dandelion greens).

  b. Vitamin K is not absorbed in the absence of bile salts.

Causes

1 Interference with flow of bile salts into gastrointestinal tract—obstructive jaudice, biliary fistula.
2 Impaired intestinal absorption (sprue, steatorrhoea, gastrocolic fistula, regional enteritis).
3 Extensive surgical resection of small bowel.
4 Dietary deprivation
5 Therapy with broad spectrum antibiotics.

Clinical Manifestations

1 Ecchymoses.
2 Epistaxis.

3   Gingival bleeding.
4   Haematuria.
5   Haematemesis and melaena.
6   Menorrhagia.
7   Operative and postoperative bleeding.

Treatment

1   Administer vitamin K via oral, subcutaneous or intramuscular route—bleeding will cease in 3–4 hours, clotting activity rises and a normal prothrombin level may be obtained in 12–14 hours.
   a. Phytonadione (Mephyton, AquaMEPHYTON).
   b. Menadiol sodium diphosphate (Synkavite, Synkamin).
2   Administer whole blood or component therapy for severe bleeding.

Bleeding Due to Ingestion of Coumarin–Indanedione Anticoagulant Drugs

Causes

Bleeding may develop from long-term use of coumarin or indanedione anticoagulant drugs that are used in the treatment of thromboembolic disorders.

Nursing Alert: Laboratory determinations of the anticoagulant status should be carried out on patients taking anticoagulant drugs who have had a change in physical condition or have had other drugs suddenly introduced or withdrawn. The anticoagulant dosage must be appropriately adjusted in these circumstances.

Clinical Manifestations

1   Bleeding in gastrointestinal tract or central nervous system.
2   Ecchymoses
3   Haematomas.
4   Epistaxis.
5   Haematuria.
6   Vaginal bleeding.

Treatment

1   Administer vitamin K (phytonadione, [Mephyton]) orally, subcutaneously or intramuscularly—will reverse the effects of the drugs.
2   Nursing precautions—pain, swelling and tenderness occasionally occur at site of subcutaneous or intramuscular injection.
3   Patient may be resistant to further anticoagulant therapy for a few days after vitamin K is given.
4   Konyne (concentrates of vitamin K-dependent factors, factors II, VII, IX and X) may be given in emergencies, even though this may increase the risk of hepatitis in some patients.

Heparin Therapy as a Cause of Bleeding

Heparin therapy is given for thromboembolic disorders.

Causes of Bleeding

1 Secondary to anticoagulant effect.
2 Overdosage of heparin.
3 Trauma (avoid intramuscular injections).
4 Surgery.

Complications

1 Cerebral haemorrhage.
2 Haemoptysis.
3 Bleeding from pre-existing gastrointestinal lesions and from sites of surgery or trauma.

Treatment

1 Stop heparin therapy immediately.
2 Give protamine sulphate as directed—neutralizes the action of heparin.

SPLENECTOMY

Splenectomy is removal of the spleen. It is useful in severe forms of autoimmune diseases (thrombocytopaenia purpura, acquired haemolytic anaemia).

Indications for Splenectomy

1 Rupture of the spleen—most common indication:
   a. History of injury.
   b. Persistent abdominal pain.
   c. Abdominal rigidity, rebound tenderness, shock.
2 Hypersplenism (premature destruction of blood cells by the spleen).
3 For haematological disorders:
   a. Idiopathic thrombocytopaenia purpura.
   b. Splenomegaly of undetermined cause.
   c. Chronic splenomegaly.
   d. Acquired haemolytic anaemia.

Nursing Management

Preoperative Care

1 Coagulation studies are performed.
   a. Platelet donor packs and fresh frozen plasma must be available.
   b. Administer vitamin K for abnormalities of prothrombin time, as ordered.
   c. Prepare for transfusion of packed red cells or fresh whole blood if patient has significant anaemia.
2 Assist with preoperative physiotherapy—to reduce incidence of pulmonary complications; patient may be debilitated from haematological disease, from immunosuppressants, etc.
3 *Preoperative preparation for patient with rupture of spleen:*
   a. Administer whole blood if rupture of spleen has occurred.

b. Empty stomach contents with nasogastric tube—to prevent aspiration.

c. Check patient for pneumothorax/haemothorax—thoracotomy tube may be in place before anaesthesia is started.

Postoperative Care

1 See p. 441 General Aspects of Nursing Management Following Abdominal Surgery.
2 Watch for the development of complications—related to location of spleen, the reason for its removal and sequelae of splenectomy.
   a. Infection—especially in children.
   b. Thrombocytopaenia—if patient had thrombocytopaenia before splenectomy, the condition may become extreme after splenectomy.
   c. Persistent or recurrent haemorrhage.
   d. Thrombosis—may follow a few days after splenectomy; platelet count of three to five times normal values may occur; this postoperative physiological thrombocytosis may be conducive to thromboembolic complications.
      (1) Abdominal discomfort and fever may be caused by thrombi lodging in branches of portal system.
      (2) Mesenteric thrombosis—watch for postprandial cramping, abdominal pain; small bowel resection is indicated.
   e. Atelectasis of left lower lobe with pneumonia; pleural effusion—operations on left upper quadrant predispose to limited diaphragmatic movement.
   f. Subphrenic abscess—observe for persistent fever.

FURTHER READING

Biggs, R (Ed) (1976) Human Blood Coagulation, Haemostasis and Thrombosis, 2nd edition, Blackwell Scientific Publications

Bloom, H J G et al. (Eds) (1975) Cancer in Children,: Clinical Management, UICC, Springer-Verlag

Bonchard, R and Owens R, (1976) Nursing Care of the Cancer Patient, C V Mosby

Cabra, L G (1972) The Care of the Cancer Patient, Heinemann

(1978) Clinical Oncology, 2nd edition. A Manual for Students and Doctors, UICC, Springer-Verlag

Laurence, D R (1973) Clinical Pharmacology, 4th edition, Churchill Livingstone

Lowry, S (1974) Fundamentals of Radiation Therapy, Uni-Books, English Universities Press

Priestman, T J (1977) Cancer Chemotherapy, An Introduction, Mouledison Pharmaceuticals Ltd, Barnet, Herts

Thompson, R B (1975) A Short Textbook of Haematology, 4th edition, Pitman Medical

Tiffany, R (Ed) (1978) Oncology for Nurses and Health Care Professionals, Vols 1 and 2, Allen and Unwin

Walker, J (1977) Cancer and Radiotherapy, 2nd edition, Churchill Livingstone

Woodliff, H J and Hermann R P (1973) Concise Haematology, Edward Arnold

Articles
Anaemias
Editorial (1975) Bone marrow grafting for aplastic anaemia, Lancet, 1, 7897: 22–23

Leukaemia
Klastersky, J (1976) The use of synergistic combinations of antibodies in patients with haematological diseases, Clin. Haematol., 5: 361–377

Malignant Lymphomas and Non-Malignant Lymphomas
Sahakian, G J (1975) Management of Hodgkin's and non-Hodgkin's lymphomas, Med. Clin. N. Am., 59: 387–397
Sutherland, R M et al. (1975) Effect of splenectomy and radiotherapy on lymphocytes in Hodgkin's disease, Clin. Oncol., 1: 275–284
Tealey, A R (1976) Radiotherapy and Hodgkin's disease, Current Pract. Oncol. Nurs. 1: 89–99

Multiple Myeloma
Rickel, L (1976) Emotional support for the multiple myeloma patient, Nursing, 76, 6: 76–80
Schumann, D et al. (1975) Multiple myeloma, Am. J. Nurs., 75: 78–81

Transfusion Therapy
Djerassi, I (1975) Editorial: transfusions of filtered granulocytes, N. Engl. J. Med., 292: 803–4
Goldman, J M (1974) Leucocyte separation and transfusion, Brit. J. Haematol, 28: 271–275
Russell, J A et al. (1976) A practical guide to granulocyte transfusion therapy, J. Clin. Pathol., 29: 369–379

Chapter 3

CONDITIONS OF THE RESPIRATORY TRACT

CONCEPTS UNDERLYING RESPIRATORY FUNCTION, DISEASE AND THERAPY

Functions of the Respiratory System

1   Uptake of oxygen.
2   Elimination of carbon dioxide, thereby helping to maintain the pH of the blood.

Anatomical Components of the Respiratory System

1   Air passages through which air passes from the external environment to the alveolar–capillary membrane, and returns.
2   Alveolar–capillary membrane—through which diffusion of carbon dioxide and oxygen occurs between the gases in the alveolar air and in the blood.
3   Respiratory muscles, which enlarge the capacity of the thoracic cavity, thereby drawing air down the air passages to the lungs. These muscles are normally the diaphragm and intercostal muscles. The accessory muscles which may be used for

forceful inspiration are the sternocleidomastoid and the anterior serratus muscles.

4   Pleura, to transmit the movement of the respiratory muscles to the lung tissue, thus varying the negative pressure within the thoracic cavity.

5   Intact nerve pathway to the muscles, i.e., intercostal nerves to the intercostal muscles and phrenic nerve to the diaphragm.

6   Respiratory centre in the medulla.

Basic Terminology

1   *Ventilation*—movement of air in and out of the lungs by means of inspiration and expiration.

2   *Tidal volume*—amount of air moved in and out of the lungs and air passages with each breath under normal conditions. In an adult this is normally about 400 ml.

3   *Vital capacity*—the maximum volume of air that can be expelled from the lungs by forceful effort following a maximum inspiration.

4   *Perfusion*—filling of the pulmonary capillaries with venous blood which has returned to the heart from the systemic circulation, and is pumped from the right ventricle via the pulmonary artery to the lungs. Normally about 2% of this blood bypasses the alveoli and does not participate in gaseous exchange. This bypass is called shunting.

For further details, see Appendix, p. 361

Abbreviations

P_ACO_2: partial pressure of alveolar carbon dioxide.
P_aCO_2: partial pressure of arterial carbon dioxide.

Control of Respiration

The rate and depth of respiration is controlled by the respiratory centre in the medulla oblongata.

The rhythmicity of respiration is controlled by the pneumotaxic centre in the pons.

Afferent Impulses Affecting the Control of Respiration

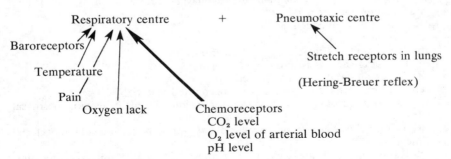

For detailed explanation of the physiology of gas exchange see Appendix, p. 361.

MAJOR MANIFESTATIONS OF BRONCHOPULMONARY DISEASE

Cough and Sputum Production

General Considerations

1   Coughing is a protective mechanism that serves to clear the airway.
2   Thick, mucopurulent sputum which is difficult to remove is more apt to cause violent coughing.
3   Violent coughing may cause bronchial obstruction and further irritation of the bronchi.
4   A severe, repeated or uncontrolled cough that is nonproductive is potentially harmful and may even cause syncope.
5   Cough-producing stimuli may be inflammatory, mechanical, chemical or thermal.
6   Clinical problems producing cough are infection, inflammation, neoplasms, cardiovascular disorders, trauma, physical agents and allergic disorders.

Nursing Management

1   Observe the character of the cough.
    a. Dry and hacking—may be due to nervousness, viral infections, bronchogenic carcinoma, early congestive heart failure.
    b. Loud and harsh—irritation in upper airway.
    c. Wheezing—associated with bronchospasm.
    d. Severe or changing in character or with position—may be bronchogenic cancer (cough, chest pain, haemoptysis).
    e. Loose—indicates problems in peripheral regions of bronchi and lung parenchyma.
    f. Painful—may indicate pleural involvement, chest wall disease.
    g. Chronic, productive—sign of bronchopulmonary disease.
2   Note time of cough and position of patient.
    a. Coughing paroxysms at night—may indicate bronchial asthma or left-sided heart failure.
    b. Cough that worsens when patient is supine—may be due to postnasal drip from sinusitis, bronchiectasis.
    c. Cough associated with food intake—may be the result of aspiration into tracheobronchial tree.
3   Relieve spasms of coughing.
    a. Vary position of the patient.
    b. Give suitable drinks, e.g., hot fruit drinks.
    c. Encourage and assist productive coughing.
    d. Drugs should be given as prescribed.
4   Observe character and quantity of expectorated material.
    a. Clear or mucoid—stems from viral infection, chronic bronchitis, postnasal drip.
    b. Thick yellow or green sputum—due to primary or secondary bacterial infections.
    c. Rusty—may indicate bacterial pneumonia (if patient not receiving antibiotics).

d. Malodorous—due to lung abscess, infection from fusospirochetal or anaerobic organisms.

e. Frothy pink sputum—indicates pulmonary oedema.

f. Note amount of sputum produced daily. A sudden decrease in the quantity of sputum may indicate inspissation (drying and thickening) in tracheobronchial tree and may lead to atelectasis, respiratory insufficiency and failure.

g. Layering of sputum in sputum cup occurs in lung abscess or bronchiectasis.

Haemoptysis

Expectoration of blood or bloodstained sputum.

Causes

1   Infections; bronchiectasis, pneumonia.
2   Neoplasm.
3   Pulmonary infarction.
4   Tuberculosis.
5   Lung abscess.
6   Blood dyscrasias.
7   Mitral stenosis.
8   Compression syndrome.

Nursing Management

1   Recognize the patient's fear and apprehension due to this threatening symptom and give him understanding and support, and ensure privacy.
2   Ascertain whether blood is coming from nose or throat, bronchi, lungs or gastrointestinal tract.
    a. Nose or throat—may flow, or may appear upon clearing of throat, without cough.
    b. Lungs—appears bright red and frothy; is accompanied by coughing and clearing of throat.
    c. Gastrointestinal tract—appears dark red, brown or black; is usually accompanied by vomiting and retching.
3   Place patient on involved side (if known).
4   Record quantity, colour, and character (mixed with mucus, pure blood).
5   Save all coughed-up blood for inspection by doctor.
6   Protect clothing.
7   Give small pieces of ice to suck.
8   Mouth care—frequent mouth washes should be given.
9   Observe pulse, blood pressure and general condition.
10 Give drugs as prescribed.

Hoarseness

Types

1   Acute hoarseness.
     When associated with febrile episode suggests viral laryngotracheobronchitis.

2 Persistent hoarseness.
   Indicates intrinsic neoplasm of vocal cord, recurrent laryngeal nerve damage, bronchogenic cancer, mediastinal lesion,, laryngeal tuberculosis.

Dyspnoea

Shortness of breath. May be acute, chronic, progressive, recurrent or paroxysmal.

Cause

In lung disease, shortness of breath is due to increase in lung rigidity, airway resistance or loss of lung elasticity. (See cardiac diseases for further causes).

Nursing Management

1 Ascertain circumstances that cause dyspnoea.
   a. How much activity provokes dyspnoea?
   b. Under what circumstances does it occur? (on exertion? when recumbent? on exposure to pollens?)
   c. Is there associated cough?
   d. Is dyspnoea associated with other symptoms?
   e. Is there expiratory wheeze?
2 Evaluate the nature of the shortness of breath.
   a. Acute dyspnoea associated with symptoms of infection (productive cough, fever, chills) suggests pneumonia.
   b. Sudden dyspnoea in ill or postoperative patient may indicate pulmonary embolus; pneumothorax.
   c. Orthopnoea—characteristic of cardiogenic pulmonary congestion.
   d. Expiratory wheeze—arises from obstructive disease in peripheral airways (asthma, chronic bronchitis, emphysema).
   e. Wheezing respirations—related to localized obstruction of major branches, tumour, foreign body.
   f. Inspiratory stridor—indicates partial obstruction at laryngeal or tracheal level.
   g. Paroxysmal wheezing unrelated to exertion—may arise from bronchial (allergic) asthma or bronchitis.
3 Relieve shortness of breath by:
   a. Removing cause if possible.
   b. Placing patient in well-supported position.
   c. Giving oxygen (if permitted).

Chest Pain

Underlying Considerations

1 Parietal pleura has rich supply of sensory nerves coming from intercostal nerves to the diaphragm. These nerve endings may be stimulated by inflammation and stretching of membranes and by respiratory movements—produces a characteristic sharp, knifelike pain.
2 Pleuropulmonary pain—bacterial pneumonia, infarction, spontaneous pneumothorax.
3 Other sources of chest pain may originate from the heart and large blood vessels, the oesophagus and chest wall.

Clinical Manifestations

1   Pleural pain is a common manifestation of inflammatory and malignant disease, but may also accompany pneumothorax and pulmonary embolism.
2   Pleural pain (usually well localized, sharp, and stabbing) occurs at end of inspiration.

Nursing Management

1   Assess quality, intensity and radiation of pain.
2   Note factors that precipitate pain.
3   Evaluate whether position of patient changes character of pain.
4   Determine the effect of inspiration and expiration on patient's pain.
5   Note other symptoms.
6   Relief measures.

Constitutional Symptoms of Bronchopulmonary Disease

1   Anorexia.
2   Fever.
3   Weight loss.
4   Fatigue, malaise, weakness. } related to duration and severity of disease.
5   Sweats.
6   Chills.

Constitutional Signs of Bronchopulmonary Disease

1   Cyanosis
2   Clubbing of fingers.
3   Wasting.

DIAGNOSTIC PROCEDURES FOR RESPIRATORY CONDITIONS

Auscultation of the Chest

A *stethoscope* is an instrument for conveying sounds from the chest wall to the ears of the listener.

Purpose

To recognize and localize abnormalities in lungs or pleura and heart and pericardium by sound.

Equipment

Stethoscope—may have bell chest piece, diaphragm chest piece, or both (Fig. 3.1)
    Bell—transmits relatively low-pitched sounds best
Diaphragm—transmits relatively high pitched sounds best

Underlying Principles

1   The doctor will need as quiet an environment as possible. All surplus clothing should be removed, so that nothing is touching the end or the tubing of the stethoscope.

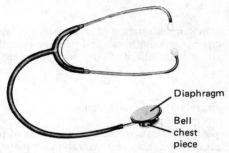

Figure 3.1.   Stethoscope with diaphragm and bell chest piece. (Courtesy: Bard Parker.)

2   If possible, have the patient sitting upright, and leaning slightly forward. A very ill patient may have to be gently turned from side to side.
3   Ask the patient to breathe with his mouth open.

Types of Sounds

Breath Sounds

1   The sound of normal breathing that is detected on the chest wall is generated by the rate at which air flows through the higher passages of the bronchial tree.
2   Since inspiration is shorter than expiration, air flows at a higher rate of speed during inspiration. The inspiratory sound is louder than the expiratory sound.
3   The character of normal breath sounds varies over different lung areas even in normal individuals.
4   A localized decrease in or absence of breath sounds may be noted in abnormal conditions.

Abnormal Breath Sounds

In diseases involving the bronchial tree and alveoli in such a way that fluid or mucus obstructs air flow, certain sounds, termed *adventitious sounds* (sounds not normally occurring), may be heard.

1   *Râles*—crackling or bubbling (discontinuous) noises; may also be called *crackles*. Râles sound like the crackling of tissue paper or the rubbing together of hairs at the end of the stethoscope. Râles may be fine, medium or coarse. Significance: pneumonia, pulmonary fibrosis or congestive heart failure.
2   *Rhonchi*—musical (continuous) sounds or vibrations, usually of longer duration; may also be called *wheezes*. Significance; airways obstruction.
    a. Generated from larger bronchi; heard in both inspiration and expiration.
    b. May vary in pitch, quality, and intensity.
3   *Pleural rub, or pleural friction rub*—leathery, grating, rough sound heard in both inspiration and expiration; induced by inflammation of pleural surfaces.
    a. Heard 'close' to the ear; sounds louder when stethoscope is pressed against the chest.
    b. Associated with breathing and unaffected by cough.

Palpation

Purpose

1   To identify areas of tenderness, masses or inflammation.
2   To assess mobility of ribs and spine.
3   To assess fremitus (palpable vibrations transmitted through the bronchopulmonary system on speaking).

Percussion

Purpose

To identify areas of dullness in the thorax, and to compare resonance on inspiration and expiration.

Diagnostic Studies

Radiography

Chest x-ray

1   Normal pulmonary tissue is radiolucent. Thus densities produced by tumours, foreign bodies, etc., can be detected.
2   Shows position of normal structures, displacement and presence of abnormal shadows.
3   Chest x-rays may reveal extensive pathology in the lungs in the absence of symptoms.

Tomography

1   Provides films of sections of lungs at different levels within the thorax.
2   Useful in demonstrating presence of small, solid lesions, calcification or cavitation within a lesion.

Computed Tomography

Computed tomography is an imaging method in which the lungs are scanned in successive layers by a narrow beam x-ray. A computer printout is obtained of the absorption values of the tissues in the plane that is being scanned.

It may be used to define pulmonary nodules, small tumours adjacent to pleural surfaces (which may be invisible on routine x-ray) and to demonstrate mediastinal abnormalities and hilar adenopathy.

Fluoroscopy

Enables radiologist to view heart, lungs and diaphragm in the dynamic (moving) state.

Barium Swallow

Outlines the oesophagus, revealing displacement of oesophagus and encroachment on its lumen, since cardiac, pulmonary and mediastinal abnormalities can be seen as deviations of the oesophagus.

Bronchography

A radiopaque medium is instilled directly into the trachea and bronchi and the entire bronchial tree or selected areas may be visualized. This is a diagnostic test for any disease that alters the calibre or patency of the bronchial tree or that causes its displacement.

1   Patient is assessed for allergic reaction to anaesthetic agent or contrast media before the test is started.
2   Topical anaesthesia is sprayed in the mouth, on tongue and posterior pharynx.
3   Local anaesthetic is injected into the larynx and tracheal tree.
    a. Extreme caution indicated in patients with respiratory insufficiency, since these patients may experience temporary problems with ventilation and diffusion.
    b. Oxygen, antispasmodic agents and cortisone should be available.
4   *Nursing responsibilities after bronchogram:*
    a. Withhold fluids and food until patient demonstrates a cough reflex.
    b. Encourage patient to cough and clear his bronchial tree; postural drainage may be required.
    c. A slight elevation of temperature is common following a bronchogram.
5   Physiotherapy is essential before and after this procedure.

Angiographic Studies of Pulmonary Vessels (radio-opacification of pulmonary blood vessels)

1   Contrast media injected into following blood vessels:
    a. Antecubital veins of one or both arms.
    b. Superior vena cava, right atrium, right ventricle or main pulmonary artery.
    c. Right or left pulmonary artery or one of its branches.
2   Films are taken in rapid sequence after injection.
    a. Useful in diagnosis of pulmonary vascular abnormalities (arterial aneurysm, thromboemboli, congenital disorders) and to detect abnormal vasculature arising from tumours.
3   Aortography—opacification studies of either thoracic aorta or abdominal aorta; taken when aneurysm of thoracic aorta is suspected.

Radioisotope Diagnostic Procedures

Perfusion Lung Scan

Following injection of a radioactive isotope, scans are made with a scintillation camera.

1   Measures blood perfusion through the lungs; evaluates lung function on a regional basis.
2   Useful in perfusion (vascular) abnormalities.

Ventilation Scan

1   Inhalation of radioactive gas (xenon), which diffuses throughout the lungs.
2   Useful in detecting ventilation abnormalities (emphysema).

Endoscopic Procedures

Bronchoscopy

The direct inspection and observation of the larynx, trachea and bronchi through a bronchoscope that is designed for passage through the trachea. It has both diagnostic and therapeutic purposes.

1 Uses
   a. Inspection of pathological changes in the bronchial tree.
   b. Removal of secretions (sputum) and tissue for cytologic and bacteriological study.
   c. Removal of a foreign body.
   d. Improvement of drainage.
   e. Treatment by application of chemotherapeutic agent.
2 Local (topical) or general anaesthesia is used.
3 *Nursing responsibilities:*
   a. Ensure that the patient understands the procedure, and that consent form is signed.
   b. Administer medication to reduce secretions and prevent vasovagal syncope and relieve anxiety. Give encouragement and nursing support.
   c. Restrict fluid and food for 6 hours before procedure—to reduce risk of aspiration when reflexes are blocked.
   d. Remove dentures, contact lenses and other prostheses.
   e. After the procedure, wait until patient demonstrates that he can cough before giving him cracked ice or fluids. A return to his usual diet is resumed in a few hours.
   f. Following bronchoscopy:
      (1) Ensure correct position before and after return of cough reflex.
      (2) Assist productive coughing.
   g. Following bronchoscopy watch patient for:
      (1) Cyanosis.
      (2) Hypotension.
      (3) Tachycardia and arrhythmia.
      (4) Haemoptysis.
      (5) Dyspnoea.
      (6) Bronchospasm.
      (7) Blocked airways.

Flexible Fiberoptic Bronchoscopy

Passage of thin, flexible and bronchofibrescope that can be directed into segmental bronchi; by its smaller size, flexibility and excellent optical system it allows increased visualization of peripheral airways.

1 May be done with patient resting in sitting or supine position.
2 Causes very little discomfort; better patient acceptance even under local anaesthetic only.
3 Allows for bronchial brush biopsy (see below).
4 Clinical applications for flexible fibreoptic bronchoscopy are similar to those for rigid bronchoscopy (see above); allows diagnostic visualization of enlarged area

for observation and biopsy; therapeutic removal of secretions, evaluation of haemoptysis.
5   Possible complications: reaction to anaesthetic agent, pneumothorax, bleeding.

Bronchial Brush Biopsy

Bronchofibrescope is introduced into the target bronchus under fluoroscopic monitoring. It is used to evaluate lung lesions and to identify pathogenic organisms.

1   Small brush attached to end of flexible wire is inserted through the fibrescope.
2   Tumour area is brushed back and forth to desquamate some of the mucosal cells.
   a. Smears and culture are made.
   b. Catheter is irrigated with saline for additional cultures and cytology material.
3   *Nursing responsibility:*
   a. See that Informed Consent has been signed.
   b. Patient may have a mild sore throat and transient haemoptysis after procedure.
   c. Possible complications: anaesthetic reactions, laryngospasm, pneumothorax (rare), haemoptysis.

Examination of Sputum

Purpose

1   Sputum is obtained for evaluation of gross appearance, for microscopic examination, for Gram staining and culture to identify the predominant organisms and for cytologic examination
   a. Direct smear—shows presence of pathogenic bacteria.
   b. Sputum culture—to make diagnosis, to determine drug sensitivity and to serve as a guide for drug treatment (choice of antibiotic).
   c. Sputum cytology (exfoliative cytology)—used to identify tumour cells.
2   Patients receiving antibiotics, steroids and immunosuppressive agents for prolonged periods may have periodic sputum examinations since these agents may give rise to opportunistic pulmonary infections.

Methods of Obtaining Sputum

Ensure patient is supported in correct position.

1   By deep breathing and coughing.
   a. Instruct patient to take several deep breaths, exhale and then clear his throat.
   b. Repeat three or four times.
   c. Cough vigorously and expectorate into sterile container.
   d. See that specimen is transported to laboratory immediately; allowing it to stand in a warm room will result in overgrowth of contaminating organisms and make culture more difficult and may alter cellular morphology.
   e. Give oral hygiene frequently especially if patient has foul sputum.
2   By ultrasonic or heated hypertonic saline nebulization.
   a. Patient inhales through mouth slowly and deeply for 10–15 min.
   b. Increases the moisture content of air going to lower tract; particles will condense on tracheobronchial tree and aid in expectoration.
3   Tracheal aspiration (see Guidelines, p. 247).

4 Bronchoscopic removal (p. 241).
5 Bronchial brushing guided by fluoroscopy (p. 241).
6 Gastric aspiration.
   a. Nasogastric tube is inserted into the stomach to siphon out swallowed pulmonary secretions.
   b. This test is useful for culture of tubercle bacilli. (See Volume 1, Chapter 6, Communicable Diseases for nursing implications.)
7 Transtracheal aspiration (Fig. 3.2).
   a. Extend the neck and place a pillow under the shoulders.
   b. Cleanse skin over cricothyroid membrane; doctor anaesthetizes area (lignocaine).

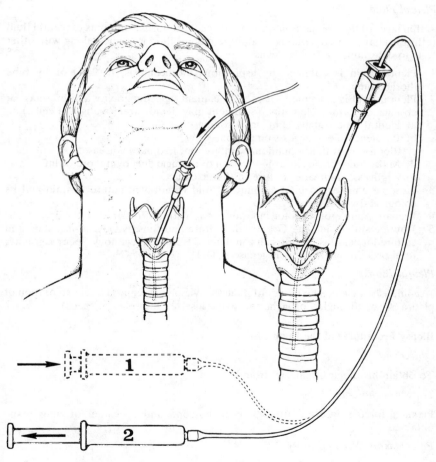

Figure 3.2.   Transtracheal aspiration.

c. A 14-gauge needle is inserted through the skin into the trachea and a polyethylene catheter is pushed through the needle into the trachea.
d. The needle is withdrawn, leaving the catheter in place.
e. Sterile saline (1–2 ml) is injected rapidly into the catheter, initiating a paroxysm of coughing.
f. Suction (by pulling back on barrel of syringe) is immediately applied and the secretions and exudates are aspirated into the catheter and syringe.
g. The catheter is withdrawn and pressure applied over the puncture site.
h. The contents of the syringe are expressed into a sterile culture tube.

Examination of Pleural Fluid and Pleural Biopsy

Pleural Fluid

A thin layer of fluid remains in the pleural space; abnormal amounts of pleural fluid (effusion) have varied aetiologies and the pleural fluid is studied along with other tests to determine underlying cause.

1 Pleural fluid is obtained by aspiration (thoracentesis, p. 248) or by tube thoracotomy.
2 Pleural fluid is examined for protein content, specific gravity and presence or absence of formed elements. (Sediment may demonstrate malignant cells.)
  a. Pleural fluid usually light straw colour.
  b. Purulent fluid—suggests empyema.
  c. Blood-tinged fluid—pulmonary infarction; neoplastic disease.
  d. Milky fluid (chylothorax)—invasion of thoracic duct by tumour or inflammatory process; traumatic rupture of thoracic duct.
3 Observe and record total amount of fluid withdrawn, nature of fluid and its colour and viscosity.
4 Prepare sample of fluid for laboratory evaluation if ordered.
5 Routine studies include Gram stain culture and sensitivity; acid-fast stain and culture for acid-fast bacilli; cell count and differential; cytology; specific gravity; total protein; lactic dehydrogenase (LDH).

Pleural Biopsy

Accomplished via needle biopsy of pleura or via pleuroscopy (visual exploration of pleural space through a bronchofibrescope inserted into pleural space).

Biopsy Procedures of the Lung

Objective

To obtain histological material from lung.

Transbronchoscopic Biopsy

Flexible forceps inserted through bronchoscope and specimen of lung tissue obtained.

Percutaneous Needle Biopsy

1 Skin site cleansed and anaesthetized.

2   Small skin incision is made and a needle is advanced under fluoroscopic control to the desired site.
3   With the needle in the periphery of the lesion, the stylet is removed, the syringe attached, and suction applied.
4   Specimen is smeared and fixed on a slide.

Open Lung Biopsy

1   Used in making a diagnosis when other biopsy methods fail.
2   Usually done by a small anterior thoracotomy; does not usually involve a rib resection.
3   Subsequent pneumothorax controlled by chest tube connected to a water-seal drainage system.

Lymph Node Biopsy (Scalene or Cervicomediastinal Nodes)

Objective

To detect lymph node spread of pulmonary disease. It is used as a diagnostic and prognostic measure.

1   Scalene lymph nodes are enmeshed in deep cervical pad of fat; these nodes drain lungs and mediastinum and may show histologic changes from intrathoracic disease.
2   Mediastinoscopy—surgery of superior mediastinum for exploration and biopsy of mediastinal nodes.
   a. Done to detect mediastinal involvement of pulmonary malignancy and to obtain tissue for diagnosis of other conditions (e.g., sarcoidosis).
   b. Biopsy usually done through a suprasternal incision.

Pulmonary Function Studies (Table 3.1).

1   Static lung volumes—low lung volumes indicate restrictive abnormalities (fibrosis, sarcoidosis, scoliosis). High residual volume (air remaining after maximal exhalation) indicates air trapping (emphysema).
2   Dynamic lung volumes (ventilatory studies)—reduction generally indicates airway obstruction (emphysema, bronchitis, asthma).
3   Diffusing capacity—reduction indicates loss of lung surface effective in transfer of gas (sarcoidosis, fibrosis, emphysema).

Essentials of Arterial Blood Gas Evaluation

Purpose

1   Are a measurement of the amount of oxygen and carbon dioxide present in arterial blood, as well as the pH of the blood.
2   Provide a means of assessing the adequacy of ventilation, i.e., the lungs supplying O_2 to the body and removing CO_2.
3   Helps assess the acid-base status in the body—whether acidosis or alkalosis is present and to what degree.

Table 3.1. Ventilatory Function Tests*

Description	Terms Used	Symbol	Remarks
The largest volume measured on complete expiration after the deepest inspiration without forced or rapid effort	Vital capacity	VC	This may be normal or even high in COLD patients and is *of little value by itself*
The vital capacity performed with expiration as forceful and rapid as possible	Forced vital capacity	FVC	This volume is often significantly reduced in COLD due to air trapping, and is an important standard measurement
Volume of gas exhaled over a given time interval during the performance of forced vital capacity	Forced expiratory volume (qualified by subscript indicating the time interval in seconds)	FEV_T ($FEV_{1.0}$)	If below predicted normal values, this is a valuable clue to the severity of the expiratory airway obstruction
FEV_T expressed as a percentage of the forced vital capacity: $\frac{FEV_T}{FVC} \times 100$	Percentage expired (in T seconds)	$FEV_{T\%}$	This time–volume relationship is another way of expressing the presence of airway obstruction
The average rate of flow for a specified portion of the forced expiratory volume, usually between 200 and 1200 ml	Forced expiratory flow	$FEF_{200-1200}$	Formally called maximum expiratory flow rate (MEFR). A slowed rate is an early manifestation of COLD
Average rate of flow during the middle half of the forced expiratory volume	Forced midexpiratory flow	$FEF_{25-75\%}$	Formerly called maximum mid-expiratory flow rate. This is slowed early in the course of ventilatory impairment
Volume of air which a subject can breathe with voluntary maximal effort for a given time	Maximal voluntary ventilation	MVV	Formerly called maximum breathing capacity. Another valuable test, usually correlating well with the patient's complaint of dyspnoea

* American Lung Association: Chronic Obstructive Pulmonary Disease, 1972, p. 42.

Clinical Uses of Arterial Blood Gas Studies

Arterial blood gas studies are helpful in diagnosis and treatment in the presence of the following:

1 Unexpected tachypnoea, dyspnoea (especially in patients with cardiopulmonary disease).
2 Unexpected restlessness and anxiety in bed patients.
3 Drowsiness and confusion in patients receiving oxygen therapy.
4 Before thoracic and other major surgery.
5 Before and during prolonged oxygen therapy and during ventilator support of patients.
6 Crically ill cardiopulmonary patients; tissue oxygenation and acid-base balance eventually affected.

GUIDELINES: Tracheal Aspiration

Purpose

To obtain a sputum specimen; to relieve obstruction.

Equipment

Tracheal aspirate specimen collection set.

Procedure

Nursing Action	Reason
NOTE: Tracheal aspiration requires education and clinical practice under expert supervision.	
1 Use sterile equipment: **a.** Sterile catheter No. 16 F, connecting tubing to tracheal aspirate specimen collection set. **b.** Sterile gloves.	1 To prevent introduction of organisms into the respiratory system.
2 Oxygenate patient before and after each passage of the catheter.	
3 Using one hand, pass the catheter (suction turned off) through the nose; place the other hand on the patient's forehead.	3 To stabilize the patient's head and to reassure the patient.
4 When the catheter reaches the larynx, coughing may be stimulated. Gently advance the catheter into the trachea.	4 At this point, coughing is unproductive.
5 Pull catheter slightly forward; this will initiate vigorous coughing. Provide tissues for patient's expectorations.	5 Irritation of trachea triggers coughing reflex.

6   Pinch off and remove catheter gently.
7   Send specimen to laboratory.
8   Comfort patient.

GUIDELINES: Assisting the Patient Undergoing Chest Aspiration

Chest Aspiration (Thoracentesis) is the aspiration of fluid or air from the pleural space. It may be a diagnostic or a therapeutic procedure (Fig. 3.3).

Purposes

1   To remove fluid and air from the pleural cavity.
2   To obtain diagnostic aspiration of pleural fluid.
3   To obtain pleural biopsy.

Equipment

Syringes: 5-20-25, 50-ml syringes
Needles: Nos. 22, 26, 16 (7·5 cm long)
Three-way tap and rubber tubing
Local anaesthetic
Biopsy needle
Antiseptic lotion for skin cleansing.

Sterile pack containing:
   Gauze swabs, gallipots,
   dissecting forceps, wool swabs,
   sterile towels, sterile jug
Three sterile specimen containers
Sterile gloves
Spencer Wells artery forceps

Procedure

Nursing Action	Reason
Preparatory Phase	
1 Ascertain in advance if chest x-rays have been ordered and completed. These should be available at the bedside.	1 Posteroanterior and lateral chest x-rays are used to localize fluid and air in the pleural cavity and to aid in determining the puncture site.
2 See if consent form has been explained and signed.	
3 Determine if the patient is allergic to the local anaesthetic agent to be used. Give sedation if ordered.	
4 Inform the patient about the procedure and indicate how he can be helpful. Explain: **a.** The nature of the procedure. **b.** The importance of remaining immobile.	4 The patient should be encouraged to ask questions before the procedure. If he wishes to speak or cough during the procedure, he should warn the doctor, before doing so, by raising the hand on the opposite side to the aspiration.

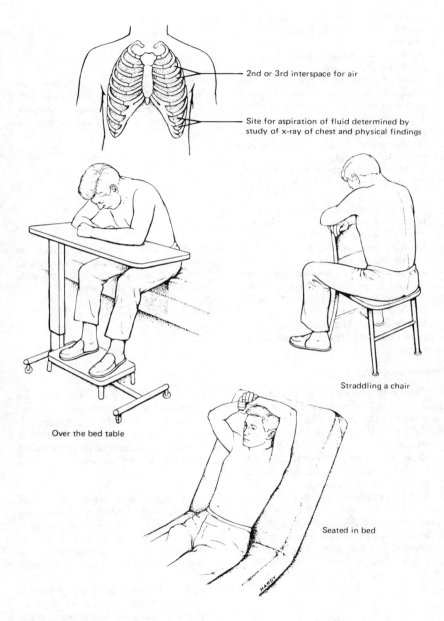

2nd or 3rd interspace for air

Site for aspiration of fluid determined by
study of x-ray of chest and physical findings

Over the bed table

Straddling a chair

Seated in bed

Figure 3.3.   Chest aspiration. Positioning patient and selecting site for chest aspiration.

c. Pressure sensations to be experienced, but he should indicate if he is in pain.

d. That no discomfort is anticipated after the procedure.

5 Make the patient comfortable with adequate supports. If possible place him upright and in one of the following positions:

a. Sitting on the edge of the bed with feet supported and head on a padded over-the-bed table.

b. Stradding a chair with his arms and head resting on the back of the chair.

If he is unable to assume a sitting position have him lie on the unaffected side.

5 The upright position facilitates the removal of fluid that usually localizes at the base of the chest. A comfortable position helps the patient to relax.

6 Support and reassure the patient during the procedure.

a. Prepare the patient for sensations of cold from skin cleanser and for pressure and sting from infiltration of local anaesthetic agent.

b. Encourage the patient to refrain from coughing. A cough linctus may be needed.

6 Sudden and unexpected movement by the patient can cause trauma to the visceral pleura with possible penetration of the lung.

Performance Phase

1 Expose the entire chest. The site for aspiration is determined from chest x-rays and by percussion. If fluid is in the pleural cavity the thoracentesis site is determined by study of the chest x-ray and physical findings, with attention to the site of maximal dullness on percussion.

1 If air is in the pleural cavity, the aspiration site is usually in the second or third intercostal space in the midclavicular line. Air rises in the thorax because the density of air is much less than the density of liquid.

2 The procedure is done under aseptic conditions. After the skin is cleansed, the doctor slowly injects a local anaesthetic with a small calibre needle into the skin, then into the deeper tissues.

2 An intradermal wheal is raised slowly; rapid intradermal injection causes pain. The parietal pleura is very sensitive and should be well in filtrated with anaesthetic before the aspiration needle is passed through it.

a. When a large quantity of fluid is withdrawn, a three-way adapter serves to keep air from entering the pleural cavity.

b. The artery forceps steady the needle on the chest wall. Sudden pleuritic pain or shoulder pain may indicate that the visceral or diaphragmatic pleura are being irritated by the needle point.

3 The doctor advances the aspiration needle with the syringe attached. When the pleural space is reached, suction may be applied with the syringe.

   a. A 20- or 50-ml syringe with a three-way adapter (stopcock) is attached to the needle. (One end of the adapter is attached to the needle and the other to the tubing leading to a receptacle that receives the fluid being aspirated.)

   b. If a considerable quantity of fluid is to be removed, the needle is held in place on the chest wall with a small pair of artery forceps.

4 After the needle is withdrawn, pressure is applied over the puncture site and a small sterile dressing is fixed in place.

5 Observe patient for faintness or shock.

Follow-up Phase

1 A chest x-ray is usually obtained following chest aspiration.

1 Chest x-ray verifies that there is no pneumonthorax.

2 Record the total amount of fluid withdrawn and the nature of the fluid and carefully label the specimen jars. A specimen container with formalin may be needed if a pleural biopsy is being performed.

2 The fluid may be clear, serous, bloody, purulent, etc.

3 Observe the patient frequently for increasing respirations, faintness, vertigo, tightness in the chest, uncontrollable cough, blood-tinged frothy mucus and rapid pulse.

3 Pneumothorax, tension pneumothorax, subcutaneous emphysema or pyogenic infection may result from an aspiration. Pulmonary oedema or cardiac distress can be produced by a sudden shift in mediastinal contents when large amounts of fluid are aspirated.

CHEST PHYSIOTHERAPY

The following exercises are normally carried out by a physiotherapist. However, nurses working in a specialized unit should fully understand the principles of these exercises, and be able to carry out basic physiotherapy in the absence of an expert.

Postural Drainage Exercise

Postural drainage is the use of specific positions so that the force of gravity can assist in the removal of bronchial secretions from the affected bronchioles into the bronchi and trachea (Fig. 3.4).

Underlying Principles

1   The patient is positioned so that the diseased area(s) are in a vertical position, and gravity is used to assist drainage of the specific segment(s).
2   The positions assumed are determined by the location, severity and duration of mucus obstruction.
3   The exercises are usually performed two to four times daily, before meals and at bedtime.

Nursing Management

1   Make the patient comfortable before the procedure starts and as comfortable as possible while he assumes each position.
   a. Bronchodilator medications may be inhaled before postural drainage to reduce bronchospasm, decrease thickness of mucus and sputum, and combat oedema of the bronchial walls.
   b. Use a back rest to prop up patient to desired height if his bed is not adjustable; have a sputum pot ready.
2   Use a stethoscope to determine the areas of needed drainage.
3   Upper lobes are generally drained by upright positions; lower and middle lobes are drained by head-down positions.
4   Place patient in left prone and left oblique positions (simultaneously)—this will give additional drainage to middle lobe and lateral segments of the right lower lobe; assuming the right prone and right oblique position (simultaneously) will give additional drainage to middle lobe and lateral segments of the left lower lobe.
5   Encourage the patient to cough after he has spent the allotted time in each position.
6   Encourage diaphragmatic breathing (p. 256) throughout postural drainage exercises; this helps widen airways so that secretions can be drained.
7   Chest wall percussion (by another person) may be desirable to loosen and propel sputum in the direction of gravity drainage.
8   Evaluate patient's colour and pulse the first few times he performs these exercises.
9   Help the patient to brush his teeth and use mouthwash after postural drainage.
10 Encourage patient to rest in bed following the procedure.

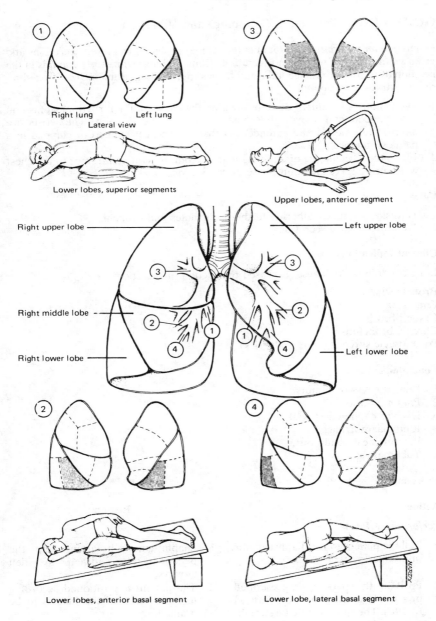

Figure 3.4.   Postural drainage.

GUIDELINES: Percussion (Clapping) and Vibration

Percussion and vibration are manual techniques designed to loosen secretions and promote drainage of mucus and secretions from the lungs while the patient is in the position of postural drainage indicated for his specific lung problem. The procedure requires trained personnel.

1 *Percussion*—Movement done by striking the chest wall in a rhythmical fashion with cupped hands over the chest segment to be drained. The wrists are alternatively flexed and extended so that the chest is cupped or clapped in a painless manner.
2 *Vibration*—Technique of applying manual compression and tremor to the chest wall during the exhalation phase of respiration.

Purposes

1 To dislodge mucus adhering to the bronchioles and bronchi.
2 To help mobilize secretions.

Clinical Indications

Lung conditions that cause increased production of secretions.

Bronchiectasis
Empyema
Cystic fibrosis
Chronic bronchitis
Postthoracic surgery (with analgesics)

Contraindications

1 Lung abscess or tumurs.
2 Pneumothorax.
3 Disease of the chest wall.
4 Lung haemorrhage.
5 Painful chest conditions.
6 Tuberculosis.

Procedure

Action

Reason

Performance Phase

1 Tell the patient to use diaphragmatic breathing (p.192).

1 Diaphragmatic breathing helps the patient to relax and helps to widen airways.

2 Position the patient in prescribed postural drainage position(s) (p.190). The spine should be straight to promote rib cage expansion.

2 The patient is positioned according to which area of the lung is to be drained.

3 Percuss (or clap) with cupped hands over the chest wall for 1 or 2 min from:
a. The lower ribs to shoulders in the back.
b. The lower ribs to top of chest in front.

3 This action helps to dislodge mucous plugs and mobilize secretions toward the main bronchi and trachea. The air trapped between the operator's hand and chest wall will produce a characteristic hollow sound.

4 Avoid clapping over the spine, liver, kidneys or spleen.

4 Percussion over these areas may cause injuries to the spine and internal organs.

5 Instruct the patient to inhale slowly and deeply. Vibrate the chest wall as the patient exhales slowly through pursed lips.
a. Place one hand on top of the other over affected area or place one hand on each side of the rib cage.
b. Tense the muscles of the hands and arms causing the arms to vibrate in a rapid motion.
c. Relieve pressure on the thorax as the patient inhales.
d. Encourage the patient to cough, using his abdominal muscles, after three or four vibrations.

5 This sets up a vibration that carries through the chest wall and helps free the mucus.
b. This manoeuvre is performed in the direction in which the ribs move upon expiration.
d. Contracting the abdominal muscles while coughing increases cough effectiveness. Coughing aids in the movement and expulsion of secretions.

6 Allow the patient to rest several minutes.

7 Listen with a stethoscope to changes in breath sounds.

7 The appearance of moist sounds (râles, rhonchi) indicates movement of air around mucus in the bronchi.

8 Repeat the percussion and vibration cycle according to the patient's tolerance and his clinical response; usually 15–20 min.

GUIDELINES: Teaching the Patient Breathing Exercises

Breathing exercises are exercises and breathing practices that are utilized to correct respiratory deficits and to increase efficiency in breathing.

Purposes
1 To relax muscles and relieve anxiety.
2 To eliminate useless unco-ordinated patterns of respiratory muscle activity.
3 To slow the respiratory rate.
4 To decrease the work of breathing.
5 To expand lower lobe and prevent hypostatic pneumonia and facilitate venous return.

General Instructions

1 Clear the nasal passages before beginning breathing exercises.
2 Always inhale through the nose—permits filtration, humidification and warming of air.
3 Breathe slowly in a rhythmical and relaxed manner—permits more complete exhalation and emptying of lungs; helps overcome anxiety associated with dyspnoea and decreases oxygen requirement.
4 Avoid sudden exertion.
5 Practise breathing exercises in several positions, since air distribution and pulmonary circulation vary according to position of the chest.

Diaphragmatic Breathing

Purpose

To increase the use of the diaphragm during breathing.

Teaching Procedure

Instruct the patient as follows:

Reason

1 Place one hand on stomach just below the ribs and the other hand on the middle of the chest.

1 This helps the patient to become aware of the diaphragm and its function in breathing.

2 Breathe in slowly and deeply through the nose, letting the abdomen protrude as far as it will (Fig. 3.5a). The abdomen enlarges during inspiration and decreases in size during expiration.

2 Slow inhalation provides ventilation and hyperinflation of the lungs.

3 Breathe out through pursed lips while contracting (tightening) the abdominal muscles.

3 Contracting the abdominal muscles assists the diaphragm in rising to empty the lung.

4 The chest should move as little as possible; attention should be directed to the abdomen, not the chest.

4 Contraction of the abdominal muscles should take place during expiration.

5 Repeat for approximately 1 min (followed by a rest period of 2 min). Work up to 10 min, four times daily.

6 Learn to do diaphragmatic breathing while lying, then sitting and ultimately standing and walking.

6 Diaphragmatic breathing should become automatic with sufficient practice and concentration. If the patient becomes short of breath have him stop the exercises until his breathing pattern comes under control.

Other Exercises

Lateral Costal Breathing

1 Place hands on sides on lower ribs.

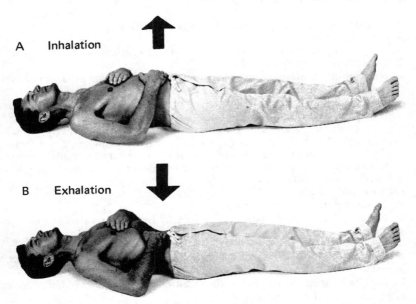

A   Inhalation

B   Exhalation

Figure 3.5.   Breathing exercises for inhalation and exhalation. (From: Living with Asthma Chronic Bronchitis, and Emphysema, Riker Laboratories, Inc., Northridge, CA).

2   Inhale deeply and slowly while sides expand, moving hands outward.
3   Exhale slowly and feel the hands and ribs move in.
4   Rest.

Posterior Basal Breathing

1   Sit in a chair. Place hands behind back; hold flat against lower ribs.
2   Inhale deeply and slowly while rib cage expands backward; the hands will move outward.
3   Keep hands in place. Blow out slowly; hands will move in.

Respiratory Failure and Insufficiency

Terminology

1   *Respiratory insufficiency*—altered function of the respiratory system which produces clinical symptoms—usually includes dyspnoea.
2   *Chronic respiratory failure:*
   a. Hypoxia (decreased P_aO_2) or hypercapnia (increased P_aCO_2).
   b. Due to disorder of any component of the respiratory system.
   c. Occurs usually over a period of months to years—allows for activation of compensatory mechanisms.
3   *Acute respiratory failure:*
   a. Hypoxia (P_aO_2 less than 6.6–8.0 kPa; 50–60 mmHg) or hypercapnia (P_aCO_2 greater than 6.6 kPa; 50 mm g).

b. Occurs rapidly, usually in minutes to hours or days.
4   *Ventilatory failure.*
   a. Respiratory failure due to decreased alveolar ventilation.
   b. Characterized by elevated $P_a\text{CO}_2$).
   c. Relationship to *minute volume* (amount of air inhaled and exhaled in 1 min).
      (1) Alveolar ventilation + *dead space ventilation* = minute volume. (Dead space is amount of air moving in and out of conducting airways and other areas of lung which are ventilated but not perfused with blood).
      (2) Ventilatory failure may be present even if minute volume is normal or even high. The lung disorder causes an increase in dead space ventilation.
      (3) In ventilatory failure due to disorders of the respiratory control centre or disorders of the thoracic cage and muscles, the minute volume and alveolar ventilation are reduced.
5   *Oxygenation failure:*
   a. Consists purely of a decreased $P_a\text{O}_2$.
   b. Found primarily in localized or diffuse infiltrative or vascular pulmonary disorders.
6   *Obstructive disorder:*
   A. Ventilatory insufficiency or failure due to impaired airflow in conducting airways.
   b. Results from airway narrowing (bronchitis, asthma) or loss of lung elasticity required to expel air (emphysema).
7   *Restrictive disorder*—ventilatory insufficiency or failure due to impaired movement of the thoracic cage or musculature or to increased lung stiffness.

Causes of Respiratory Failure

1   Disorders of the respiratory control centre.
   a. Drug intoxication (general anaesthetics, narcotics, barbiturates, hypnotics, excessive oxygen administration to patients with chronic obstructive lung disease).
   b. Vascular disorders (brainstem infarction and haemorrhage, decreased perfusion due to shock).
   c. Trauma (head injury, increased intracranial pressure).
   d. Infection (meningitis, encephalitis).
   e. Others ('primary alveolar hypoventilation', myxoedema coma, status epilepticus).
2   Disorders of impulse transmission.
   a. Drug intoxication (curariform drugs, anticholinesterases).
   b. Degenerative disorders (amyotrophic lateral sclerosis, multiple sclerosis).
   c. Infection (poliomyelitis, Guillain-Barré syndrome, tetanus, rabies).
   d. Trauma (transection of the spinal cord).
   e. Others (myasthenia gravis).
3   Disorders of the thoracic wall and musculature.
   a. Skeletal (scoliosis, flail chest, multiple rib fractures, thoracotomy).
   b. Muscular (polymyositis, muscular dystrophies).
   c. Pleural (effusion, haemothorax, empyema, fibrothorax, pneumothorax).
4   Disorders of conducting airways.

a. Upper airways (foreign body, epiglottitis, laryngitis, smoke and noxious gas inhalation, acute laryngeal oedema, tumour).

b. Peripheral airways (chronic bronchitis, emphysema, asthma).

5   Disorders involving the alveolar-capillary membrane.

a. Infection (lobar, aspiration or interstitial pneumonia).

b. Vascular (thromboemboli, fat emboli, polyarteritis, Wegener's granulomatosis, pulmonary oedema).

c. Neoplasm (lymphogenous spread of carcinoma).

d. Others (interstitial fibrosis, uraemic pneumonitis, shock lung, noncardiac pulmonary oedema).

Clinical Manifestations of Respiratory Failure

Nursing History	Interpretation
Cough, dyspnoea, wheezing, sputum production and colour.	*Any* recent *change* should point to an abnormality of the lung and raise suspicion of respiratory insufficiency or failure.
Drug usage.	May point to depression of the respiratory control centre and raise the likelihood of ventilatory failure.
Oxygen administration	Oxygen administration, particularly in patients with chronic bronchitis or emphysema who are dependent on hypoxaemia as a stimulus to breathing and who have grown insensitive to carbon dioxide as a stimulus to breathing, may bring about ventilatory failure.
Weakness or paralysis	Weakness or paralysis in any other part of the body indicates the possibility of weakness or paralysis of the thoracic muscles and actual or impending ventilatory failure.
State of responsiveness	Coma occurs early in disorders of the respiratory control centre but may be a late manifestation of other causes of respiratory failure; *any otherwise unexplained change in the level of consciousness should raise the possibility of respiratory failure.*
Respiratory rate	Reduced in disorders of the respiratory control centre; rapid respiratory rate occurs early in disorders of the thoracic cage and musculature and of the lung proper.

Nursing History	Interpretation
Pattern of respiration	Abnormalities of rhythm (Cheyne–Stokes respiration, Biot's respiration) are found in disorders of the respiratory control centre.
Depth of respiration	Shallow in disorders of the respiratory control centre, disorders of impulse transmission and weakness of the thoracic musculature; *may be deceptively normal* in disorders of the lung.
Use of accessory muscles of breathing (scalene, sternomastoid and pectoralis) and intercostal retraction.	Laboured breathing usually seen in disorders of the lung parenchyma, skeletal deformities.
Pulse	Usually rapid in acute respiratory failure, but may be deceptively normal in disorders of the respiratory control centre (drug intoxication) and disorders of impulse transmission (Guillain—Barré syndrome).
Cyanosis	Useful only when present; absence of cyanosis, however, does not exclude respiratory failure.
Chest Auscultation	Abnormalities may indicate lung disease; *breath sounds may be decreased in intensity or deceptively 'normal' in severe airway obstruction.*

Nursing Alert:
1 **Any of the abnormalities outlined above should point to the possibility of actual or impending respiratory failure.**
2 **Arterial blood gases should be obtained whenever the nursing history or patient assessment suggests respiratory insufficiency or failure.**
3 **Even if arterial blood gas studies are normal, respiratory insufficiency may still be present and may progress to respiratory failure.**
4 **Bedside measurement of the vital capacity at frequent intervals is helpful in following the progress of patients with disorders of the respiratory control centre, or impulse transmission, or of the thoracic musculature.**

Treatment of Respiratory Insufficiency and Failure
1 Ventilatory insufficiency and failure.
   a. *Without lung disease:*
      (1) Specific treatment for cause of respiratory failure (i.e., narcotic antagonist for narcotic or narcotic analogue intoxication, pyridostigmine for myasthenia gravis).
      (2) Ventilatory support with mechanical ventilator if P_aCO_2 is elevated, or if vital capacity is 1 l or less, *or if there is rapid progression of signs and symptoms.*

b. *With underlying lung disease* (usually emphysema or chronic bronchitis).
  (1) Treat the cause of exacerbation (i.e., antibiotics for respiratory infection).
  (2) Restore airflow in conducting airways.
    (a) Bronchodilators for bronchospasm.
    (b) Mucolytics to liquefy mucus plugs.
    (c) Chest physiotherapy to remove mucus plugs.
  (3) Increase alveolar ventilation.
    (a) Remove respiratory depressants such as drugs or excessive oxygen.
    (b) Encourage deep breathing.
    (c) Administer intermittent positive pressure breathing with monitoring of tidal volume.
  (4) Give ventilatory support with mechanical ventilator *if*:
    (a) pH is less than 7.25 and P_aCO_2 is greater than 8 kPa (60 mmHg) *or* if tidal flow is less than 230 l/min *or* if
    (b) P_aCO_2 rises by 0.6 kPa (5 mmHg) or more per hour—*or* if
    (c) Patient cannot co-operate with other therapeutic methods.
2 Oxygenation failure.
  a. Give specific treatment for underlying disorder (i.e., antibiotics for pneumonia; diuretics for pulmonary oedema due to left ventricular failure).
  b. Administer oxygen to maintain P_aO_2 of 60 mmHg using devices that provide increased oxygen concentrations (cannula, aerosol mask, partial rebreathing mask, nonrebreathing mask).
  c. If P_aO_2 of 60 mmHg cannot be achieved with devices described above or if inspired oxygen concentration required is greater than 60% for 24 hours, patient may require intubation and the use of intermittent positive pressure ventilation (IPPV) with mechanical ventilation or Continuous Positive Airway Pressure (CPAP) without mechanical ventilation.

Pharmacology

For commonly used nebulized drugs see Table 3.2.

OXYGEN THERAPY

General Considerations

1 Oxygen is an odourless, tasteless, colourless transparent gas that is slightly heavier than air.
2 Oxygen supports combustion, so there is always danger of fire when oxygen is being used.
  a. Avoid using oil or grease around oxygen connections.
  b. Eliminate antiseptic tinctures, alcohol and ether in immediate oxygen environment.
  c. Do not permit any electrical devices (radios, heating pads, electric razors) in or near an oxygen tent.
  d. Keep the oxygen cylinder (if used) secured in an upright position away from heat.
  e. Post NO SMOKING signs on the patient's door and in view of the patient's visitors.

Table 3.2. Commonly Used Nebulized Drugs

	Pharmacological Effect	Indications	Side-Effects
Bronchodilators and Decongestants			
Salbutamol (Ventolin)	Sympathomimetics with selective Beta 2 activity	Bronchospasm	Rare
Terbutaline (Bricanyl)	Sympathomimetics with selective Beta 2 activity	Bronchospasm	Rare
Orciprenaline (Alupent)	Sympathomimetics with selective Beta 2 activity	Bronchospasm	Rare
Mucolytic			
N-Acetylcysteine (Airbron)	Lowers viscosity of mucus. Action occurs after 1 min	Abnormally thick or inspissated secretions in airways	May cause bronchospasm, and a bronchodilator drug may be needed. If patient has difficulty coughing up secretions, vigorous suction may be needed
Tyloxapol (Alevaire)	Lowers viscosity of mucus. Action occurs after 1 min	Abnormally thick or inspissated secretions in airways	
Corticosteroids			
Beclamethasone (Becotide)	Synthetic corticosteroid with potent anti-inflammatory action	Steroid dependent asthma	Oral moniliasis. N.B.: Should not be used in status asthmaticus, C.I., pulmonary tuberculosis (old lesions)
Miscellaneous			
Disodium Chromoglycate (Intal) plain *or* with Isoprenaline	Inhibits release of histamine from mast cells in the respiratory tract when inhaled as a dry powder; prevents acute attacks *only*, and must be used *regularly* for 2–4 weeks to demonstrate effectiveness	Allergic asthma	Cough, bronchospasm. N.B.: Not used in patients with status asthmaticus

f. Have fire extinguisher available.
3   Oxygen is dispensed from a cylinder or piped-in system and requires:
    a. *Reduction gauge*—reduces pressure to that of the atmosphere.
    b. *Flow meter* (flow gauge, flow control)—regulates control of oxygen in litres per minute.
4   Oxygen is given to relieve hypoxia, either local or generalized.
    a. *Hypoxia*—a state in which there is an insufficient amount of oxygen available in the tissue cells to meet the requirements of an organ or tissue at that moment.
    b. *Hypoxaemia*—a decrease in the oxygen content of the blood.
5   Measurement of the arterial blood gases is the best method of determining the need for and adequacy of oxygen therapy (p. 183).

Clinical Assessment

1   A change in the patient's respiration is often evidence of the need for oxygen therapy.
2   Other signs of hypoxia, such as cyanosis, may or may not be present.
3   The *goal* in administering oxygen is to treat the hypoxia while decreasing the work of breathing and stress on the myocardium.
4   The appropriate form of oxygen therapy is best ascertained after obtaining arterial blood gases, which will indicate the patient's oxygenation status and acid-base balance.
5   Oxygen must be given with extreme caution to some patients. In certain conditions (chronic obstructive lung disease) the administration of a high oxygen concentration will remove the respiratory drive that has been created largely by the patient's low oxygen tension.
    a. Ventilation is reduced.
    b. Acute acidosis and carbon dioxide narcosis may follow.

NOTE: Oxygen toxicity should always be of concern in the patient receiving inspired concentrations over 60% for over 24 hours.

Oxygen Delivery Systems

1   Oxygen may be administered by nasal cannula, oropharyngeal catheter (nasal catheter), various types of face masks and tent. It may also be applied directly to endotracheal or tracheal tube via T-piece or hyperinflation bag.
2   The method selected depends on the concentration of oxygen required.

Monitoring Oxygen Therapy

Nursing Alert:

1   **Arterial blood gas evaluations are the best means of gauging the effectiveness of oxygen therapy and guiding appropriate changes. Of particular importance is the effect of oxygen therapy on the patient who has chronic obstructive lung disease and who may retain carbon dioxide if given too much oxygen. Frequent blood gas evaluations may be necessary in this type of patient to make sure that his respiratory drive is not suppressed. Also continue clinical observations, as above.**
2   **Various types of oxygen analysers are available which allows the nurse to measure the concentration of oxygen delivered to the patient. Oxygen analysers are**

especially useful in measuring the amount of oxygen delivered by the various types of masks.

GUIDELINES: Administering Oxygen by Nasal Cannula (Fig. 3.6)

Purpose

To administer a low-to-medium concentration of oxygen, when precise accuracy is not essential.

Equipment

Oxygen source
Plastic nasal cannula with connecting tubing (disposable)
Humidifier filled with sterile distilled water to indicated level
Flowmeter
NO SMOKING signs (2)

Procedure

Preparatory Phase

1   Post NO SMOKING signs on patient's door and in view of patient and visitors.
2   Show the nasal cannula to the patient and explain the procedure.
3   Make sure the humidifier is filled to the appropriate mark. If the humidifier bottle is too full, the bubbling water will overflow into the gauges.
4   Attach the connecting tube from the nasal cannula to the humidifier outlet.
5   Set the flow rate at 2 l/min. Feel to determine if oxygen is flowing through the nasal tips of the cannula.

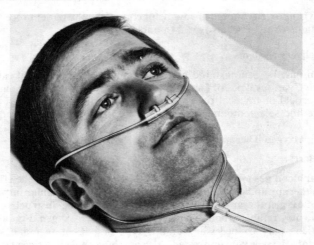

Figure 3.6.   Administering oxygen by nasal cannula. (Courtesy: Hudson Oxygen Therapy Sales Company.)

Nursing Action	Reason

Performance Phase

1 Place the tips of the cannula in the patient's nose.

2 Adjust flow rate to prescribed rate.

Nursing Alert: Patients who require low, constant concentrations of oxygen and whose breathing pattern varies greatly may need to use the venturi mask particularly if they are carbon dioxide retainers.

If higher concentrations are required, consider an alternate form of therapy.

3 Fasten tubing to the pillow and bed clothing.

Follow-up Phase

1 Change cannula, humidifiers, tubing and other equipment exposed to moisture daily.

2 Assess patient's condition and the functioning of equipment at regular intervals.

1 Position the cannula so that the tips do not extend more than 2.5 cm (1 in) into the nares.

2 A flow of 0.5–5 l/min should provide an inspired oxygen concentration of 22–35%, depending on the patient's breathing pattern. (The greater the minute volume, the less the oxygen enrichment).

Flow rates in excess of 6 l/min may lead to air swallowing and cause irritation to the nasal and pharyngeal mucosa.

1 Contaminated equipment may cause virulent infections in debilitated patients.

2 Assess the patient for mental aberration, disturbed consciousness, abnormal colour, perspiration, changes in blood pressure and increasing heart and respiratory rates.

GUIDELINES: Administering Oxygen by Oropharyngeal Catheter*

Purpose

To administer moderate to moderately high concentrations of oxygen.

Equipment

Oxygen source
Flowmeter
Humidifier filled with sterile distilled water to appropriate mark
Oropharyngeal catheter
   No. 8–10 F for children
   No. 10–12 F for women
   No. 12–14 F for men.

Connecting tubing
Tongue depressor, water-soluble lubricant, gauze squares
Flashlight
Hypoallergenic tape
NO SMOKING signs.

* Oropharyngial catheters are used infrequently.

Procedure

Preparatory Phase

1   Post NO SMOKING signs on door of room and in view of patient and visitors.
2   Explain the advantages of oxygen therapy to the patient.
3   Attach flowmeter to humidifier and then to wall outlet or oxygen cylinder.
4   Attach tubing to humidifier and the catheter to the connecting tube.

Nursing Action	**Reason**

Performance Phase

1 To measure the depth of catheter insertion:	
a. Measure the catheter from the tip of the patient's nose to the tragus (lobe) of the ear. Mark this with tape.	**a.** This is only an approximation of the correct distance to insert the catheter.
2 To insert oropharyngeal catheter:	
a. Lubricate the catheter with a small amount of water-soluble lubricant.	
b. Start the flow of oxygen at 2–3 l/min.	**b.** This assures the patency of the catheters and its apertures. If some of the holes in the catheter become plugged, the stream of oxygen flowing on a localized area of mucous membrane will cause a burning sensation.
c. Determine the natural droop of the catheter.	
d. Hyperextend the patient's head.	
e. Clean nostrils with sodium bicarbonate solution if necessary.	
f. Slide the lubricated catheter along the floor of either nare into the oropharynx.	
g. Inspect the oropharynx, using the tongue depressor and flashlight to see the position of the catheter.	**g.** The tip of the catheter should rest approximately opposite the uvula.
h. *Pull the catheter back slightly until the tip cannot be seen.*	**h.** This is done to prevent aspiration of oxygen.
3 Use the opposite nare if insertion is difficult.	3 Nasal pathology (deviated septum, mucosal oedema, mucus drainage, polyps) may interfere with catheter insertion.
4 Adjust flow rate to prescribed rate.	4 A flow rate of 4–8 l/min should provide an ispired oxygen concentration of 30–50%.
5 Secure the catheter to the bridge of	5 Proper fixation is essential to prevent

Nursing Action	Reason
the nose or the side of the face with 1.25 cm (0.5 in) hypoallergenic tape.	downward displacement of the catheter.
6 Attach the connecting tube to the bed, leaving enough slack so that the patient can move about comfortably.	
7 Observe and palpate the epigastrium to see if distension develops.	7 In patients with depressed glottal reflexes or epiglottal paralysis (coma, post stroke, etc.) the oxygen stream may be directed into the oesophagus and may cause gastric distension or rupture (if the catheter is positioned too deeply).
8 Stay with the patient for a period of time to make sure he does not swallow, gag or cough.	

Follow-up Phase

1 Remove old catheter and insert a fresh catheter into opposite nostril every 8–12 hours.	1 Frequent changes of the oro-pharyngeal catheter are necessary to prevent catheter encrustation and ulceration of the nasal mucosa.
2 Observe and examine the patient hourly to see if: **a.** Catheter is unobstructed and positioned correctly (use flashlight). **b.** Oropharynx is free from irritation. **c.** Humidifier bottle contains water.	**c.** Oxygen dehydrates tissues unless moistened.
d. Leaks are occurring around humidifier and tubing connections. **e.** Oxygen cylinder contains enough oxygen.	
3 Assess the patient's condition frequently.	3 Assess the patient for mental aberration, disturbed consciousness, abnormal colour, perspiration, changes in blood pressure and increasing heart and respiratory rates.

GUIDELINES: Administering Oxygen by Venturi Mask (Fig. 3.7)

A *venturi mask* is a face mask designed to administer precisely controlled low oxygen concentrations (24, 28, 32, 35 and 40%). It is used primarily to increase the comfort and breathing efficiency of the patient with chronic lung disease, but may safely be used by other patients if they need it and if their oxygen need is met.

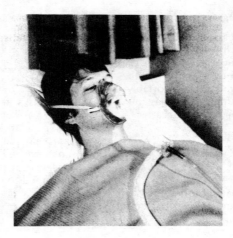

Figure 3.7.   Venturi mask with humidity enrichment.

Underlying Principles (Fig. 3.8)

1   The venturi mask mixes a fixed flow of oxygen with a high but variable flow of air so as to produce a constant oxygen concentration regardless of breathing rate.
2   Excess gas leaves the mask through the perforated cuff, carrying with it the expired carbon dioxide; this virtually eliminates rebreathing of carbon dioxide.
3   This mask maintains an oxygen concentration sufficient to relieve the hypoxia of patients with chronic lung disease without inducing hypoventilation and CO_2 retention.

Equipment

Oxygen source
Flowmeter
O_2 nipple adapter to attach connecting tubing to flowmeter
   If high humidity is desired:
      Nebulizer with sterile distilled water
      Large bore tubing
      Compressed air source and flowmeter to power nebulizer
Venturi mask with lightweight tubing and correct concentration adapter if the venturi mask with interchangeable colour-coded adapters is used.
NO SMOKING signs.

Procedure

Preparatory Phase

1   Post NO SMOKING signs on the door of patient's room and in view of patient and visitors.

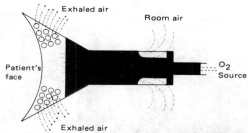

Figure 3.8.   The principle of high airflow with oxygen enrichment (HAFOE).

2   Explain the benefits of therapy to the patient.
3   Connect the mask by lightweight tubing to the oxygen source.
4   Turn on the flowmeter and adjust to the prescribed rate (usually indicated on the mask). Check to see that oxygen is flowing out the vent holes in the flexible face piece.

Nursing Action	Reason
Performance Phase	
1 Place venturi mask over patient's nose and mouth and under the chin. Mould the mask to fit the patient's face.	
2 Adjust elastic strap around the patient's head and position strap below the ears and around the neck.	
3 If high humidity is used, attach large bore tubing to nebulizer and connect it to the fitting for high humidity at the base of the venturi mask.	
Follow-up Phase	
Assess patient's condition at frequent intervals.	Assess the patient for mental aberration, disturbed consciousness, abnormal colour, perspiration, changes in blood pressure and increasing heart and respiratory rates.
1 Change mask and tubing daily.	

GUIDELINES: Administering Oxygen by Aerosol Mask (Fig. 3.9).

Purpose

To provide oxygen in concentrations of 35% or greater with high humidity by administering aerosol mist either heated or unheated, or when high humidity compressed air therapy is desired.

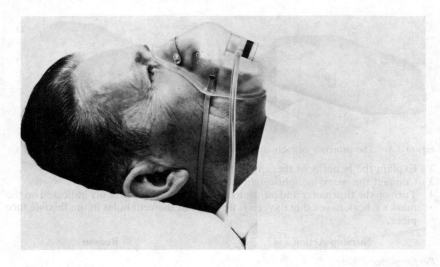

Figure 3.9.   Disposable face mask which is anatomically sculptured for patient comfort. There is a flexible aluminium strip at the nose portion of the mask that prevents oxygen leakage into the patient's eyes. (Courtesy: Hudson Oxygen Therapy Sales Company).

Equipment

Oxygen source
Nebulizer bottle with sterile distilled water
Plastic aerosol mask
Large bore tubing
Flowmeter
NO SMOKING signs

For heated aerosol therapy:
Nebulizer heating element
Thermometer

Procedure

Preparatory Phase

1   Post NO SMOKING signs on patient's door and in view of patient and visitors.
2   Show the aerosol mask to the patient and explain the procedure.
3   Make sure the nebulizer is filled to the appropriate mark.
4   Attach the large bore tubing from the mask to the nebulizer outlet.
5   Set desired oxygen concentration of nebulizer bottle and adjust thermostat if heating element is used.

Nursing Action	Reason
Performance Phase	
1 Adjust the flow rate until the desired mist is produced (usually 8–10	1 This assures the patient of receiving flow sufficient to meet his inspiratory

Nursing Action	Reason

l/min). The oxygen (or air) flow should be adjusted to that point at which the column of aerosol mist in the tubing is not completely withdrawn on the inspiratory phase.

demand and maintains a constant accurate concentration of oxygen.

2 Apply the mask to the patient's face and adjust the straps so that the mask fits securely and there are no leaks.

Follow-up Phase

1 Change mask, tubing, nebulizer and other equipment exposed to moisture daily.

1 Contaminated equipment may cause virulent infections in debilitated patients.

2 Assess patient's condition and the functioning of equipment at regular intervals.

2 Assess the patient for mental aberration, disturbed consciousness, abnormal colour perspiration, changes in blood pressure and increasing heart and respiratory rates.

3 Drain the tubing frequently. If a heating element is used, the tubing will have to be monitored and drained more often.

3 The tubing must be kept free of condensate. Condensate allowed to accumulate in the delivery tube will block flow and alter oxygen concentration.

4 If a heating device is used, the temperature must be checked often.

4 Excessive temperatures can cause airway burns; patients with elevated temperatures should be humidified with an unheated device.

5 If the patient appears tachypnoeic, increase flow rate and monitor the oxygen concentration with an oxygen analyser.

5 Inadeqate flow rates may cause inaccurate oxygen concentrations in patients who are tachypnoeic.

GUIDELINES: Administering Oxygen by Partial Rebreathing Mask

A *rebreathing bag* permits the patient to inhale a moderately high concentration of oxygen from a reservoir bag. Perforations on both sides of the mask serve as exhalation ports. High concentrations of oxygen are indicated in the acute phase of some diseases (pneumonia, pulmonary oedema, pulmonary embolism).

Purpose

To administer a moderately high oxygen concentration (50–60%).

Equipment

Oxygen source
Plastic face mask with reservoir bag and
  tubing

Humidifier with distilled water
Flowmeter
NO SMOKING signs

Procedure

Preparatory Phase

1 Post NO SMOKING signs on patient's door and in view of patient and visitors.
2 Fill humidifier with sterile distilled water.
3 Attach tubing to outlet on humidifier.
4 Attach flowmeter.
5 Explain the benefits of the oxygen therapy to the patient.
6 Flush the reservoir bag with oxygen to partially inflate the bag and adjust
   flowmeter to 6–10 l/min.

Nursing Action

Performance Phase

1 Place the mask on the patient's face and adjust litre flow so that the rebreathing bag will not collapse during the inspiratory cycle, even during deep inspiration.

Reason

1 Be sure the mask fits snugly since there must be an airtight seal between the mask and the patient's face.
   With a well-fitting rebreathing bag adjusted so that the patient's inhalation does not deflate the bag, inspired oxygen concentrations of 50–60% can be achieved. Some patients may require flow rates higher than 10 l/min to ensure that the bag does not collapse on inspiration.

2 Attach the tubing to the pillow and bed clothes. Keep the tubing free of kinks.

3 Stay with the patient for a period of time to make him comfortable and observe his reactions.

3 Be sure that oxygen is not escaping from the top of the mask and blowing into the patient's eyes.

Follow-up Phase

1 Remove mask periodically (if patient's condition permits) to dry the face around the mask. Powder skin and massage face around the mask.

1 These actions reduce moisture accumulation under the mask. Massage of the face stimulates circulation and reduces pressure over the area.

2 Observe for change of condition. Assess equipment for malfunction-

2 Assess the patient for mental aberration, disturbed consciousness, ab-

ing and low water level in humidifier.

normal colour, perspiration, change in blood pressure and increasing heart and respiratory rates.

GUIDELINES: Administering Oxygen by Nonrebreathing Mask

Purpose

To administer a high oxygen concentration when ordered by the doctor. (This method can deliver close to 100% oxygen at flows of 10 l/min or higher when correct technique is used.) The same method is used when tanked gases of precise composition are delivered (e.g., helium–oxygen or carbon dioxide–oxygen mixtures).

NOTE: Constant observation of the patient is necessary.

Equipment

Oxygen source

Plastic face mask with reservoir bag and tubing

The nonrebreathing mask differs from the partial rebreathing mask in that it has a one-way valve between the bag and mask which insures that the patient receives only 100% oxygen from the reservoir bag. The mask has two flapper valves which allow the patient to exhale but which do not allow him to inhale room air and thereby dilute the oxygen concentration.

Humidifier with sterile distilled water

Flowmeter

NO SMOKING sign

Procedure

Preparatory Phase

1 Post NO SMOKING signs on patient's door and in view of patient and visitors.
2 Show the mask to the patient and explain the procedure.
3 Make sure the humidifier is filled to the appropriate mark.

Nursing Action	**Reason**

Performance Phase

1 Place the mask on the patient's face and adjust litre flow so that the reservoir bag will not collapse during the inspiratory cycle, even during deep inspiration.

1 Since the patient is receiving all of his ventilation from the reservoir bag, the flow rate must be sufficient to provide the patient's minute ventilation.

Nursing Alert: If oxygen flow is not sufficient to keep reservoir bag filled, oxygen concentration will be reduced as room air is drawn in through flapper valves.

2 Be sure the mask fits snugly since there must be an airtight seal be-

Nursing Action	Reason
tween the mask and the patient's face.	

Follow-up Phase

1 Remove mask periodically (if patient's condition permits) to dry the face around the mask. Powder skin and massage face around the mask.

1 These actions reduce moisture accumulation under the mask. Massage of the face stimulates circulation and reduces pressure over the area.

2 Pay particular attention to see that the reservoir bag never completely collapses as the patient's ventilatory pattern varies.

2 Assess the patient for mental aberration, disturbed consciousness, abnormal colour, perspiration, change in blood pressure and incresing heart and respiratory rates

3 Observe for change of condition. Assess equipment for malfunctioning and low water level in humidifier.

GUIDELINES: Administering Oxygen via Endotracheal and Tracheostomy Tubes.

A T-tube is a device which connects directly to the patient's endotracheal or tracheostomy tube; it delivers oxygen and humidity from a nebulizer source (see Fig. 3.20, p. 310

Purpose

To administer oxygen in conjunction with humidity to the patient whose upper airway (and its humidification) has been bypassed either by a tracheostomy or by an endotracheal tube.

Equipment

Oxygen or compressed air source
Flowmeter
Nebulizer and sterile distilled water (heating element may be used as described in aerosol masks)
Large bore tubing
T-piece and 15·2–30·5 cm (6–12 in) reservoir tubing (a venturi tube system may be substituted for the T-piece and nebulizer if precise O_2 concentrations are required, but it is always used with humidity enrichment in patients with a tracheostomy or endotracheal tube)
NO SMOKING signs

Procedure

1 Post NO SMOKING signs on the patient's door and in view of patient and visitors.

2   Show the T-tube or venturi tube to the patient and explain the procedure.
3   Make sure the nebulizer is filled to the appropriate mark.
4   Attach the large bore tubing from the T-tube to the nebulizer outlet.
5   Set desired oxygen concentration of nebulizer bottle and adjust thermostat if heating element is used.

Nursing Action	**Reason**
Performance Phase	
1 Adjust the flow rate until desired mist is produced and meets the patient's inspiratory demand.	1 The aerosol mist in the reservoir tube should not be completely withdrawn on the patient's inspiration.
2 The tubing should be positioned so that it is not pulling on the tracheostomy tube and so that it allows a comfortable range of movement for the patient.	
Follow-up Phase	
1 Change mask, tubing, nebulizer and other equipment exposed to moisture daily.	1 Contaminated equipment may cause virulent infections in debilitated patients.
2 Assess patient's condition and the functioning of equipment at regular intervals.	2 Assess the patient for mental aberration, disturbed consciousness, abnormal colour, perspiration, changes in blood pressure and increasing heart and respiratory rates.
3 Drain the tubing frequently. If a heating element is used, the tubing will have to be monitored and drained more often.	3 The tubing must be kept free of condensate. Condensate allowed to accumulate in the delivery tube will block flow and alter oxygen concentration.
4 If a heating device is used, the temperature must be checked often.	4 Excessive temperatures can cause airway burns; patients with elevated temperatures will be better humidified with an unheated device.
5 If the patient appears tachypnoeic, increase flow rate and monitor the oxygen concentration with an oxygen analyser.	5 Inadequate flow rates may cause inaccurate oxygen concentrations in patients who are tachypnoeic.

GUIDELINES: Administering Oxygen by Tracheostomy Collar (Fig. 3.10)

A *tracheostomy collar* is a device that fits over the tracheostomy and delivers humidity and oxygen.

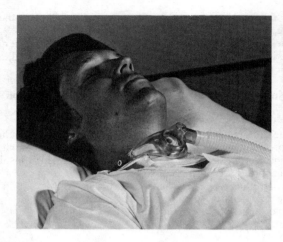

Figure 3.10.   Administering oxygen by tracheostomy collar.

Purpose

To administer humidity (either with or without oxygen) to the tracheostomized patient. If the patient does not require either precise or high concentrations of oxygen he is usually more comfortable with a tracheostomy collar than with a T-tube (blow-by) or venturi tube.

Equipment

Oxygen or compressed air source
Flowmeter
Nebulizer and sterile distilled water
   (heating element may be used as
   described in aerosol masks)

Large bore tubing
Tracheostomy collar
NO SMOKING signs

Procedure

Nursing Action	Reason
Performance Phase	
1 Adjust the flow rate until the desired mist is produced and meets the patient's inspiratory demand.	1 The aerosol mist in the tracheostomy collar should not be completely withdrawn on the patient's inspiration.
Follow-up Phase	
1 Change mask tubing, nebulizers and other equipment exposed to moisture daily.	1 Contaminated equipment may cause virulent infections in delibitated patients.

GUIDELINES: Administering Oxygen by Tent*

An *oxygen tent* is a device that circulates filtered and cooled air within the environment of a plastic canopy (tent).

Purpose

To provide a low-to-moderate concentration of oxygen in a temperature-controlled environment.

Procedure

Oxygen source	Wrench
Oxygen tent	NO SMOKING signs (2)
Special tent call bell	Draw sheet

Equipment

Preparatory Phase

1 Place NO SMOKING signs on patient's door and on equipment in view of patient and visitors.
2 Explain the benefits of oxygen therapy. To allay anxiety offer this explanation before bringing the equipment into the room.
3 Support the patient in upright position, using back rest and pillows.
4 Connect regulator to oxygen tank or wall outlet.
   a. Plug cord into wall.
   b. Turn on motor.
   c. Adjust temperature control to 18.5–22.2°C (65–70°F).
   d. Turn on oxygen tank and flush with high litre rate until desired concentration is reached.

Nursing Action	Reason
Performance Phase	
1 Extend the rod. Drape canopy over patient and over a half to two-thirds of bed.	
a. Tuck top and side edges of canopy under mattress.	**a.** A tight seal must be made between the canopy and bed to prevent oxygen leaks.
b. Use a folded drawsheet across patient's legs to improve the seal.	
c. Tuck drawsheet under mattress.	
2 Turn flowmeter to 12–15 l/min.	
3 Give the patient the special call bell.	3 Sparks from an electrical call bell are exceedingly dangerous since oxygen supports combustion.
4 Plan nursing care so that the patient	4 Oxygen is lost by displacement of

* Oxygen tents are used infrequently.

Nursing Action	**Reason**
and tent are disturbed as little as possible.	incoming gas when the canopy is opened and by diffusion of gas molecules through minute leaks around the console.
a. When bathing patient, slide the canopy towards the patient's neck.	
b. Flood the tent with oxygen after readjusting the canopy.	**b.** The oxygen environment is disrupted when the canopy is opened. The patient thereby receives only room air.
c. Wrap the patient's head and shoulders if the circulating air causes an uncomfortable draught.	
d. Take the patient's temperature via rectum.	
5 Use an oxygen analyser to determine oxygen concentration within the tent every 4 hours.	5 An oxygen analyser monitors oxygen concentration and permits the nurse or therapist to evaluate the operating efficiency of the tent.

Follow-up Phase

1 N.B.: Assess the patient every 30–45 min to determine his condition and to check the following: **a.** Temperature of the tent. **b.** Litre flow. **c.** Amount of oxygen in the tank. **d.** If oxygen vent is unobstructed.	1 Assess the patient for drowsiness, mental aberration, disturbed consciousness, abnormal colour, perspiration, changes in blood pressure and increasing heart and respiratory rates.

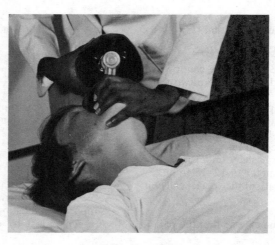

Figure 3.11   Technique of using resuscitator bag with a mask.

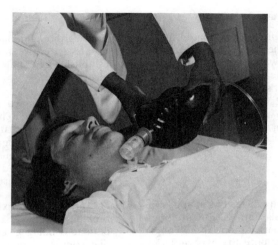

Figure 3.12.   Bag airway: the patient who is on a ventilator, is hyperventilated with a resuscitator bag directly attached to the tracheostomy prior to suctioning.

GUIDELINES: Administering Oxygen by Ambu-bag and Bag-airway Systems

An *Ambu-bag* is used when a patient is not intubated. This situation usually occurs only during a cardiopulmonary arrest episode (Fig. 3.11).

Bag-airway systems are used on an intubated patient and commonly are used to hyperinflate ventilator patients during suctioning and when being transported. (Fig. 3.12).

Equipment

Oxygen source
Resuscitation bag and mask
O_2 connecting tubing

Nipple adapter to attach flowmeter
  to connecting tubing
Flowmeter

Procedure

Nursing Action	Reason
Performance Phase	
1 Attach connecting tubing from flowmeter and nipple adapter to resuscitation bag.	1 A humidifier bottle is not used since the high flow rates of oxygen required would force water into the tubing and clog it.
2 Turn flowmeter to 'flush' position.	2 A high flow rate or 'flush' position is necessary to meet the minute ventilation of the patient.

Nursing Action	Reason
3 If the patient is not intubated, attach mask to the bag, insert an oral airway, and while hyperextending the patient's head, place the mask over the patient's face.	3 In a cardiopulmonary arrest situation, every effort should be made to establish a patent airway in the comatose patient.
4 Squeeze resuscitation bag with sufficient force and at the rate necessary to maintain adequate minute ventilation.	4 If cardiac massage is being given, breaths will have to be quickly interposed between cardiac compressions. If the patient needs only respiratory assistance, watch for chest expansion and listen with the stethoscope to ensure adequate ventilation.
5 Continue squeezing bag at appropriate intervals until CPR (cardiopulmonary resuscitation) is no longer required or until the hyperinflation accompanying suctioning has ceased.	5 A rate of approximately 14–18 breaths per minute is used unless the patient is being given external cardiac compressions.

GUIDELINES: Using Oxygen with CPAP

Continuous positive airway pressure (CPAP) is used in the spontaneously breathing patient in conjunction with oxygen. It maintains the alveoli in an 'open' state to allow adequate oxygenation of the patient (Fig. 3.13).

Equipment

O_2 source—usually an oxygen blender
Large bore tubing
Reservoir bag
T-piece→system→patient's endotracheal or tracheostomy tube
Nebulizer with sterile distilled water
CPAP valves or premeasured water bottle and underwater CPAP of desired pressure is used
Pressure manometer
One-way valve.

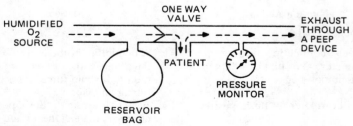

Figure 3.13. CPAP schematic.

Procedure

Nursing Action	Reason

Performance Phase

1 Connect various pieces of equipment as shown in illustration.

2 Turn on oxygen source and adjust flowrate so that it is sufficient to meet the patient's inspiratory demand.

    2 The patient will be receiving all of his minute ventilation from this 'closed system', so it is essential that the flowrate be adequate to meet changes in the patient's breathing pattern.

3 Connect the T-piece to the patient and observe the patient's respiratory rate and effort.

    3 If the CPAP level is too high for a particular individual (CPAP is usually not used in levels above 10 cm), the patient's work of breathing may actually be increased rather than diminished.

        In this case, lower levels of CPAP may be needed.

Follow-up Phase

1 Change tubing, nebulizer and other equipment exposed to moisture daily.

    1 Contaminated equipment may cause virulent infections in debilitated patients.

2 Assess patient's condition and functioning of equipment at regular intervals.

    2 The pressure manometer should be checked frequently to determine that the correct level of CPAP is being maintained. Tubing should be drained frequently so that condensate does not build up and block flow to the patient. The patient's respiratory rate and effort of breathing should be assessed regularly to determine adequacy of the therapy.

OTHER RESPIRATORY THERAPEUTIC METHODS

GUIDELINES: Assisting the Patient Undergoing Intermittent Positive Pressure Breathing (IPPB)*

The intermittent positive pressure breathing unit is a piece of equipment that supplies air or oxygen under positive pressure (above atmospheric) during inspiration.

---

* IPPB is being supplanted by other forms of therapy, e.g., slipstream nebulizer and incentive spirometer.

Purposes

1 To administer aerosolized medication.
2 To mobilize secretions and aid expectoration.
3 To improve alveolar ventilation and prevent atelectasis.
4 To assist respiration via positive pressure on inspiration.

Contraindications

1 Uncompensated pneumothorax.
2 Mediastinal and subcutaneous emphysema.
3 Untreated active tuberculosis.
4 Use with caution in patients with gastrointestinal surgery, haemoptysis, bullous disease.

Equipment

According to the type of machine used (each machine has different controls and settings)
NO SMOKING signs.

Procedure

Nursing Action	Reason
Preparatory Phase	
1 Post NO SMOKING signs. Explain the procedure to the patient.	1 Proper explanation of the procedure helps to ensure the patient's co-operation.
2 Measure the heart rate before and after the treatment for patients using bronchodilator drugs for the first time.	2 Bronchodilators may accelerate cardiac action. They may produce precordial distress, palpitation, dizziness, nausea and excessive perspiration.
3 Place the patient in a comfortable sitting or semi-Fowler's position.	3 The diaphragmatic excursion is greater in this position, and the upright position helps prevent air-swallowing.
4 Turn on the pressure source (oxygen, compressed air).	
5 Place the prescribed medication in the nebulizer/or sterile distilled water.	5 An IPPB treatment should not be given with dry gas.
6 Adjust all controls on tentative settings (usually 15). Select the inspiratory flowrate according to the machine being used (and doctor's request).	6 Positive pressure is measured in centimetres of water pressure; the pressure delivery is usually in the range of 10–20 cm H_2O. Each unit should be tested to see whether the predetermined setting is accomplished before treating the patient.

Nursing Action	Reason
7 Check the nebulizer for mist.	7 Adequate fog and particle size is essential to effective distribution of medication.

Performance Phase

1 Instruct the patient to bite down gently on the mouthpiece and to seal the mouthpiece with his lips.	1 The mouthpiece (or mask) must constitute a closed circuit if the unit is to cycle. (If the patient exhales through his nose while using the mouthpiece the unit will not reach the desired pressure).
2 Tell the patient to breathe slowly and normally and let the machine do the work.	2 A slight inspiratory effort will activate the positive pressure phase, and the lungs will be inflated with a rapid rate of flow until the predetermined pressure is reached and pressure expiration takes place.
3 Observe expansion of the patient's chest and measure exhaled tidal volume to ensure adequate ventilation.	3 Measurement of tidal volumes is particularly useful in the patient who has a high arterial P_{CO_2} and needs high tidal volumes to lower it.
a. Patient should breathe at own rate.	a. The machine will exert a regulated pressure on inhalation, helping him to breathe more deeply.
b. Instruct him to hold his breath 3–4 s at the end of each inspiration.	b. This ensures settling of aerosol particles on bronchiolar mucosa.
4 Remind the patient to exhale completely and slowly in a relaxed manner. The patient controls exhalation.	4 This type of breathing encourages good diaphragmatic motion and reduces residual air volume.
5 After several breaths, tell the patient to push all the air out, count 1, 2, 3, and stop inhaling (on the machine) for a few seconds to assess extent of improvement.	5 The treatment should take 10–20 min depending on the clinical problem.
6 Encourage the patient to continue this type of breathing until all the medication is given.	6 The medication should be completely nebulized to ensure effectiveness of treatment.

Follow-up Phase

1 Record medication used, patient's respiratory rate and effort and description of secretions expectorated (also pressure limit and flow rate).	1 Note the patient's tolerance of the treatment.

Nursing Action	Reason
2 Disassemble and clean the exhalation unit and nebulizer after each use. Keep this equipment in the patient's room. This equipment is changed every 24 hours.	2 Each patient has his own breathing circuit (exhalation valve, nebulizer, tubing, mouthpiece and mask). By proper cleaning, sterilization and storage of equipment infection can be prevented from entering already diseased lungs.

GUIDELINES: Assisting the Patient Undergoing Nebulizer Therapy Without Positive Pressure (Slipstream Nebulizer)

The *slipstream nebulizer* is a piece of equipment which allows for the nebulization of medication without positive pressure. The nebulizer is powered by either oxygen or compressed air (air compressor or piped compressed air at 4–5 l/min).

Purposes

1 To administer aerosolized medication.
2 To mobilize secretions and aid expectoration.

Contraindications

1 Inability of patient to co-operate in taking deep breaths.
2 Adverse reactions encountered with medication.

Equipment

Air compressor or oxygen or air flow meter
O_2 nipple adaptor

O_2 connecting tube
Nebulizer manifold

Procedure

Nursing Action	Reason
1 Explain the procedure to the patient.	1 Proper explanation of the procedure helps to ensure the patient's co-operation. This therapy depends on patient effort.
2 Measure the heart rate before and after the treatment for patients using bronchodilator drugs for the first time.	2 Bronchodilators accelerate cardiac action. They may produce precordial distress, palpitation, dizziness, nausea and excessive perspiration.
3 Place the patient in a comfortable sitting or semi-Fowler's position.	3 The diaphragmatic excursion is greater in this position.
4 Connect the nebulizer and connecting tubing to flowmeter and set flow at 4–5 l/min.	

Nursing Action	Reason

Performance Phase

1 Instruct the patient to exhale.

2 Tell the patient to take in a deep breath from the mouthpiece.

3 Nose clips are sometimes used if the patient has difficulty breathing only through his mouth.

4 Instruct the patient to breathe slowly and deeply until all of the medication is nebulized.

5 Observe expansion of the patient's chest to ascertain that he is taking deep breaths.

6 Encourage the patient to cough after several deep breaths.

2 This will ensure that medication is deposited below the level of the oropharynx.

4 Medication usually will be nebulized in 10–15 min at a litre flow of 4–5 l/min.

6 The deep lung inflation may loosen secretions and facilitate their expectoration.

Follow-up Phase

1 Record medication used, patient's respiratory rate and effort and description of secretions.

2 Disassemble and clean nebulizer after each use. Keep this equipment in the patient's room. This equipment is changed every 24 hours.

1 Note the patient's tolerance of the treatment.

2 Each patient has his own breathing circuit (nebulizer manifold, tubing and mouthpiece). By proper cleaning, sterilization and storage of equipment, infections can be prevented from entering already diseased lungs.

GUIDELINES: Assisting the Patient Using an Ultrasonic Nebulizer

An *ultrasonic nebulizer* delivers very small aerosolized particles into the lungs at atmospheric pressure.

Purpose

The ultrasonic nebulizer increases deposition of moisture in the bronchopulmonary tree to allow for mobilization of secretions. Ultrasonic nebulizers may be used in-line with intermittent positive pressure breathing (IPPB) treatments (Fig. 3.14).

Equipment

This depends on the type of nebulizer. Examples may include:

Ultrasonic nebulizer and nebulizer cup

Large bore tubing 30.4 cm (12 in)

Large bore tubing 1.8 m (6 ft).

One-way valve (placed between blower and nebulizer cup)

Disposable aerosol mask

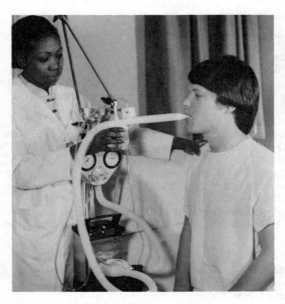

Figure 3.14.   IPPB treatment with ultrasonic nebulizer in line.

Procedure

Nursing Action	Reason
Preparatory Phase	
1 Fill the couplant compartment of the machine with distilled water.	
2 Place nebulizer cup in couplant compartment and fill with prescribed fluid.	2 Sterile distilled water or normal saline is used.
3 Connect 30.4 cm (12 in) large bore tubing to blower, add one-way valve to the other end, and connect to the nebulizer cup.	3 If oxygen source is desired, connect large bore tubing from oxygen powered nebulizer to the ultrasonic nebulizer cup.
4 Connect 1.8 m (6 ft) large bore tubing to the other side of the nebulizer cup.	
5 Connect the mask to the other end of the 1.8 m (6-ft) tubing.	
6 Plug in the machine and adjust the setting until the desired amount of mist is obtained.	

Nursing Action	Reason

Performance Phase

1 Instruct the patient to breathe in slowly through his mouth and to exhale the same way.

1 This allows maximum particle deposition.

2 Have the patient continue to breathe in this manner for the prescribed length of the treatments.

2 The procedure lasts usually 15–30 min.

3 Observe the patient for any adverse reactions to the treatment.
   a. Wheezing (bronchospasm)
   b. Excessive fluid deposition ('drowning') causing suffocation.

3 The patient may develop wheezing or may not be able to expectorate delivered fluid or his secretions. He may need assistance in draining his secretions by suctioning or postural drainage.

4 Encourage the patient to periodically expectorate loosened secretions during the treatment.

Follow-up Phase

1 Record medication used, patient's respiratory rate and effort and description of secretions expectorated.

1 Note any adverse reactions.

2 Keep this equipment in the patient's room. The equipment should be changed every 24 hours.

2 Ultrasonic nebulizers have a high contamination rate when not used properly. It is desirable that each patient have his own machine in his room.

ARTIFICIAL AIRWAY MANAGEMENT

GUIDELINES: Endotracheal Intubation

NOTE: This procedure is only undertaken by trained nurses who have received postregistration instruction, and who are working in a special unit, and with the consent of the medical staff, according to hospital policy.

Purpose

An endotracheal tube may be inserted via the nose or mouth to facilitate suctioning, to bypass an upper airway obstruction and to permit connection of the patient to a resuscitation bag or mechanical ventilator.

Equipment

1 Laryngoscope with curved or straight blade and working light source. (Check batteries and bulb periodically).
2 Endotracheal tubes with low-pressure cuffs and adapter to connect tube to ventilator or bag.

3   Stylet to guide endotracheal tube.
4   Oral airway (assorted sizes), tongue blade to keep patient from biting into and occluding endotracheal tube.
5   Adhesive tape.
6   Lubricant jelly.
7   Syringe.

Procedure

Preparatory Phase

1   Remove dental bridgework and plates.
2   Remove headboard of bed.
3   Make sure light source of laryngoscope is working.
4   Select endotracheal tube of appropriate size (7.5–9 mm for average adult).
5   Inflate and deflate cuff to make sure it is intact.
6   Lubricate endotracheal tube.
7   Insert stylet if tube is very flexible.

Nursing Action	Reason

Performance Phase (Fig. 3.15)

1 If cervical spine is not injured, place head in a 'sniffing' position, flexed at the junction of the neck and thorax and extended at the junction of the spine and skull.	1 Upper airway is open maximally in this position and mouth of unconscious patient will often open.
2 Ventilate and oxygenate the patient with resuscitation bag before intubation.	2 This decreases the likelihood of cardiac arrhythmias secondary to hypoxia.
3 Hold the handle of the laryngoscope in the left hand and hold patient's mouth open with the right hand by crossing fingers.	3 Leverage is improved by crossing thumb and index fingers when opening the patient's mouth.
4 Insert blade of laryngoscope along the right side of the tongue, pointing tongue to the left, and use right thumb and index finger to pull patient's lower lip away from lower teeth.	4 Rolling lip away from teeth prevents injury by being caught between teeth and blade.
5 Lift laryngoscope forwards (towards ceiling) to expose epiglottis.	
6 Lift laryngoscope upwards and forwards at 45° angle to expose glottis (vocal cords).	6 This stretches the hypoepiglottis ligament, folding the epiglottis upwards and exposing the glottis.
7 As the epiglottis is lifted forwards (towards ceiling) the vertical opening of the larynx between the vocal cords will come into view.	7 Do not use wrist; use shoulder and arm to lift epiglottis—to avoid using teeth as a fulcrum, which could lead to dental damage.

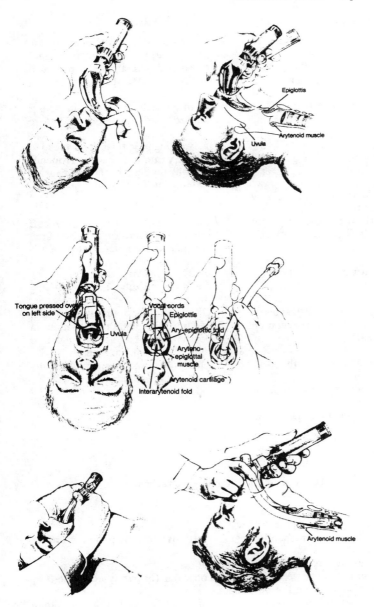

Figure 3.15.   Sequence of steps for endotracheal intubation. (From: Patient Care, 15 June 1871. Copyright 1971, Miller and Fink Corp., Darien, CT. All rights reserved.)

Nursing Action	Reason
8 Once vocal cords are visualized, insert tube into the right corner of the mouth and pass the tube—guided by blade but keeping cords in constant view.	8 Make sure you do not insert tube in oesophagus; the oesophageal mucosa is pink and the opening is horizontal rather than vertical.
9 Gently push the tube through the triangular space formed by the vocal cords.	9 If the vocal cords are in spasm (closed), wait a few seconds before passing tube.
10 Stop insertion just after the tube cuff has disappeared from view beyond the cords.	10 Advancing tube further may lead to its entry into a mainstem bronchus (usually the right bronchus) causing collapse of the unventilated lung.
11 Withdraw laryngoscope, holding endotracheal tube in place.	
12 Inflate cuff with the minimal amount of air required to occlude trachea.	12 The amount of air used for cuff inflation depends on the size of the cuff and the diameter of patient's trachea.
13 Insert oral airway or bite block.	13 This keeps patient from biting down on the tube and obstructing the airway.
14 Observe expansion of both sides of the chest by observation and auscultation of breath sounds.	14 Observation and auscultation help in determining that tube remains in position and has not slipped into right mainstem bronchus.
15 Mark proximal end of tube with marking pen or tape.	15 This will allow for detection of any later change in position.
16 Secure tube with adhesive tape to the patient's face.	
17 Take chest x-ray to verify tube position.	

Tracheostomy

A *tracheostomy* is an external opening made into the trachea.

Purposes

1 To provide and maintain a patent airway.
2 To enable the removal of tracheobronchial secretions when the patient is unable to cough productively.
3 To permit the use of positive pressure ventilation.
4 To prevent aspiration of secretions in the unconscious (or paralysed) patient by closing off the trachea from the oesophagus.
5 To replace an endotracheal tube when such an airway is needed for more than 5–7 days.
6 To reduce dead space.

Kinds of Tracheostomy Tubes

1   Plastic (nylon, polyvinyl chloride or silastic) tracheostomy tubes are available with or without inner tubes and usually with attached low pressure cuffs.
2   Silver tracheostomy tube consists of three parts: obturator (pilot), inner cannula and outer cannula.
3   Jackson silver tracheostomy tube with Morch adapter—similar to No. 1 with a screw-on swivel adapter (on the inner cannula) to connect with a ventilator. Suction is permitted without disturbing ventilator.
4   Endotracheal cuff may be attached to the cannula to provide a closed system (Fig. 3.16).

Performing a Tracheostomy

A tracheostomy may have to be performed as an emergency measure, or as planned surgery. It is necessary for the nurse to understand the basic steps of the procedure so that she can assist the doctor in an emergency.

Sterile tracheostomy instruments are usually kept prepacked in theatre, accident and emergency departments and intensive care units. In addition to the pack, the following equipment is needed:

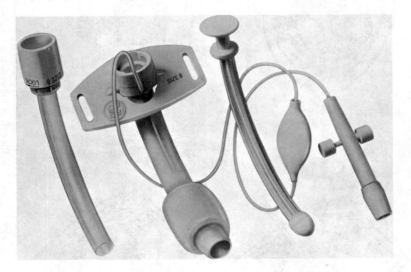

Figure 3.16.   The disposable low pressure cuff tracheostomy tube consists of several parts: on the left is the translucent inner cannula that locks into the next piece, the outer cannula. Note the inflatable cuff encircling the outer cannula; this cuff is connected to an airline which emerges at the top of the tube and lead to an inflatable bag which is in turn connected to a pressure retention clamp. The clamp has a syringe connector at the extreme right of the illustration. The ribbed piece to the right of the tracheostomy tube is an obturator. (Courtesy; Shiley Laboratories, Inc.)

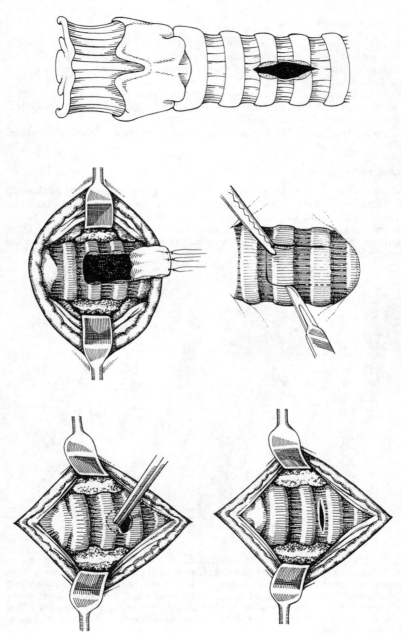

Figure 3.17. Left. Horizontal incision of trachea, and conversion of horizontal incision into stoma. Centre. The Bjorn flap. Initial incision, and securing flaps to subcutaneous tissue. Right. Vertical incision of trachea. Reproduced with permission of Portex Ltd.

Sucker with sterile suction catheters
Sterile gloves and towels
Syringes and needles
Local anaesthetic
Skin cleansing lotion
Good lighting

Procedure

The patient is placed in the supine position; a small pillow may be placed under the shoulders but the neck should not be overextended. The incision is usually between the second and third rings of cartilage. It may be horizontal or vertical and may incorporate a flap (see Fig. 3.17). The appropriate tube is inserted and the introducer withdrawn. The tube is secured in place by tapes going round the neck of the patient (see Fig. 3.18).

Nursing Management

Physical Care of Patient

1   Provide adequate humidity since natural humidifying pathway of the oropharynx is no longer used.
2   Aspirate secretions since the patient's own cough mechanism is not as effective.
3   Suction gently to avoid injuring the epithelium; limit each suctioning time to between 10–15 s.
4   Introduce *sterile* aspirating tubes to prevent infection.
5   Recognize patient's ability to breath comfortably; if he has difficulty, assess need for ventilatory assistance.
6   Elevate him to semi-Fowler's or sitting position if he contraindicated since this is usually more comfortable and makes breathing easier.
7   Observe stomal site for bleeding or irritation; when the outer tracheostomy tube is changed (by doctor for first 4 or 5 days), apply small amount of antibiotic ointment before reinserting tube. Place unfrayed sterile dressing around collar of tracheostomy tube (Fig. 3.18).

Psychological Care of Patient

1   Recognize that the patient is usually apprehensive, particularly about choking, about being unable to remove secretions and about his ability to communicate.
2   Explain and demonstrate the procedure carefully, using tracheostomy equipment; proceed according to the patient's ability to absorb information and his desire to learn; instruction may be divided into several sessions.
3   Inform the patient and his family that he will not be able to speak; determine with the patient the best method of communication, e.g., sign language, writing, etc.; supply him with note paper, pencil, 'Magic slate' and call bell.
4   Anticipate some of his questions by providing the answer to "Is it permanent?" "Will it hurt to breathe?" "Will someone be with me?"
5   A nurse should stay constantly by the patient for the first 24–48 hours, particularly if patient is fearful.

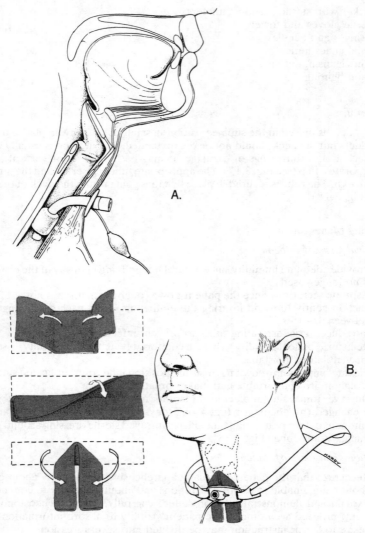

Figure 3.18.   a. This shows how the cuff of the tracheostomy tube fits smoothly within the tracheal wall. Pressure should be great enough to ensure a snug fit but not so great as to produce a stenosis. b. The lower illustration shows how to unfold a 3 × 3 gauze square and refold it so that it need not be cut (cut frayed threads could be aspirated) and yet will provide a comfortable neck pad. Change as often as necessary. Note the manner in which the neck twill tapes are fastened to the openings in the neck plate of the tracheostomy tube. This eliminates a knot which could create pressure on the neck. Twill tape ends should be tied to the side of the neck rather than at the back. (A knot at the back would not be comfortable to lie on.)

Equipment

1   Sterile gloves and duplicate sterile tracheostomy set including Trousseau dilator and two tracheal retractors (or hooks), one tissue forceps, one grooved director, two haemostats, petrolatum gauze or antibiotic ointment, sterile dressing.
2   Humidifying equipment.
   a. For the room—a heated aerosol machine.
   b. For the patient—ultrasonic mist unit, nebulizer attached to tracheostomy tube, or a high humidity tracheal collar.
3   Suction equipment (see below, Guidelines: Aspirating Through the Tracheostomy Tube).
4   Communication materials; pencil, paper, etc., call bell.
5   Mirror—for use when patient is beginning self-care.

GUIDELINES: Aspirating Through the Tracheostomy Tube

NOTE: For high-risk patient, see procedure immediately following.

Purpose

To remove secretions when audible in the tracheobronchial tree, so that a patent airway is maintained.

Equipment

Aseptic Technique
Sterile disposable catheter
   No. 14 or 16 (adult)
   No. 8 or 10 (child)

Sterile gloves, individually wrapped
Sterile saline
Sterile syringe—5 ml
The nurse wears a mask for this procedure.

General Nursing Considerations

1   Administer analgesics and sedatives with caution so that the respiratory centre is not depressed.
2   Suction trachea when necessary (may be every 5 or 10 min for the first several postoperative hours and less frequently when need is less).

Nursing Alert: Need for aspiration is expressed by noisy, moist respirations, increased pulse and respirations. Encourage patient to cough to bring up and expel secretions; use suction if coughing is not productive.

3   Use stethoscope to check patency of airway.
4   Avoid unnecessary suctioning which is irritating to mucosa and may initiate infection.

Procedure (Fig. 3.19)

Nursing Action	Reason
1 Lubricate catheter with normal saline.	1 To facilitate passage of tube.

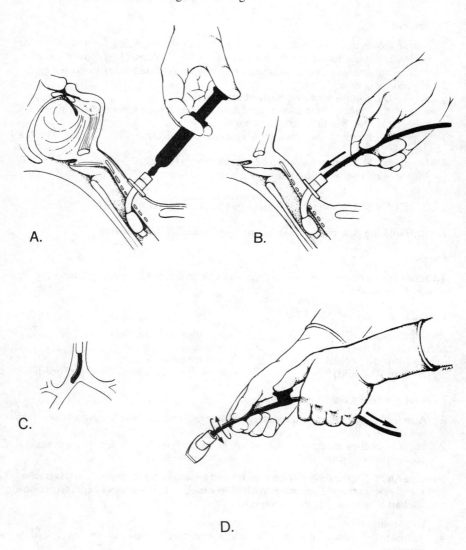

Figure 3.19. Care of the tracheostomy patient. a. After the tracheostomy cuff is deflated (note that the cuff does not touch the sides of the trachea) 3–5 ml of sterile saline can be instilled into the tube to loosen secretions. b. After donning sterile gloves, the nurse introduces a sterile catheter without applying suction. c. To remove secretions from the bronchus, insert tube 20–30 cm (7.5–11.5 in). d. Suction is applied by sealing the button outlet with the thumb. Gradually withdraw the catheter with a rotating motion.

Nursing Action	Reason
2 Insert catheter with suction turned off.	2 So as not to suction the wall of the cannula or irritate the mucous membrane wall.
3 Pass tube into bronchus from 20 to 30 cm (8–12 in), unless contraindicated, and then gradually open suction.	3 To stimulate coughing and to loosen secretions even beyond the cannula.
4 Remove catheter when patient coughs.	4 Catheter obstructs cannula and interferes with expulsion of secretions.
5 For tenacious secretions, instil sterile saline solution as prescribed (usually 3–5 ml).	5 Saline aids in dissolving mucus. It is helpful to have patient take a deep breath.
6 Have tissue or container ready to receive expelled secretions.	
7 Rotate catheter between thumb and forefinger; move it up and down gently as it is withdrawn with suction on.	
8 Do not suction patient more than 15 s at a time (rest at least 3 min between suctionings). Administer oxygen and ventilate patient between aspirations to relieve hypoxia and prevent arrhythmias.	8 There is the danger of hypoxia if suctioning is prolonged.
9 Use a stethoscope along bronchial tree to detect gurgling mucous sounds.	9 Auscultation will determine effectiveness of suctioning; respiration should be quiet and essentially effortless at end of aspiration.

Aftercare of Equipment

1 When inner silver cannula is clogged with mucus, remove to clean.
2 Soak in a cold solution of half water and half hydrogen peroxide to loosen adhering particles (some prefer 2% sodium bicarbonate solution). Hot water would cause protein in mucus to coagulate.
3 A brush may be used to scrub interior of tube with soap and water. A pipe cleaner may be used for small tubes.
4 Disinfect tube by boiling for 5 min; cool.
5 Suction outer cannula in patient before reinserting cleaned inner cannula.
6 Dispose of catheter. Replace with new (covered) catheter.
7 Carry out care of suction bottle.

GUIDELINES: Caring for the Patient with a Cuffed Tube (Tracheostomy or Endotracheal)

A *cuff* is the inflatable balloon of a tracheostomy or endotracheal tube which is designed for providing the snug fit required for ventilators. It prevents leakage of air and of secretions around the tube and aspiration of vomitus and oropharyngeal secretions.

General Nursing Considerations

1   Inform the patient that he will not be able to talk normally when the endotracheal cuffed tube is in place because no air passes over the larynx. (Speaking may be resumed when the tube is removed.)
2   Maintain the neck in a comfortable position of extension.
3   Recognize the importance of frequent and adequate mouth care.

Procedure

May require a doctor's request: Usually the cuff is initially inflated by the doctor.

Action	Reason
Deflating a Cuff	
1 Suction pharynx—oral and nasal.	1 Removes secretions which could be aspirated during the process of deflation.
2 Deflate cuff slowly.	2 On endotracheal tube, a small test balloon at end of tubing remains inflated as long as cuff is inflated.
3 Suction through the tracheostomy or endotracheal tube.	3 Removes secretions which may have been present above inflated cuff and around exterior of tube and may now have seeped downwards. The coughing reflex may be stimulated during deflation, which helps to mobilize secretions.
4 Provide adequate ventilation while cuff is deflated.	
a. If the patient does not require assisted ventilation: provide humidified warm air.	**a.** Continue observation of patient: pulse, colour, etc. If any signs of distress, place patient back on mechanical ventilator.
b. If the patient requires assisted ventilation; provide a manually inflating breathing bag or respirator if patient has been on a mechanical ventilator.	**b.** If patient is apnoeic, cuff should not be deflated more than 30 or 45 s.
Inflating a Cuff (slowly)	
1 Stipulations:	
a. To be done when patient requires mechanical ventilation or is being fed.	**a.** To prevent aspiration of food into lungs.
(1) Semi-Fowler's position is	(1) Gravity assists in moving food

Action	Reason
most comfortable if permissible, and is required for half an hour after feeding. (2) On right side.	into the stomach. (2) To prevent regurgitation of feeding.
b. Inflate cuff during inspiration (positive pressure phase). 2 Method A: **a.** Inject air into cuff until complete seal is achieved or to selected pressure, following doctor's orders. By listening with a stethoscope placed just below chin (submental) one may determine that no leak exists. **b.** Clamp tube leading to cuff.	**a.** The pressure-cycled ventilator will turn off; air will not escape around tube or from nose or mouth. In the conscious patient, a leak-free system is present when he is aphonic.
3 Method B (minimal leak inflation): **a.** Inject air until full seal is acquired; withdraw 0.5 ml of air and clamp tube. **b.** Note and record amount of air required to inflate cuff.	**a.** A partial leak is purposely created so that ventilator can be set to compensate for it. **b.** If at subsequent times more air is required to inflate cuff, tracheal dilatation or other serious problem (erosion of a large blood vessel or tracheo-oesophageal diverticulum or fistula) may be the cause.
Suctioning (done with *Sterile* equipment)	*To minimize possibility of infection*
1 Tracheobronchial secretions are suctioned as frequently as necessary—5 or 10 s at a time and not more often than once every 3 min. 2 Via endotracheal tube. **a.** Insert catheter (for an adult) approximately 45–50 cm (18–20 in). (1) If impossible to pass suction tube this distance, a mucus plug may be in the way; inject 5 ml saline.	1 This is a nursing judgement based on recognition of signs suggesting accumulation of secretions. **a.** Tube inserted deep since this patient has difficulty mobilizing deep secretions. (1) Injecting saline helps in liquefying mucus.
3 Via tracheostomy tube (See Guidelines, p. 294). 4 Oropharyngeal with endotracheal tube in place. Suction oropharynx frequently. (Patient is taking nothing by mouth).	4 Volume of secretions is greater due irritation of mucous membrane.

5   Oropharyngeal with cuffed tracheostomy tube in place. (Patient is able to swallow and have a normal intake).

Maintaining Humidified Warm Inspired Air

1 Provide continuous flow of mist.	1 To prevent drying of secretions and irritation of mucuous membrane.

Complications	*Means of Avoiding Complications*
1 Laryngeal irritation and damage to vocal cord due to movement of endotracheal tube.	1 Prevent movement or jarring of tube.
2 Laryngeal oedema.	2 Supply mist during and after extubation.
3 Tracheal stenosis.	3 Proper nursing care includes humidity, suction, etc.
4 Haemorrhage.	

GUIDELINES: Preparing for Tracheostomy Tube Removal

Purposes

To preserve tracheostomy while training the patient to breathe through his mouth.

Procedure

Nursing Action	Reason
1 Determine patient's ability to breathe deeply and cough effectively.	1 Clinical assessment of respiratory exchange over a period of time helps in determining time of weaning.
2 Check the patient's reflexes for swallowing, gagging, coughing.	
3 Observe patient's ability to bring up tracheobronchial secretions without assistance for 24 hours.	
4 Cork tracheostomy tube intermittently with cuff deflated.	4 Increase the time of occlusion as much as patient can tolerate.
5 Remove tracheostomy tube as soon as safe.	5 This is determined by tolerance of the individual patient with no respiratory difficulties.
6 Tape skin edges together.	6 Tract closes spontaneously in a few days.

MECHANICAL VENTILATION

A *mechanical ventilator* is a positive pressure breathing device which can maintain respiration automatically for prolonged periods of time. It is indicated when the patient is unable to maintain safe levels of arterial carbon dioxide or oxygen by spontaneous breathing.

Types of Ventilators

1 *Pressure-cycled*—the ventilator delivers a predetermined pressure, then turns off.
   a. Gas flows result from this pressure and increases lung volume.
   b. Volume delivered is dependent on lung compliance and varies from breath to breath.
   c. Blockage at any point between machine and lungs will not stop the on–off cycling of the ventilator—but the patient will receive *no volume*.
   d. Volume-based alarms should always be used with this ventilator.
2 *Volume-cycled*—the ventilator delivers a predetermined volume of air to the patient regardless of any changing lung condition.
   If machine is unable to deliver such volume, the operator is alerted by an audible and visible alarm.

Modes of Operation

Ventilators are used as assistors, controllers or as assist-controllers.

1 *Assist mode*—used for patient who is making an inspiratory effort, but who, for various reasons, cannot achieve an adequate tidal volume.
   The patient initiates each breath, which is then augmented by the ventilator to achieve a preset volume.
2 *Control mode*—used for patient whose respiratory drive is absent or excessive.
   a. If respiratory effort is absent, machine initiates breaths at a predetermined rate.
   b. If rate is excessive for maintenance of adequate acid-base status, the rate can be controlled—machine will not respond to any attempt by the patient to breathe spontaneously.
3 *Assist-control mode*—used for patient whose respiratory rate is erratic.
   a. If patient maintains adequate rate, the ventilator functions as an assistor.
   b. If respiratory rate falls below a preset level, machine takes over and initiates breathing at a predetermined rate.
   c. The patient can resume regulation of his own respiratory rate at any time.

Special Mechanical Ventilator Techniques

Intermittent Positive Pressure Ventilator (IPPV)

1 Purpose:
   IPPV prevents collapse of alveolar units during exhalation and thus increases the surface for oxygen transfer.
2 Mechanisms of operation:
   a. Mechanical ventilation and spontaneous ventilation are exactly alike—each allows a passive exhalation phase.
   b. The diaphragm relaxes (or ventilatory pressure is removed), intrapulmonary pressure falls until it *equals* atmospheric pressure, and gas flow out of the lung ceases.

c. IPPV prevents intrapulmonary pressure from falling to atmospheric level—*a positive intrapulmonary pressure is maintained during inhalation and exhalation*.

3   Benefits:

a. Positive intrapulmonary pressure may be helpful in reducing the effects of pulmonary oedema by diminishing the rate of transudation of fluid from the pulmonary capillaries to the alveoli.

b. Since a greater surface area for diffusion is available and shunting is reduced it is often possible to use inspired oxygen concentrations much lower than would otherwise be required to obtain adequate arterial oxygen levels. This reduces the risk of oxygen toxicity.

4   Hazards:

a. Since the mean intrathoracic pressure is increased by IPPV, venous return and cardiac output may be impeded.

b. High IPPV levels (above 15–20 cm H_2O) may possibly cause alveolar rupture with a resulting tension pneumothorax.

5   Precautions:

a. Chest auscultation must be performed very frequently. Diminished or absent breath sounds require immediate notification of the doctor in charge.

b. Suctioning must never exceed 15 s from disconnection to reconnection of the ventilator. Presuctioning hyperventilation should be done on the ventilator with 100% oxygen or by a hand resuscitator capable of providing IPPV.

Continuous Positive Airway Pressure (CPAP) (see Fig. 3.13)

1   Gives the same end result as IPPV but without the use of a ventilator.

2   Generally used if a patient is capable of maintaining an adequate rate and tidal volume but has some pathology which prevents maintenance of adequate levels of tissue oxygenation.

3   CPAP has the same purposes, benefits, hazards and precautions noted with IPPV.

Underlying Principles

1   Variables that control ventilation and oxygenation:

a. The ventilator *rate*—measured with a watch. (Some ventilators have respiratory rate marked on respirator and adjusted by a rate knob.)

b. The *tidal volume*—measured as expired volume with a gas meter.

c. The *inspired oxygen concentration*—measured with an oxygen analyser.

2   Tidal volume and rate together control the elimination of carbon dioxide.

3   The inspired oxygen concentration is controlled to produce normal arterial oxygen tension.

4   The duration of inspiration should not exceed expiration. Obstruction of venous return by prolonged inspiration lowers cardiac output and decreases the rate of oxygen transport to body tissues.

5   The inspired gas delivered to the patient must be fully saturated with sterile, distilled water at body temperature to prevent thickening of tracheobronchial secretions. Water is added by either a heated humidifier or nebulizer.

Clinical Indications

1   Respiratory failure (see p. 258).

2 Chronic obstructive lung disease.
3 Administration of respiratory depressants.
4 Neuromuscular disorders.
5 Drug intoxication.
6 Cardiac arrest.
7 Chest injury.
8 Left ventricular failure and pulmonary oedema.
9 Pulmonary embolus.

Complications

Airway obstruction (secretions, inadequate humidification)
Damage to the trachea (necrosis or malacia)
Infection
Gastrointestinal bleeding
Tension pneumothorax
Inability to wean from ventilator
Pulmonary oxygen toxicity.

GUIDELINES: Managing the Patient Requiring Mechanical Ventilation

Procedure

Nursing Action	Reason
Performance Phase	
1 Obtain baseline samples for blood gas determinations (see Appendix) (pH, PO_2, PCO_2, HCO_3) and chest x-ray.	1 Baseline measurements serve as a guide in determining progress of therapy.
2 Give a brief explanation to the patient.	2 Emphasize that mechanical ventilation is a temporary measure. The patient should be prepared psychologically for weaning the day the ventilator is first used.
3 Establish the airway by means of a cuffed endotracheal tube.	3 Endotracheal intubation provides access to the lower part of the airway for removal of secretions. The cuffed tube prevents leakage of air into mouth during ventilation and permits control of pressure and lung inflation.
a. Inflate the cuff to the pressure prescribed by the doctor to achieve a proper seal. Inflation pressure should not normally exceed 20 mmHg as measured by a cuff pressure manometer. (See Cuff Inflation, p. 298).	**a.** Pressure greater than 20 mmHg can compromise circulation in the trachea. Insufficient cuff pressure may allow gas leakage and a diminished volume of air may be delivered to the patient.

Nursing Action	Reason

b. Secure the tube in place with surgical adhesive. Insert an oral airway as a bite block to prevent the patient from occluding an orotracheal tube.

b. Securing the tube prevents dislodgment into the right or left mainstem bronchus.

4 Prepare ventilator according to manufacturer's directions:
a. Turn on machine.
b. Adjust volume control; establish tidal and minute volumes as determined by the doctor.
c. Set the oxygen concentration.

4 Maintenance of ventilation depends on correct machine settings.

b. Arterial blood pH, carbon dioxide and oxygen tensions serve as guides in adjusting the ventilator.
c. This is generally based on the arterial oxygen levels obtained as a baseline.

d. Adjust respiratory rate of ventilator to 12–14 respirations/min.

d. This setting approximates normal respiration. The patient who has respiratory stimulus will cycle machine by himself; set the control to a rate slightly lower than the patient's actual rate. These machine settings are subject to change according to patient's condition and response and the make of the machine being used.

e. Adjust flow state (velocity of gas flow during inspiration) to 30–40 l/min.

e. The slower the flow rate the lower will be the pressure required to deliver the patient's gas volume. This results in a lower intrathoracic pressure and less impedance of venous return and cardiac output.

f. Couple the patient's endotracheal tube to the ventilator.

f. Be sure connections are secure. Watch for accidental disconnection between the patient's airway and the ventilator; observe for separation of ventilator tubings from nebulizer, electrical wall-plug slippage, etc.

5 Carry out arterial blood gas determinations approximately 20 min after patient is on ventilator. Arterial blood sampling is carried out repeatedly during the acute period.

5 The only effective way to attain and maintain normal oxygen and carbon dioxide tensions is to measure these tensions frequently in arterial blood and adjust the settings of the ventilator accordingly. Arterial blood gases are monitored to assess the effectiveness of therapy. There are no reliable clinical signs of CO_2 retention or alkalosis.

Nursing Action	Reason

6 The patient is never left unattended or unobserved.

Positioning

1 Turn patient from side to side hourly.
2 Lateral turns of 120° are desirable; from right semiprone to left semiprone.
3 Sit the patient upright at regular intervals.

    3 Upright posture increases ventilation of lower lobes.

4 Position the patient in postural drainage positions as requested (pp. 252–253).

    4 Adequate postural drainage decreases the need for deep tracheobronchial catheter aspiration by preventing retention of secretions in the periphery of the lungs.

5 Carry out passive range of motion exercises of all extremities.

Deep Breaths

1 Augment the patient's spontaneous tidal volume by periodically giving him six to eight deep breaths with a hand resuscitator bag or use sigh mechanism available on some ventilators. Provide patient with adequate oxygenation during this manoeuvre.

    1 Periodic sighing with greater than normal tidal volumes helps to prevent alveolar collapse. Provision of deep breaths by mechanical hyperinflation also helps to promote coughing and reveals the presence of retained secretions.

Aspiration of Secretions

1 Aspirate secretions from the trachea using sterile technique (p. 294).

    1 Ventilation and nebulization liquefy secretions, causing them to rise into the upper airways.

2 Oxygenate patient for 1–2 min prior to each suctioning episode and before second passage of the catheter.

    2 Do not prolong aspiration more than 15 s because cardiac arrest may ensue in patients with borderline oxygenation.

3 Note the amount, colour, and consistency of tracheal secretions obtained.
4 Inform the doctor if there is appreciable change.

Chest Auscultation

1 Listen with a stethoscope to the chest from bottom to top on both sides (hourly).

    1 Auscultation of the chest is a means of assessing airway patency and ventilatory distribution. It also con-

Nursing Action	Reason

firms the proper placement of the endotracheal or tracheostomy tube.

2   Determine whether breath sounds are present or absent, normal or abnormal, and whether a change has occurred.

3   Observe the patient's diaphragmatic excursions and changes in the use of accessory muscles of respiration.

Humidification

1   Check the water level in the humidification reservoir to ensure that the patient is never ventilated with dry gas. Empty the water that condenses in the delivery tubing.
    Humidifier or nebulizer and tubing must be changed every 24 hours.

1   Water condensing in the delivery tubing may cause obstruction and sudden flooding of the trachea.
    Warm, moist tubing is a perfect breeding area for bacteria.

Airway Pressure

1   Check the airway pressure gauge at frequent intervals in patients on volume-limited ventilators.

1   Since these ventilators deliver a fixed volume, a sudden drop in pressure indicates a leak in the system. A sudden rise in pressure indicates obstruction of the delivery of gas to the patient. Could indicate (1) blockage by secretions; (2) tube slippage into a mainstem bronchus; (3) pneumothorax; or (4) pulmonary oedema.

Tidal Volumes

1   Measure the tidal volume with a respirometer for patients on pressure-limited ventilators.

1   An abrupt fall in tidal volume indicates increase in airway resistance (e.g., bronchospasm or other obstruction), an increase in tissue resistance (pulmonary oedema) or a leak in the patient circuit of the ventilator.

Cuff Inflation

1   Clean the pharynx and larynx of accumulated secretions by either suction or postural drainage.

2   Release air slowly from the cuff, using a syringe, while maintaining positive pressure via the ventilator or a self-inflating manual resuscitator.

1   If the tube becomes blocked the patient will not be able to breathe.

2   The cuff is deflated periodically to prevent necrosis of the tracheal mucosa. However, with soft cuffs or atmospheric seal cuffs, deflation of

Nursing Action	Reason
	cuffs is not usually necessary.
3 Reinflate the cuff with just enough air to prevent gross leakage when positive pressure is again applied to airway.	3 Excessive cuff inflation may cause pressure necrosis over a period of time.

Tracheostomy

1 Tracheostomy care should be given as needed, using sterile technique.	1 To continue ventilation while the inner cannula is removed, a substitute sterile inner cannula or adapter should be inserted into the outer cannula and connected to the ventilator.

Bacteriologic Specimens

1 Aspirate tracheal secretions into a sterile container and send to laboratory for culture and sensitivity tests.	1 This technique allows the earliest detection of infection or change in infecting organisms in the tracheobronchial tree.
a. This is done immediately after endotracheal intubation. **b.** Daily Gram staining of secretion is also done.	

Circulatory Measurements

1 Monitor pulse rate and arterial blood pressure; intra-arterial pressure monitoring may be carried out.	1 To accomplish intra-arterial pressure monitoring a catheter is introduced into an artery, usually the radial or femoral, and the pressure at the catheter tip is transmitted to a pressure transducer that converts the pressure wave into an electrical signal that is displayed for continuous visual observation on an oscilloscope.
2 Measure the central venous pressure as directed.	2 This measurement provides a guide for the administration of blood and other intravenous fluids and is also a criterion for determining the presence of right ventricular failure.

Sedation and Muscle Relaxants

1 Administer sedatives and muscle relaxants as directed.	1 Sedatives and muscle relaxants eliminate spontaneous breathing efforts between ventilator cycles and reduce oxygen consumption. Mor-

Nursing Action	Reason

| | phine and curare (or similar drugs) produce vasodilation. Measure arterial blood pressure before their administration to detect hypotension. |

2   Explain procedures to patient and provide reassurance.

2   The patient may be awake although not capable of any motor response while these drugs are being given.

Fluid Balance

1   Record intake and output precisely and obtain an accurate daily weight.

1   Positive fluid balance resulting in increase in body weight and interstitial pulmonary oedema is a frequent problem in patients requiring mechanical ventilation. Prevention requires early recognition of fluid accumulation. Average adult who is dependent on parenteral nutrition can be expected to lose 0.25 kg (0.5 lb)/per day; therefore, *constant body weight indicates positive fluid balance*.

Nutrition

1   Offer patient oral fluids and food if he is able to swallow. If aspiration occurs, stop the feeding and place patient in a semiprone position with head down; tilt and institute chest physiotherapy to remove aspirated material.
   a. Start nasogastric feeding if oral intake is not adequate.

1   Starvation is a frequent and serious complication of patients in respiratory failure.

Abdominal Complications

1   Test all stools and gastric drainage for occult blood.

1   About a quarter of patients requiring mechanical ventilation develop gastrointestinal bleeding; many of these patients require blood transfusions.

2   Measure abdominal girth daily.

2   Abdominal distension occurs frequently with respiratory failure and further hinders respiration by elevation of the diaphragm. Measurement of abdominal girth provides objective assessment of the degree of distension.

Communication

1 Provide writing paper and pad. A patient on mechanical ventilation with tracheostomy tube is unable to talk.
2 Establish some form of nonverbal communication if patient is too sick to write. Give patient the call light.
3 Reassure patient and family that normal speech will return upon removal of tracheal tube.
4 Ensure that the patient has adequate rest and sleep.
5 Keep the patient in touch with reality; explain that mechanical ventilation is only temporary.

Recording

Maintain a flow sheet to record ventilation patterns, arterial blood studies, venous chemical determinations, haematocrit, status of fluid balance, weight and assessment of patient's condition.

Weaning the Patient from the Mechanical Ventilator

Weaning—the process by which the patient is gradually allowed to resume the responsbility for regulating his own breathing.

Weaning Modalities

Intermittent Mandatory Ventilation (IMV)

A process in which the rate of ventilator-delivered breaths/min decreases. The patient is allowed to breathe spontaneously from a reservoir bag connected in line with the ventilator circuit between machine-controlled breaths.

Nursing Action	Reason
1 Install IMV setup in ventilator circuit.	1 Explain procedure to patient.
2 Set ventilator to control mode.	2 This is done to assure that the patient's tidal volume will be the result of his inspiratory effort instead of simply initiating a machine-delivered breath.
3 Set IMV interval.	3 This determines the time period between machine-delivered breaths during which the patient will breathe on his own from the reservoir bag.
4 Observe reservoir bag.	4 The gas flow rate into the bag must be adequate to prevent the patient from collapsing it during inspiration. Flow rates of 4–6 l/min are usually adequate.
5 Stay with patient.	5 Constant reassurance, especially during initial weaning stages, is crucial.

Nursing Action	Reason

6   Observe respiratory rate and pulse rate.

6   Dramatic increases in either respiration or pulse could indicate that the patient is not yet ready for weaning.

7   Obtain arterial blood gas analysis.

7   Blood gas analysis, especially the parameters of carbon dioxide and oxygen, are direct indicators of the ability of the patient to adequately ventilate himself. A dramatic rise in carbon dioxide levels indicates inadequate ventilation.

8   With each increase of IMV interval or decrease in FIO_2, blood gases should be obtained.

Briggs Adapter (T-tube)

This system provides oxygen enrichment and humidification to a patient with an endotracheal or tracheostomy tube while allowing completely spontaneous respiration (see Fig. 3.20). For further amplification see Oxygen Therapy section.

Nursing Action	Reason

1   Explain the procedure to patient.

2   Install the equipment.

2   Oxygen levels are usually those used during IMV.

A.   IMV reservoir bag
B.   Oxygen supply
C.   Cascade humidifier
D.   Inspiratory tubing
E.   Thermometer
F.   Manifold
G.   Tracheostomy connector (T-tube)
H.   Expiratory tubing
I.   Blender
J.   Flowmeter
K.   Spirometer

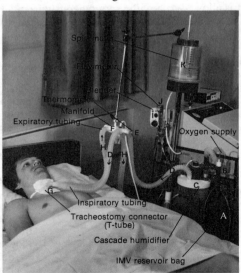

T-tube

Figure 3.20   Mechanical ventilation with IMV modality. Detail of T-tube.

3   Observe patient closely.

3   Dramatic increases in pulse and respiratory rate may indicate the patient is not ready for this stage of weaning.

4   Obtain arterial blood gases in 20–30 min.

4   Same as step 7 under IMV.

5   If step 4 above produces adequate blood gases the oxygen levels may be gradually decreased until the patient is breathing room air.

5   Repeat blood gas analysis after each change.

NOTE: It is not within the scope of this book to establish criteria for the use of one weaning method as opposed to another.

Stages of Weaning

Preweaning Assessment

1   Tidal volume—about 300–400 ml.
2   Forced vital capacity.
    It is desirable to have a forced vital capacity of 1 litre or two times tidal volume.
3   Inspiratory effect.
    a. This measures the ability of the respiratory muscles to develop subatmospheric pressure within the respiratory system.
    b. 20 cm H_2O is generally deemed adequate.
4   Respiratory drive.
    Patient must be breathing spontaneously.
5   Blood gas analysis.
    a. Patient should be close to what is for him a 'normal' acid-base state.
    b. Arterial CO_2 levels should also be close to 'normal' for the patient.

NOTE: Steady-state values for a young, healthy adult are not the same as those of a 75-year-old person with severe COLD.

    c. Failure to adhere to guidelines **a** and **b**, above, may result in rapid alterations of pH and unsuccessful weaning attempts.

Weaning from Mechanical Ventilator

1   IMV (see p. 309).
2   T-tube (see p. 310).

Weaning from Tracheostomy or Endotracheal Tube

1   The patient must be able to maintain adequate blood gases when breathing spontaneously.
2   Sit patient upright and deflate tracheostomy or endotracheal cuff.
3   Test patient's ability to swallow without aspiration before cuff is deflated.
    a. Clear trachea, nasopharynx and oropharynx of secretions.
    b. Deflate the cuff.

c. Have the patient drink dilute methylene blue solution (0.5 ml in 60 ml of water).

d. Aspirate the trachea immediately; absence of blue dye in tracheal aspirate indicates the ability to swallow without aspiration.

Weaning from the Tracheostomy Stoma

1   A fenestrated tracheostomy tube (uncuffed tube with window in greater curvature to decrease resistance to air flow) may be used after mechanical ventilator has been discontinued.

2   Plug the external orifice of fenestrated tracheostomy tube.

   a. Evaluate the patient's ability to breathe spontaneously for long periods.

   b. Assess ability to cough and mobilize secretions without aid of tracheal aspiration.

   c. Have the patient drink dilute methylene blue solution ($0 \cdot 5$ ml in 60 ml of water).

   d. Aspirate the trachea immediately; absence of blue dye in tracheal aspirate indicates the ability to swallow without aspiration.

3   The tube is usually removed when tracheal aspiration has been unnecessary for 24 hours.

4   Cover the stoma with a sterile dressing; stoma is allowed to close.

Weaning from Supplementary Inspired Air

Supplementary inspired oxygen may be required for an additional period until patient can maintain adequate O_2 and CO_2 tensions while breathing room air.

Patient Education for Prevention of Recurrences of Respiratory Failure

Instruct the patient as follows:

1   Avoid and treat respiratory infections promptly.

2   Avoid respiratory irritants, particularly smoking.

3   Take oral and nebulized bronchodilators on prescribed basis.

4   Ensure adequate hydration.

5   Carry out a programme of gradually increasing exercise tolerance.

CLINICAL CONDITIONS

The Pneumonias

Pneumonia is an infection of the lung parenchyma. (See Table 3.3, pp. 246–249).

Characteristics of Pneumonia

1   Pathogens producing pneumonia may be carried in nasopharynx of a healthy person.

2   Pathogens may invade tissues when the host's natural resistance is lowered.

3   Colds and upper respiratory tract infections lead to more serious illnesses by allowing bacterial invasion of lower respiratory tract.

4   A wide variety of pulmonary infections may develop in patients receiving

corticosteroids or other immunosuppressive drugs (aerobic and anaerobic Gram-negative bacilli, *Staphyloccocus, Nocardia*, fungi, *Candida*, viruses (including cytomegalovirus), *pneumocystis carinii*, reactivation of tuberculosis and others).

5   Patients on high dosages of corticosteroids have a reduced resistance to infections.

6   Any condition interfering with normal drainage of the lung will predispose the person to pneumonia (e.g., cancer of the lung).

7   Postoperative patients may develop bronchopneumonia, since anaesthesia impairs respiratory defenses and decreases diaphragmatic movement.

8   Therapy of pneumonia depends on laboratory identification of the agent causing the infection and on drainage of purulent secretions.

Nursing Alert: Recurring pneumonia often indicates underlying disease (cancer of the lung, multiple myeloma).

Pneumonia

Pneumonia is an inflammatory reaction of lung tissues to infection or irritants, causing consolidation of the alveoli. This is due to an exudate which contains erythrocytes, as well as many leucocytes. This exudate may become purulent.

Type of Pneumonia

1   Infective—bacterial, mycoplasmal, rickettsial, viral.
2   Aspiration:
   a. Inhaled chemical irritants, gases and vapours, e.g. ammonia.
   b. Inhaled vomit.
   c. Inhaled oily or fatty material.
   d. Hypostatic pneumonia.
3   Suppurative:
   a. A type of aspiration pneumonia, due to the inhalation of infected material during a period of unconsciousness.
   b. Infection with *Staphylococcus pyogenes*.

Predisposing Causes

1   Lowered resistance of host, e.g., old age, with a reduction of effectiveness of the coughing mechanism in clearing secretions.
2   Chronic systemic disease, e.g., diabetes mellitus, glomerulonephritis, multiple myelomatosis.
3   Corticosteroid therapy, causing depression of the normal immune response.
4   Viral infections of the upper respiratory tract, e.g., Influenza. Also, measles particularly in the first 2 years of life.
5   Chronic infection of the upper respiratory tract, e.g., chronic sinusitis.
6   Decreased diameter of the air passage:
   a. In infancy.
   b. In chronic airway obstruction due to chronic bronchitis, bronchiectasis, cystic fibrosis.

7 Impairment of drainage of bronchial secretions.
   a. Distal to local obstruction, e.g., bronchial carcinoma or inhaled foreign body
   b. Retained sputum leading to infected secretions.
8 Prolonged immobilization, e.g. patients postoperatively.

Preventive Measures for susceptible persons

1 Natural resistance should be maintained (adequate nutrition, rest, exercise).

Table 3.3. Commonly Encountered Pneumonias

Type (Nonbacterial)	Organism Responsible	Manifestations
Mycoplasmal pneumonia	*Mycoplasma pneumoniae*	Gradual onset, severe headache, irritating hacking cough productive of scanty, mucoid sputum Anorexia; malaise Low grade fever
Viral pneumonia	Influenza viruses Parainfluenza viruses Respiratory syncytial viruses Adenovirus Varicella, rubella, rubeola, herpes, simplex, cytomegalovirus, Epstein–Barr virus	Cough Constitutional symptoms may be pronounced (severe headache, anorexia, fever and myalgia)
Pneumocystis carinii pneumonia	*Pneumocystis carinii*	Insidious onset Increasing dyspnoea and nonproductive cough Tachypnoea; progresses rapidly to intercostal retraction, nasal flaring and cyanosis Lowering of arterial oxygen tension Chest x-ray will reveal diffuse, bilateral interstitial pneumonia
Legionnaire's disease	Legionella pneumophilia	Cough Toxaemia Gastro-intestinal symptoms Hyponatraemia

2   Avoid contact with people who have upper respiratory infections.
3   Obliteration of cough reflex and aspiration of secretions should be avoided.
4   Highly susceptible persons (elderly and chronically ill) should be immunized against influenza.
5   Adequate bronchial hygiene should be employed.
6   Immobilized patients should be turned every 2 hours and encouraged to breathe deeply, sigh and cough.

Clinical Features	Treatment	Complications

Occurs most commonly in children and young adults
Cold agglutinin antibody titre elevated
	Tetracycline	Rare:
		  pleural effusion
		  meningoencephalitis
		  myelitis
		  Guillain–Barré syndrome

In majority of patients influenza begins as an acute coryza; others have bronchitis, pleurisy, etc., while still others develop gastrointestinal symptoms Risk of developing influenza related to crowding and close contact of groups of individuals	Treat symptomatically Does not respond to treatment with presently available antibiotics Prophylactic vaccination recommended for high risk persons (over 65; chronic cardiac or pulmonary disease, diabetes and other metabolic disorders)	May develop a superimposed bacterial infection Bronchopneumonia Pericarditis; endocarditis
Usually seen in host whose resistance is compromised Organism invades lungs of patients who have suppressed immune system (from cancer, leukaemia) or following immunosuppressive therapy for cancer, organ transplant or collagen disease Frequently associated with concurrent infection by viruses (cytomegalovirus), bacteria and fungi Diagnosis made by lung biopsy	Pentamide isethionate	Patients are critically ill Death may be due to asphyxia
	Eurythromycin	

Type (Bacterial)	Organism Responsible	Manifestations
Streptococcal pneumonia*	*Streptococcus pneumoniae*	May be history of previous respiratory infection Sudden onset, with shaking and chills Rapidly rising fever Cough, with expectoration of rusty or green (purulent) sputum Pleuritic pain aggravated by cough Chest dull to percussion; râles, bronchial breath sounds
Staphylococcal pneumonia	*Staphylococcus aureus*	Often prior history of viral infection Insidious development of cough, with expectoration of yellow, blood-streaked mucus Onset may be sudden if patient is outside hospital Fever Pleuritic chest pain Pulse varies; may be slow in proportion to temperature
Klebsiella pneumonia	*Klebsiella pneumoniae* (Friedländer's bacillus —encapsulated Gram-negative aerobic bacillus)	Onset sudden with high fever, chills, pleuritic pain, haemoptysis Dyspnoea, cyanosis Pink, gelatinous or loose, thin sputum expectorated Profound prostration and toxicity
Pseudomonas pneumonia	*Pseudomonas aeruginosa*	Apprehension, confusion, cyanosis, bradycardia, reversal of diurnal temperature curve

Clinical Features	Treatment	Complications
Herpes simplex lesions often present Usually involves one or more lobes	Penicillin G Alternate drug therapy in penicillin-allergic patient (erythromycin, clinda-mycin, cephalothin)	Shock Pleural effusion Superinfections Pericarditis
Frequently seen in hospital setting Staphyloccocal pneumonia is a necrotizing infection Treatment must be vigorous and prolonged due to disease's tendency to destroy the lungs Organism may develop rapid lung resistance Prolonged convalescence usual	Methicillin, nafcillin, clindamycin, lincomycin	Effusion/pneumothorax Lung abscess Empyema Meningitis
Tends to attack chronically ill, debilitated, alcoholic and elderly men or those with chronic obstructive pulmonary disease Tissue necrosis occurs rapidly in lungs May be rapidly fulminating, progressing to fatal outcome High mortality rate	Gentamicin, cephalothin, cefazolin, kanamycin	Multiple lung abscesses with cyst formation Persistent cough with expectoration remains for prolonged period Empyema Pericarditis
Susceptible persons: those with pre-existing lung disease, cancer (particularly leukaemia); those with homograft transplants, burns; debilitated persons; patients receiving prolonged courses of antibiotics Positive pressure breathing equipment may be contaminated with these organisms	Gentamicin, carbenicillin	Multiple lung abscess formation High fatality rate

Clinical Manifestations

See Table 3.3, pp. 314–317).

Diagnosis

1 Chest auscultation and percussion—listen for dullness to percussion, decreased breath sounds, râles.
2 Lateral and posteroanterior chest x-rays—to localize the process and determine presence or absence of fluid.
3 Gram stain, culture and sensitivity studies of sputum.
4 Blood culture—to recover causative organism.
5 Aspiration—if pleural effusion is present.
6 Testing for cold agglutinin antibody titre—persons with atypical pneumonia will have elevated titre.

Overall Objectives of Nursing Care for a Patient with Pneumonia

1 To provide good nursing care, including constant observation and prevention of complications.
2 The patient will be nursed in a quiet, warm, draught free room, well supported in a upright position in bed, and spared unnecessary exertion.
3 Full nursing care of a febrile patient: encourage fluids by mouth, bed baths, frequent mouth washes, light, warm bedclothes.
4 Very careful nursing is needed, particularly for extreme ages, e.g., very young children or very old people.

Objectives of Treatment and Nursing Management

For patient with bacterial pneumonia.

To Take a Careful History to Help Establish Aetiologic Diagnosis

1 What was the mode of onset?
2 Number and frequency and duration of chills.
3 Description of chest pain.
4 Patient taking any recent antibiotic drugs?
5 Any family illness?
6 Alcohol, tobacco, drug abuse?

To Identify the Aetiologic Agent Causing the Pneumonia and to Determine the Drug Sensitivity

1 Obtain freshly expectorated sputum for direct smear (Gram stain) and culture.
2 Be sure patient *coughs* up sputum, not saliva.
3 Instruct patient to expectorate into sterile container for culture.
4 Utilize percussion (p. 254) with or without IPPB treatment as directed; tenacious sputum may be liquefied by inhaling nebulized aerosol of water or saline solution by mask.
5 Aspirate trachea with catheter if patient is too ill to raise sputum (See Guidelines, p. 247).
6 Sputum may also be collected by transtracheal aspiration (p. 243).

To Listen for Râles, Signs of Consolidation or Pleural Effusion

1 Blood may be taken for bacterial culture (for predominant organism) and for sedimentation rate, white blood count and differential cell count.
2 Elevated leucocyte count seen in bacterial pneumonia; leucopaenia indicates inability of body to maintain an immune response.
3 Differential cell count assesses body's ability to combat foreign particles.

To Clear the Bronchi of Collected Secretions—Retained Secretions Interfere with Gas Exchange and may Cause Slow Resolution (subsidence).

1 Encourage high-level of fluid intake within limits of patient's cardiac reserve—adequate hydration thins mucus and serves as an effective expectorant.
2 Humidify air to loosen secretions and improve ventilation.
3 Encourage patient to cough; avoid suppressing the cough reflex, especially in patients who sound 'bubbly'.
4 Arrange for physiotherapist to give appropriate therapy to loosen secretions.
5 Utilize tracheal aspiration in patients with poor cough response.
6 Assist in bronchoscopic removal of inspissated (thickened) mucus plugs if patient is too weak to cough effectively.
7 Control cough when coughing paroxysms cause serious hypoxia; give moderate doses of linctus codeine as prescribed.
8 Avoid hypoxia especially in patients with existing heart disease.

To Observe the Patient Carefully and Continuously Until Clinical Condition Improves

1 Remember that lethal complications may develop during the early period of antibiotic treatment.
2 Monitor temperature, pulse, respiration and blood pressure at regular intervals to assess patient's response to therapy.
3 Listen to lungs and heart—heart murmurs or friction rub may indicate acute bacterial endocarditis, pericarditis or myocarditis.
4 Assess for resistant fever or return of fever from:
   a. Drug allergy. Usually skin eruptions appear 7–10 days after the beginning of treatment.
   b. Drug resistance or slow response to therapy.
   c. Inadequate or inappropriate antibiotic therapy.
   d. Superinfection (infection with a second organism resistant to antibiotics used).
   e. Failure of pneumonia to resolve; raises suspicion of underlying carcinoma of bronchus.
   f. Pneumonia caused by unusual bacteria, fungi, tuberculosis or *Pneumocystis carinii*.
5 Obtain chest x-rays to follow resolution (subsidence) of pneumonic process.

To Utilize Supportive Methods of Treatment

1 Do blood gas analysis to determine oxygen need, give precise oxygen guidance and evaluate oxygen effectiveness.
   An arterial oxygen tension (Po_2) below 7.3 kPg (55 mmHg) indicates hypoxaemia.

2   Administer oxygen at concentration to maintain Po_2 at acceptable level.
3   Avoid high concentrations of oxygen in patients with chronic obstructive lung disease (chronic bronchitis, emphysema(—*the use of high oxygen concentrations may worsen alveolar ventilation by removing patient's only remaining ventilatory drive*.
4   Observe patient for cyanosis, dyspnoea, hypoxaemia.
5   Patients with pneumonia with coexisting chronic ventilatory insufficiency may require mechanical ventilation.
6   Relieve the pleuritic pain.
   a. Avoid suppressing a productive cough.
   b. Avoid narcotics in patient with history of chronic obstructive lung disease (COLD)
   c. Administer moderate doses of analgesics to relieve pleuritic pain.
   d. Treat dry cough and laryngospasm with aerosolized water produced by an ultrasonic nebulizer.
   e. Give semiliquid diet to avoid aspiration when patient is coughing.
   f. Observe level of response before administering sedatives or tranquillizers to assess for signs and symptoms suggestive of meningitis.

Nursing Alert: Restlessness, confusion, aggressiveness may be due to cerebral hypoxia. In such instances sedatives are inappropriate.

7   Maintain adequate hydration since fluid loss is high from fever, dehydration, dyspnoea and diaphoresis.
8   Encourage modified bed rest during febrile period.
9   Treat abdominal distension which may be due to swallowing of air during intervals of severe dyspnoea.
   a. Pass nasogastric tube for acute gastric distension.
   b. Use a rectal tube and give neostigmine methylsulphate to facilitate intestinal decompression.
   c. Allow patient to breathe high concentrations of oxygen, since oxygen may be rapidly absorbed from intestines (except for patients with COLD).

To Observe for Complications

1   Patients should respond to treatment within 24–48 hours. However, be on the alert for complications such as the following:
   a. Pleural effusion.
   b. Sustained hypotension and shock, especially in Gram-negative bacterial disease, particularly in the elderly.
   c. Meningitis; look for nuchal rigidity.
   d. Atelectasis (may occur at any stage of acute pneumonia).
   e. Toxic delirium (*this is considered a medical emergency*).
   f. Lung abscess; brain abscess.
   g. Congestive heart failure, cardiac arrhythmias, pericarditis, myocarditis.
   h. Peripheral thrombophlebitis, with or without pulmonary emboli.
   i. Petechiae in skin—possible bacterial endocarditis.
   j. Empyema.
2   Employ special nursing surveillance for patients with the following conditions:
   a. Alcoholism or chronic obstructive lung disease; these persons as well as

elderly patients may have little or no fever.

b. Chronic bronchitis. It is difficult to detect subtle changes in condition, since patient may have seriously compromised pulmonary function.

c. Epilepsy; pneumonia may result from aspiration following a seizure.

d. Delirium, which may be caused by hypoxia, meningitis, delirium tremens of alcoholism.

  (1) Prepare for lumbar puncture; meningitis may be lethal.

  (2) Assure adequate hydration and give mild sedation.

  (3) Give oxygen.

  (4) Delirium must be controlled to prevent exhaustion and cardiac failure.

3   Assess these patients for *unusual behaviour*, alterations in mental status, stupor, and congestive heart failure.

Discharge Planning and Health Teaching

1   Fatigue and weakness may be prolonged after pneumonia.

2   Encourage chair rest after fever subsides; gradually increase activities to bring energy level back to preillness stage.

3   Encourage breathing exercises (p. 255) to clear lungs and promote full expansion and function after the fever subsides.

4   Explain that a chest x-ray is taken 2–4 weeks after discharge; should show cleared lungs.

5   It is wise to stop smoking. Cigarette smoking destroys tracheobronchial cilial action, which is first line of defence of lungs; also irritates mucous cells of bronchi and inhibits function of alveolar scavenger cells (macrophages).

6   Advise patient to keep up natural resistance with good nutrition, adequate rest—one episode of pneumonia may make the individual susceptible to recurring respiratory infections.

7   Instruct patient to avoid overfatigue, sudden changes in temperature and excessive alcohol intake, which lowers resistance to pneumonia.

8   Encourage patient to obtain influenza vaccine at prescribed times. Influenza increases susceptibility to secondary bacterial pneumonia.

Aspiration Pneumonia

Aspiration is the inhalation of oropharyngeal secretions and/or stomach contents into the lungs. It may produce an acute form of pneumonia.

Aetiology

Patients at risk; factors associated with risk:

1   Loss of protective airway reflexes—swallowing, laryngeal, cough.

  a. Altered state of consciousness (general anaesthesia, head injury, stroke, coma, convulsions).

  b. Drugs, alcohol.

  c. During resuscitation procedures.

  d. Seriously ill, debilitated patients.

2   Nasogastric tube feedings.

3 Obstetrical patients—from general anaesthesia, lithotomy position, delayed emptying of stomach from enlarged uterus, labour contractions.
4 Oesophageal disease—motility disease, hiatal hernia.
5 Delayed emptying time of stomach—intestinal obstruction, abdominal distension.
6 Prolonged endotracheal intubation/tracheostomy—can depress glottic and laryngeal reflexes from disuse.

Clinical Manifestations

1 Depends on volume and character of aspirated contents.
   a. Food particles—mechanical blockage of airways and secondary infection.
   b. Pathogenic bacteria—from oropharyngeal secretions containing bacteria.
   c. Gastric juice—destructive to alveoli and capillaries; results in outpouring of protein-rich fluids into the interstitial and intra-alveolar spaces—impairs exchange of oxygen and carbon dioxide producing, hypoxaemia and respiratory insufficiency and failure.
   d. Faecal contamination—endotoxins may be absorbed or thick proteinaceous material found in the intestinal contents may obstruct airway, leading to atelectasis and secondary bacterial infection.
2 Tachycardia.
3 Dyspnoea.
4 Cyanosis.
5 Râles, rhonchi, wheezing.
6 Pink, frothy, sputum (may simulate acute pulmonary oedema).
7 Fever.

Prevention

1 Be on guard constantly and monitor patients at risk as described above.
2 Elevate head of bed for debilitated patients, for those receiving tube feedings and for those with motility diseases of the oesophagus.
3 Place patients with impaired reflexes in a lateral position.
4 Be sure that nasogastric tube is functioning.
5 Give tube feedings slowly with patient sitting up in bed.
   a. Check position of tube in stomach before feeding.
   b. Check seal of cuff of tracheostomy or endotracheal tube before feeding.
6 Keep patients in a fasting state before anaesthesia (at least 6 hours).

Treatment and Nursing Care

Objective

To remove the factor(s) interfering with adequate gas exchange.

1 Clear the obstructed airway.
   a. If foreign body becomes lodged in throat, perform the Heimlich manoeuvre or remove with forceps.
   b. Place patient in tilted head-down position on right side (right side more frequently affected if patient has aspirated solid particles).
   c. Suction trachea/endotracheal tube.

d. Prepare for laryngoscopy/bronchoscopy if patient is asphyxiated by solid material.
2   Correct hypoxia by immediate ventilation.
   a. Give oxygen.
   b. Place patient on assisted ventilation—if adequate PO_2 cannot be maintained with other means of administering oxygen (see p. 303).
   c. Give intravenous aminophylline or bronchodilators by nebulizer—to help relieve bronchospasm.
3   Correct hypotension (usually the result of hypovolaemia and hypoxia) by fluid volume replacement.
4   Give supportive therapy as indicated.
   a. Corticosteroids—may diminish inflammatory response.
   b. Antibiotics—to prevent secondary bacterial infection.
   c. Correct acidosis—respiratory acidosis and metabolic acidosis indicate a severe reaction due to gastric contents.
   d. Monitor arterial blood gases.

Pleurisy

Pleurisy (pleuritis) is inflammation of the pleura.
   Fibrinous pleurisy is deposition of a fibrinous exudate on the pleural surface.

Causes

May occur in the course of many pulmonary diseases:

1   Pneumonia (bacterial, viral).
2   Tuberculosis.
3   Pulmonary infarction, embolism.
4   Pulmonary abscess.
5   Upper respiratory tract infection.
6   Pulmonary neoplasm.

Clinical Manifestations

1   Chest pain—becomes severe, sharp and knife-like upon inspiration.
   a. Pain may become minimal or absent when breath is held.
   b. Pain may be localized or radiate to shoulder or abdomen.
2   Intercostal tenderness.
3   Pleural friction rub—grating or leathery sounds heard in both phases of respiration; heard low in the axilla or over the lung base posteriorly; may be heard only a day or so.
4   Evidence of infection; fever, malaise, increased white cell count.

Diagnosis

1   Chest x-ray.
2   Sputum examination.
3   Examination of pleural fluid obtained by thoracentesis for smear and culture.
4   Pleural biopsy (selected patients).

Treatment and Nursing Management

Objective

To discover underlying condition.

1   Treat the underlying primary disease (pneumonia, infarction, etc.). Inflammation usually resolves when the primary disease subsides.
2   Relieve the pain.
   a. Give prescribed analgesics.
   b. Splint the rib cage (Fig. 3.21, p. 352) when the patient coughs.
   c. Apply heat or cold—to provide symptomatic relief.
   d. Instruct patient to lie on affected side occasionally—to splint chest wall.
   e. Assist with procaine intercostal block.
3   Watch for signs of development of pleural effusion (collection of fluid in pleural space): shortness of breath, pain, local decreased excursion of chest wall.

Pleural Effusion

Pleural effusion refers to a collection of fluid in the pleural space. It is rarely a primary disease, but is usually secondary to other diseases.

Aetiology

Complication of:
1   Disseminated cancer (particularly lung and breast); lymphoma.
2   Infection: tuberculosis, bacterial pneumonia, pulmonary infection.
3   Congestive heart failure.

Clinical Manifestations

1   Increasing dyspnoea.
2   Dullness or flatness to percussion (over areas of fluid) with minimal or absent breath sounds.

Diagnosis

1   Chest x-ray.
2   Aspiration—biochemical, bacteriologic and cytologic studies of pleural fluid.
3   Physical examination.
4   Pleuroscopy (p. 242) done occasionally.

Treatment and Nursing Management

Objectives

To determine the cause.
To remove fluid in order to relieve discomfort and dyspnoea.
To prevent fluid collection from recurring.

1   The treatment depends on the cause. Give specific treatment related to the underlying disease.

2 The following modalities of treatment have been advocated for malignant effusions.
   a. Thoracentesis (aspiration) for fluid removal and relief of dyspnoea.
      (1) In malignant diseases, aspiration may provide only transient benefits since effusion may return within a few days.
      (2) Repeated aspiration results in pain, depletion of protein and electrolytes, pneumothorax.
   b. Tube drainage (chest catheter) connected to underwater seal drainage system or suction; single or daily irrigation of pleural space with cytotoxic or other chemically irritating drugs.
      (1) Chest catheter helps to evacuate pleural space and re-expand lung.
      (2) Drug is introduced into catheter; tube is clamped; patient is helped to assume the following positions for at least 1 min each to ensure uniform distribution of the drug and maximize drug contact with pleural surfaces: prone, left side down, supine, right side down, knee to chest (if able).
      (3) Tube is unclamped as prescribed.
      (4) Nitrogen mustard may require aspiration within 24 hours—causes inflammatory reaction.
      (5) Chest drainage continued several days longer.
   c. Radioactive isotopes added to pleural space (gold, yttrium, yttrium/gold combinations).
   d. Radiation of chest wall.
   e. Surgical pleurectomy.
   f. Diuretics.

Empyema

Empyema refers to a pleural effusion that contains pus.

Aetiology

1 Secondary to infection of the lung, most commonly bacterial pneumonias and tuberculosis.
2 Infected penetrating injuries of the chest wall.
3 Rupture of a subphrenic abscess through the diaphragm (rare).

Clinical Manifestations

1 Patient with a chest infection who fails to respond to normal therapy.
2 Systemic features: Pyrexia—usually high—rigors, sweating, malaise, anorexia, loss of weight.
3 Local features: cough and purulent sputum, chest pain.
4 Clubbing of the fingers may develop within 3–4 weeks.

Diagnosis

1 Chest x-ray.
2 Chest aspiration.

Treatment and Nursing Management

1   Identification of causative organism—from sputum specimens and pleural fluid, followed by treatment with appropriate antibiotic.
2   Acute stage. If the pus is thin in consistency, aspiration with a fairly wide bore needle can be carried out. If fluid tends to reaccumulate, an intercostal tube may be inserted, and attached to an underwater-seal drainage (see Fig. 3.22, p. 356).
3   If the pus becomes thicker, and fibrosis of the lung is present, it may be necessary to replace the underwater-seal by a suction type. (see Fig. 3.22, p. 356).
4   Chronic stage. Fibrosis of the pleura in the affected area, and loculation of the empyema cavity occurs. Thoracotomy and decortication may be necessary. If the pulmonary function is poor, or the patient unfit for major surgery, an open pleural drain may be inserted into the localized fibrosed cavity. This is rarely needed these days.
5   Arrange for chest physiotherapy.
6   Maintain general health. Because of prolonged infective focus, rest, good nutrition, with a high protein intake and suitable environment are essential.

Lung Abscess

A *lung abscess* is a localized, pus-containing, necrotic lesion in the lung characterized by cavity formation.

Aetiology

1   Aspiration of infected material from upper respiratory tract.
    a. Blood after tonsillectomy.
    b. Dental deposits, mucoid or purulent nasopharyngeal secretions.
    c. Foreign body aspirated into lung—during drug overdose, alcoholic stupor, coma, epileptic seizure, children inhaling peanut during exercise.
2   Bronchial obstruction (usually a tumour causes obstruction to the bronchus, causing distal stasis and infection of secretions, or there is necrosis within the tumour mass).
3   Necrotizing pneumonias.
4   Tuberculosis.
5   Pulmonary embolism.
6   Chest trauma.

Clinical Features and Manifestations

1   The right lung is involved more frequently than the left—owing to dependent position of the right bronchus, the less acute angle which the right main bronchus forms within the trachea and its larger size.
2   In the initial stages, the cavity in the lung may or may not communicate with the bronchus.
3   Eventually the cavity becomes surrounded or encapsulated by a wall of fibrous tissue, except at one or two points where the necrotic process extends until it reaches the lumen of some bronchus or pleural space and establishes a communication with the respiratory tract, the pleural cavity (bronchopleural fistula), or both.

Symptoms

1 Cough.
2 Fever and malaise—from segmental pneumonitis and atelectasis.
3 Headache, asthenia, weight loss.
4 Pleuritic chest pain—from extension of suppurative pneumonitis to pleural surface.
5 Production of sputum—foul, yellow, green mucopurulent material which becomes profuse after abscess ruptures into bronchial tree.
6 Clubbing of fingers and toes—may signify underlying bronchogenic carcinoma.

Diagnosis

1 History of patient.
2 X-ray of chest—for diagnosis and location of lesion.
3 Bronchogram—may be necessary to differentiate between lung abscess and bronchiectasis.
4 Direct bronchoscopic visualization—to exclude possibility of tumour or foreign body.
5 Leucocytosis in acute stage.
6 Sputum culture and sensitivity—to determine causative organism(s) and antibiotic sensitivity.
7 Dullness and bronchial breath sounds—may be heard over diseased segment.

Treatment and Nursing Management

Objectives

To establish adequate drainage.
To eradicate the infection.

1 Give appropriate antibiotic based upon sensitivity of organisms cultured—mixed infections are common and may require multiple antibiotics.
2 Carry out drainage procedures.
   a. Postural drainage (hastens resolution)—positions to be assumed depend on the segmental localization of the abscess (see p. 252).
   b. Therapeutic bronchoscopy—to drain abscess.
3 Measure and record the volume of sputum—to follow the course of healing.
4 Utilize supportive measures during the acute phase of illness.
   a. Give a high protein, high calorie diet—significant protein loss may occur when the patient is expectorating large quantities of sputum.
   b. Care of the patient having blood transfusions—anaemia may be advanced in patient with infection.
5 Prepare for surgical intervention if indicated—done only if patient fails to respond to adequate medical treatment.
   a. Excision—usually lobectomy (occasionally segmental resection); done because infiltrative pneumonitis surrounding the lung abscess pocket usually extends beyond the segmental confines of the lung.
   b. Thoracotomy tube drainage—usually done for patients who cannot tolerate major thoracotomy (elderly patients, alcoholics, patients with low pulmonary functional reserve).
   c. See p. 348 for care of the patient having thoracic surgery.

Discharge Planning and Health Teaching

1 Encourage the patient to have patience—it may take 10 days to several months for the chest x-ray to be clear and for the cavity to close.
2 Encourage patient to assume responsibility for attaining and maintaining an optimum state of health through a planned programme of good nutrition, rest and exercise.

Bronchial Asthma

See Allergy Problems, Volume 1, Chapter 8

Bronchiectasis

Bronchiectasis is a chronic dilatation of the bronchi, usually peripheral.

Causes

1 Pulmonary infections and obstruction of bronchi.
2 Aspiration of foreign bodies, vomitus or material from upper respiratory tract.
3 Extrinsic pressure from tumours, dilated blood vessels, enlarged lymph nodes.

Altered Physiology

Bronchial obstruction→infection→progressive fibrosis of involved areas→weakening of bronchial wall→stenosis of involved segments→stasis of infected secretions→bronchial dilatation

Clinical Manifestations

The patient experiences symptoms when he has superimposed infection.

1 Productive cough.
2 Mucopurulent sputum.
3 Haemoptysis.
4 Râles over involved portion of lungs.
5 Recurrent bouts of localized pulmonary infection.
6 Dyspnoea (depending upon amount of lung tissue involved).
7 Clubbing of fingers.
8 Wheezing.

Diagnosis

1 Chest x-ray (may reveal areas of atelectasis with widespread dilatation of bronchi).
2 Bronchogram (to map the entire bronchial tree to determine the extent of bronchial dilation).
3 Bronchoscopy (usually shows purulent secretions from involved area).

Treatment and Nursing Management

Objective

To rid the affected portion(s) of the lungs of excessive secretions.

1 Treat the patient during periods of acute infection.
   a. Employ judicious antibiotic therapy guided by sensitivity studies upon organisms cultured from sputum.
   b. Patients with repeated infections may be given small doses of antibiotic prophylactically during the winter months.
2 Empty the bronchi of their accumulated secretions.
   a. Use postural drainage suitable to segment(s) involved to drain the bronchiectatic areas by gravity, thus reducing degree of infection and amount of secretions (see p. 252).
      (1) Postural drainage should be done for 20 min twice daily or more frequently as clinical condition indicates.
      (2) Affected chest area may be percussed or 'cupped' to assist in raising secretions (see p. 254).
   b. Encourage copious fluid intake to reduce viscosity of sputum.
   c. Utilize vaporizer to provide humidification and to keep secretions liquid.
   d. Eliminate smoking and dusts, which are bronchial irritants that increase secretions.
   e. Give expectorants and bronchodilator drugs when indicated. (See treatment of patient with emphysema, p 332.)
   f. Prepare patient for bronchoscopy when necessary to drain sputum and remove foreign body.
3 Employ surgical intervention when conservative treatment is inadequate.
   a. Segmental resection to spare as much healthy, functioning lung parenchyma as possible. (See p. 350) for principles of nursing following chest surgery).
   b. Evaluate for postoperative complications.
      (1) Pneumonia.
      (2) Empyema.

Discharge Planning and Health Teaching

1 Instruct the patient to avoid noxious fumes, pulmonary irritants (cigarette smoking) and dust.
2 Encourage regular dental care.
3 Instruct patient in postural drainage exercises. See pp. 335–336 for other health teaching aspects (patient with emphysema).

Chronic Obstructive Lung Disease (COLD)

Chronic obstructive lung disease (COLD) is a term that refers to a group of conditions associated with chronic obstruction of airflow in the lungs. It includes:

1 Bronchitis.
2 Emphysema.
3 Asthma.

Altered Physiology

1   Basically, the person with COLD has:
    a. Excessive secretion of mucus within the airways not due to specific causes (bronchitis).
    b. An increase in size of air spaces distal to the terminal bronchioles with loss of alveolar walls and elastic recoil of the lungs (emphysema).
    c. Narrowing of the bronchial airways that changes in severity (asthma; see Volume 1, Chapter 7 since the triggering device in asthma is allergic in origin).
    d. There may be an overlap of these conditions.
2   As a result of these conditions there is a subsequent derangement of airway dynamics—e.g., obstruction to airflow.

Causes of COLD (Emphysema-Bronchitis Complex)

1   Cigarette smoking.
2   Air pollution.
3   Occupational exposure.
4   Allergy.
5   Autoimmunity.
6   Infection.
7   Genetic predisposition.
8   Aging.

Chronic Bronchitis

Chronic bronchitis is a clinical syndrome which develops as a result of repeated irritation or infection of the bronchical mucosa.

It may vary from a simple type, in which there is cough and sputum for several months of the year, to a complicated type, in which acute exacerbations may cause severe airway obstruction and ventilatory failure.

A World Health Organization (WHO) definition of chronic bronchitis is 'cough and sputum on most days of over 3 months over two consecutive years, in the absence of other major lung disease'.

Altered Physiology

Infection, irritation, hypersensitivity→local hyperaemia→hypertrophy.

Clinical Manifestations

Usually insidious, developing over a period of years.

1   Recurrent bouts of coughing and sputum production.
2   Recurrent acute respiratory infections followed by persistent cough.
3   Production of thick, gelatinous sputum (greater amounts produced during superimposed infections).
4   Wheezing and dyspnoea as disease progresses.

Clinical Features

1   Acute exacerbations of chronic bronchitis are most apt to occur during winter months—patients have bronchospasm due to inhalation of cold air.
2   A wide range of viral, bacterial and mycoplasmal infections can produce acute exacerbations of bronchitis.
3   Secretions must be expelled; otherwise they produce chronic bronchial obstruction, air trapping, hypoxaemia, carbon dioxide retention and localized infection.
4   Chronic bronchitis often progresses to emphysema.

Diagnosis

1   Chest x-ray—to exclude other diseases of the chest.
2   Lung function studies.
3   Arterial blood gas analysis.

Treatment and Nursing Management

Objectives

To maintain patency of peripheral bronchial tree.
To facilitate removal of bronchial exudates.
To prevent disability.

See p. 00 (emphysema) for treatment.

Pulmonary Emphysema

Pulmonary emphysema is a complex lung disease characterized by loss of lung elasticity due to alveolar destruction.

Causes

See Causes of Chronic Obstructive Lung Disease, above.

Diagnosis

1   Clinical assessment of patient.
2   Timed vital capacity.
3   Chest x-ray.
4   Arterial blood gas analysis (with exercise if possible) to detect hypoxaemia.
5   Alpha$_1$–Antitrypsin Assay—useful in identifying person at risk.

Clinical Manifestations

1   *Dyspnoea;* slow in onset and steadily progressive.
2   Weakness, lethargy, anorexia, weight loss—due to hypoxia, increased respiratory muscular effort and respiratory acidosis.
3   Cough may be minimal except with respiratory infection.

Complications

1   Respiratory acidosis.
2   Cor pulmonale.
3   Congestive heart failure.
4   Spontaneous pneumothorax.
5   Overwhelming respiratory infections.
6   Cardiac arrhythmias.
7   Profound depression.
8   Malnutrition.

Objectives of Treatment and Nursing Management

To Remove Bronchial Secretions—Retained Mucopurulent Secretions Perpetuate the Problem

1   *Eliminate all pulmonary irritants, particularly cigarette smoking.*
    a. Cessation of smoking usually results in decreased pulmonary irritation, sputum production and cough.
    b. Avoid outside physical activities when air pollutants are high.
    c. Keep bedroom as dust-free as possible.
    d. Consider the use of air filters to remove particles and pollutants from air in areas where this is a problem.
    e. Use a room humidifier—allows dust particles to settle and makes air less irritating.
    f. Keep constant room temperature throughout the house.
2   Control bronchospasm—nearly all patients with chronic obstructive pulmonary disease have some degree of bronchospasm.
    a. Bronchospasm is detected by auscultation with a stethoscope.
    b. Administer prescribed bronchodilators, which dilate airways by combating both bronchial mucosal oedema and smooth muscle contraction.
    (1) See p. 262 for table of bronchodilators.
    (2) Drugs may be administered orally, subcutaneously, intravenously or rectally; or via nebulization (by pressurized aerosols, hand-held nebulizers, pump-driven nebulizers or IPPB).
    (3) Assess patient for cardiovascular side-effects—tremor, tingling of extremities, tachycardia and excessive perspiration.
    (4) Avoid excessive use of bronchodilators.
    (5) Assess effectiveness of bronchodilators by use of Peak Flow Meter.
3   Keep secretions liquid.
    a. Encourage a high level of fluid intake (10–12 glasses; 2.5–3 l daily) within level of cardiac reserve.
    b. Administer expectorants as directed to alter bronchial secretions.
    c. Administer inhalations of nebulized water to humidify bronchial tree and liquefy sputum.
4   Give IPPB treatments to deliver nebulized medications, increase alveolar ventilation, moisten secretions and relieve respiratory insufficiency.
    a. See p. 281 for technique of IPPB.
    b. Patient may be given simultaneous nebulization of a sympathomimetic bronchodilator and a mucolytic agent.

c. Use gentle inspiration with prolonged expiratory phase.

d. IPPB treatments with oxygen must be given with extreme caution to patients who have chronically elevated carbon dioxide tensions and who are breathing on hypoxic stimulus. Use compressed air to drive machine if patient retains CO_2

5 Use postural drainage positions to aid in clearance of secretions, since mucopurulent secretions are responsible for airway obstruction.

a. Positions that drain lower and middle lobes appear to be most helpful in patients with COLD.

b. Other patients achieve effective cough and sputum clearance while seated and leaning forward.

c. Vigorous physiotherapy will help to loosen tenacious sputum.

6 Prepare patient for bronchoscopic removal of secretions if he is unable to cough and raise his sputum.

7 Prepare patient for endotracheal intubation or tracheostomy if indicated, to permit more effective suctioning of secretions and to provide ventilatory assistance.

To Control Infections in Order to Diminish Inflammatory Oedema and Allow Bronchial Mucosa to Recover Normal Ciliary Action—Repeated Respiratory Infections Contribute to Progress of COLD

1 Recognize early manifestations of respiratory infection—increasingly marked shortness of breath; fatigue; change in colour, amount and character of sputum; nervousness; irritability; low grade fever.

2 Obtain sputum for smear and culture.

3 Give prescribed antibiotics to control secondary bacterial infection in the bronchial tree, thus clearing the airways (tetracycline, erythromycin, ampicillin).

4 Periodic sputum cultures for possible superinfection should be done for patients on long-term antibiotic therapy.

5 Advise patient to avoid exposure to persons with respiratory tract infections.

6 Corticosteroid drugs may be prescribed; these drugs have an anti-inflammatory effect, and thus help to relieve airway obstruction.

a. Short course of corticosteroids may be beneficial to persons who have acute attacks of bronchial obstruction, severe wheezing or marked eosinophilia in sputum or blood.

b. Antacids may be ordered to prevent development of an ulcer.

Nursing Alert: Watch for increased susceptibility to infections, for gastrointestinal ulceration and for bleeding tendencies.

To Maintain Nutrition, Since Anorexia is a Common Problem

1 Dyspnoea, with accompanying air swallowing, cough and sputum production combined with intake of medications, promotes loss of appetite.

2 Offer high protein diet with between meal snacks to improve caloric intake and counteract weight loss.

3 Avoid foods producing abdominal discomfort.

4 Give supplemental oxygen while patient is eating (when directed).

To Relieve Severe Hypoxaemia and Related Symptoms

1   Give low-flow oxygen to selected patients with severe, chronic, obstructive pulmonary disease—to increase exercise tolerance, relieve effects of hypoxaemia, decrease secondary erythrocytosis, reduce right ventricular strain.
2   The aim of low-flow oxygen therapy is to relieve dangerous tissue hypoxia without depressing overall ventilation:
    a. In patients with COLD, poor exchange of gases may result in chronically elevated CO_2 (which is then a less effective stimulus to respiration). Giving a high concentration of oxygen may remove the hypoxic drive—leading to increased hypoventilation, respiratory decompensation, and the development of a worsening respiratory acidosis.
    b. Low-flow oxygen dosage is individualized and is given after analysis of arterial blood gases.
    c. Usual O_2 flow rate is 1–3 l/min at rest or 1–4 l/min with exercise, depending on PO_2.
    d. Graded exercise with low-flow oxygen may be given to increase exercise capacity.
3   Avoid narcotics, sedatives, and tranquillizers. Watch for excessive somnolence, restlessness, aggressiveness or confusion.

To Utilize Techniques of Breathing Retraining to Strengthen Diaphragm and Muscles of Expiration and to Decrease the Work of Breathing

1   Teach lower costal, diaphragmatic and abdominal breathing (p. 256), using a slow and relaxed breathing pattern to lessen airway resistance and dyspnoea.
2   Use pursed-lip breathing (p. 256) at intervals and during periods of dyspnoea—prevents collapse of air passages which lack elastic support during expiration.

To Recondition Patient and Increase his Physical Activity.

1   Employ graded exercise and physical conditioning programmes—walking, stationary bicycle.
    Portable oxygen cylinder for low-flow oxygen may be used for ambulation in selected patients.
2   Encourage patient to carry out regular exercise training programme to increase physical endurance and promote sense of well-being and independence.
3   Train patient in energy-saving methods.

To Support the Patient Emotionally

1   Demonstrate a positive and interested approach to the patient.
    a. Be a good listener and show that you care.
    b. Be sensitive to his fears, anxiety and depression; helps give emotional relief and insight.
2   Strengthen the patient's self-image.
3   Allow the patient to express his feelings and retain (within a controlled degree) the mechanisms of denial and repression.

Discharge Planning and Health Teaching

Objective

To improve the quality of life.

1   Give the patient a clear explanation of his disease, what to expect, how to treat and live with it.
    Reinforce by frequent explanations, reading material, demonstrations and question and answer sessions.
2   Review with patient the objectives of treatment and nursing management (pp. 332–333).

Instruct the patient and his family:

1   Avoid exposure to respiratory irritants—e.g., smoke, fumes, dust, cold.
    a. Stop smoking!
    b. Stay out of extremely cold weather or keep a scarf over nose and mouth to warm inspired air; this avoids provoking airway irritation.
    c. Try to avoid abrupt environmental changes.
    d. Have a home humidifier system.
2   Prevent and eliminate bronchial infections.
    a. Report any evidence of respiratory infection to the doctor *promptly*.
    b. Take prescribed antibiotic at first sign of infection.
    (1) Have a home supply available.
    (2) Have periodic sputum cultures when receiving long-term antibiotic therapy.
3   Reduce bronchial secretions.
    a. Maintain an adequate fluid intake (10–12 glasses daily); mark down the amount of liquid consumed daily.
    b. Take bronchodilators only as directed.
    c. Follow postural drainage exercises as ordered.
    (1) Stay in each position 5–15 min.
    (2) Utilize controlled cough after each position.
    d. Take medications prescribed for cough and expectoration.
4   Increase pulmonary ventilation:
    Use nebulization treatment consistently and faithfully.
    a. Do the procedure immediately upon arising in the morning and before meals when indicated.
    b. Inhale and exhale as evenly as possible during the treatment.
    c. Try to cough *productively* (with *controlled coughing*) after the treatment.
    (1) Breathe slowly and deeply, using diaphragmatic breathing.
    (2) Hold breath several seconds.
    (3) Cough—two short, forceful coughs with the mouth open; the first cough loosens mucus and the second cough moves it.
    (4) Pause and inhale by sniffing quietly. (Inhaling vigorously may initiate unproductive coughing, which is energy consuming.)
    (5) Rest.
    d. Practice oral hygiene after each treatment.
    e. Clean respiratory therapy equipment daily.

5   Do breathing exercises to strengthen muscles of expiration and to strengthen and co-ordinate muscles of breathing.
   a. Practise diaphragmatic breathing and pursed-lip breathing (p. 256).
   b. Consciously use pursed-lip breathing during episodes of dyspnoea and stress.
   c. Maintain muscle tone of the body by regular exercise.
6   Maintain general health at as high a level as possible.
   a. Exercise to improve physical condition.
   b. Have rest periods before and after meals if eating produces dyspnoea.
   c. Avoid overfatigue, which is a factor in producing respiratory distress.
   d. Obtain immunization for influenza—influenza may precipitate acute respiratory insufficiency.
7   Study own life style and avoid energy-wasting activities.
   a. Live within the limits that emphysema imposes.
   b. Adjust activities to individual fatigue pattern.
   c. Breathe in a slow and relaxed manner during periods of physical activity.
8   Supplementary Social Security Benefits may be needed if income is not sufficient to supply necessary nutrition and warmth.

Pulmonary Heart Disease (Cor Pulmonale)

Pulmonary heart disease (cor pulmonale) is an alteration in the structure or function of the right ventricle resulting from disease affecting lung structure or function or its vasculature (except when this alteration results from disease of the left side of the heart or from congenital heart disease).

Aetiology

1   Chronic obstructive lung disease—chronic bronchitis, emphysema most common.
2   Conditions that restrict ventilatory function—kyphoscoliosis.
3   Pulmonary vascular disease—pulmonary emboli.

Pathophysiology

Chronic obstructive lung disease→hypoxia→hypercapnia→acidosis→circulatory complications→pulmonary hypertension→right heart enlargement→right heart failure.

Clinical Manifestations

1   Peripheral oedema.
2   Respiratory insufficiency; progressive dyspnoea (orthopnoea, paroxysmal nocturnal dyspnoea), chronic cough.
3   Right heart enlargement demonstrated by:
   a. Physical examination.
   b. ECG changes.
   c. Chest x-ray—shows change in heart size.
4   Manifestations of carbon dioxide narcosis—headache, confusion, somnolence, coma.
5   Central cyanosis.

Clinical Evaluation

1   Arterial blood gas analysis.
2   Pulmonary function tests.

Treatment and Nursing Management

Objectives

To treat underlying lung disease.
To correct hypoxaemia.
To treat manifestations of heart disease.

1   Improve ventilation.
    a. Employ IPPB, with bronchodilators
    or, if the patient shows signs of respiratory failure, employ endotracheal intubation, bronchial aspiration, and/or mechanical ventilation.
    b. Monitor arterial blood gases as a guide in assessing adequacy of alveolar ventilation.
    c. Use continuous nasal low-flow oxygen for patients with chronic hypoxia and acidosis.
    d. Avoid central nervous system depressants (narcotics, barbiturates, hypnotics;—have depressant action on respiratory centres.
    e. See p. 257 for management of respiratory failure.
2   Combat respiratory infection, which commonly precipitates pulmonary heart disease—respiratory infection causes carbon dioxide retention and hypoxia, resulting in constriction of pulmonary arterioles and subsequent pulmonary hypertension.
3   Treat heart failure when it exists.
    a. Reverse the patient's hypoxaemia and hypercapnia. (See above treatment first in order to improve cardiac action.)
    b. Limit physical activity.
    c. Restrict sodium intake.
    d. Give diuretics to reduce peripheral oedema and reduce circulatory load on right heart.
    e. Give digitalis as directed. Digitalis is given with caution, since digitalis toxicity is a serious problem in management of respiratory failure because of hypoxia, acidosis and electrolyte abnormalities.
    f. Employ ECG monitoring when necessary—high incidence of arrhythmias in these patients.

Discharge Planning and Health Teaching

1   Emphasize the importance of stopping cigarette smoking; cigarette smoking is a major cause of pulmonary heart disease.
    a. Query patient about his smoking habits.
    b. Inform patient of risks of smoking and benefits to be gained when smoking is stopped.

2   Teach patient to treat infections immediately.
3   Inform the patient of inter-relationship between infection, air pollution and cardiopulmonary disease.

Pulmonary Embolism

Pulmonary embolism generally refers to the obstruction of one or more pulmonary arteries by a thrombus (or thrombi) originating somewhere in the venous system or in the right side of the heart. It may also be caused by air, amniotic or fat embolism.

Predisposing Factors

1   Stasis of venous circulation, especially in blood vessels with injury to the endothelial lining—leads to intravascular clotting.
2   Intimal damage.
3   Hypercoagulability of the blood.
4   Most emboli originate in veins of the lower extremities or pelvic area where they become detached and are carried to the lungs.
     Bed rest, sitting, prolonged standing contribute to venous stasis of lower extremities.

Preventive Measures

1   Assess each patient with a high index of suspicion for pulmonary embolism.
2   Be aware of high-risk patients—trauma to pelvis (especially surgical) and lower extremities (especially hip fracture), obesity, varicose veins, pregnancy, congestive heart failure, myocardial infarction, malignant disease, postoperative patients. Preventative measures should be taken in the operating theatre—suitable padding on the table and supports, and the use of alternating pressure mattresses or leggings.
3   Prevent stasis of blood in extremities due to dependent position of legs, prolonged sitting, immobility, constricting clothing.
     a. Elevate legs 15–20° at intervals—to minimize stasis and increase venous return.
     b. Apply fitted elastic stockings—to increase blood flow to deep leg veins.
     c. Instruct patient to wiggle toes, move feet, raise and lower legs frequently—to increase venous return.
     d. Do not allow patient's legs and feet to dangle in a dependent position; have the patient place his feet on a chair when sitting on the edge of the bed (if bed is in high position). Instruct patient to avoid crossing the legs.
4   Avoid haemoconcentration and immobilization of patients confined to bed.
5   Encourage higher levels of fluid intake during periods of immobility.
6   Avoid leaving catheters in veins (parenteral therapy, measurement of central venous pressure) for prolonged periods.
7   Use prophylactic low dose anticoagulant therapy for high-risk patients.
8   Assess for positive Homan's sign. (While patient is in supine position, lift leg and dorsiflex foot. Pain in the calf during this manoeuvre may indicate deep vein thrombosis).

Clinical Manifestations

1 Underlying principles:
   a. The size and location of the embolus determines the physiologic effect. Symptoms therefore vary from none to cardiovascular collapse.
   b. The physiological effects develop from pulmonary artery obstruction.
   c. Small emboli tend to be multiple and recurrent.
2 Dyspnoea and tachypnoea.
3 Subtle deterioration in patient's condition with no explainable cause.
4 Substernal pain with apprehension and a sense of impending doom; occurs when most of the pulmonary artery is obstructed.
5 Pallor, cyanosis, tachyarrhythmias, clinical shock.
6 Engorgement of neck veins.
7 Pleural friction rub, accentuated pulmonic second sound, gallop rhythm.

Nursing Alert: Have a high index of suspicion if there is a subtle deterioration in the patient's condition and unexplained cardiovascular and pulmonary findings.

Diagnosis

1 Physical findings.
2 Chest x-ray.
3 Pulmonary angiogram (most definitive).
4 Lung scan.
5 ECG.
6 Arterial blood gases—indicate degree of respiratory insufficiency.
7 Contrast phlebography or impedance phlebography—for detecting deep vein thrombosis.

Objectives of Treatment and Nursing Management

Objectives

To support life during acute episode.
To promote resolution and prevent recurrence.

To Restore Cardiopulmonary Function

1 Provide respiratory assistance to eliminate hypoxia.
   a. Oxygen via face mask or nasal catheter.
   b. Tracheal intubation if necessary (see p. 287).
2 Monitor vital signs, ECG and arterial blood gases.
3 Treat patient for heart failure when present.
4 Give analgesics and sedatives as directed for pain control and apprehension.

To Give Anticoagulant Therapy to Prevent Recurrence and Extension of Thromboembolism

1 Administer heparin (intravenously)—heparin extends the clotting time of blood; it is anticoagulant and antithrombotic.
2 Heparin may also be given by continuous intravenous infusion (drip or pump), a reliable method of obtaining and controlling the desired extended clotting time.

3 Dosage adjusted to maintain the clotting tests at 2–2.5 times the control level an hour prior to the next dose.
4 Assess patient for untoward bleeding.
5 Have protamine available to neutralize heparin during episodes of acute bleeding.
6 Give warfarin sodium as anticoagulant; may be given simultaneously at the beginning or at the end of heparin therapy.
   a. Anticoagulants may be proscribed (prohibited) in certain situations: recent brain, spinal cord, joint or urinary surgery; certain bleeding tendencies; fracture of pelvis or extremity; recent bleeding from peptic ulceration.
   b. Have phytonadione (Mephyton) available to counteract effects of prothrombin depressant drugs (warfarin sodium).
7 Be aware that many drugs interact with anticoagulants.

To Prepare Patient for Surgical Intervention when Anticoagulation is Contraindicated or has Failed, or when Patient has a Major Embolization

1 Inferior vena cava interruption—reduces channel size to prevent passage of emboli and at the same time permits some blood to flow. One of the following may be done:
   a. Plication with suture or slips.
   b. Intraluminal obstruction achieved with umbrella filters, balloon catheters, trapping catheters.
   c. All methods of venacaval interruption may produce venous insufficiency of lower extremities with subsequent stasis and oedema.
2 Pulmonary embolectomy—direct removal of embolus from pulmonary artery.
   Performed with cardiopulmonary bypass in patients with massive embolism with shock.

Discharge Planning and Health Teaching

1 See Preventive Measures, p. 338.
2 Patient may have to continue taking anticoagulant therapy for 3–6 months following his initial episode.
3 Female patients who have experienced thromboembolism should be advised against taking oral contraceptives.
4 Instruct the patient to watch for signs of overanticoagulation: bleeding gums, nosebleeds, bruising, haematuria, blood in stools, etc.
5 Patient should avoid taking *any* medications unless approved by doctor, since many drugs interact with anticoagulants.
6 Patient should notify the dentist that he is on an anticoagulant.

Sarcoidosis

Sarcoidosis is a systematic granulomatous disease of unknown cause. It may involve almost any organ or tissue but most commonly the lungs, lymph nodes, liver, spleen, skin, eyes, phalangeal bones and parotid glands.

Clinical Features

1 Patients with sarcoidosis may show altered immunological reactivity.
2 The onset usually occurs during third or fourth decade.
3 First clinical manifestations are usually thoracic, with hilar and mediastinal lymph node enlargement; may progress to diffuse involvement of lungs and then to fibrosis.

Clinical Manifestations

Depend on size and extent of lesions and degree of fibrosis

1 Pulmonary manifestations—dyspnoea and cough (may appear late).
2 Skin lesions—nodules and infiltrations of face, ears, nose, extensor surfaces.
3 Hypercalciuria and hyperglobulinaemia.
4 Uveitis, joint pain, fever—depending on whether acute or slowly progressive.

Diagnosis

1 Kveim test:
   a. Intradermal injection of saline suspension of sarcoid tissue obtained from spleen or lymph nodes of patients with active sarcoidosis.
   b. Produces a nodule at injection site (in 4–8 weeks).
   c. Area is biopsied and tissue examined.
2 Biopsy of skin and lymph nodes (most definitive diagnostic procedure) reveals noncaseating granulomas.
3 Elevated serum globulin, calcium and alkaline phosphatase.
4 Chest x-ray—reveals hilar adenopathy; causes smooth hilar enlargement.
5 Pulmonary function tests—give an indication of the degree of functional impairment.

Treatment

1 There is no specific treatment; the natural course of the disease is towards resolution.
2 Corticosteroid therapy in selected patients; has anti-inflammatory effect; used in patients with hypercalcaemia, ocular and myocardial disease, extensive pulmonary disease with compromise of pulmonary function.
3 Isoniazid may be given to patients with positive tuberculin test.

Health Teaching

1 The majority of persons do not require treatment. Most patients improve spontaneously.
2 Measurements of pulmonary function are made at intervals to follow physiological impact of disease.

Cancer of the Lung (Bronchogenic Cancer)

Bronchogenic cancer refers to a malignant tumour of the lung arising within the wall or epithelial lining of the bronchus. The lung is also a common site of metastasis from cancer elsewhere in the body via venous circulation or lymphatic spread. Primary cancer of the pleura is uncommon, except in asbestos workers.

Classification (according to cell type)

1 Squamous cell—most common.
2 Undifferentiated (includes variety of anaplastic or poorly differentiated cells).
   a. Small cell undifferentiated carcinoma (oat cell).
   b. Large cell undifferentiated carcinoma.
3 Adenocarcinoma.
4 Bronchiolar or alveolar carcinoma.

Predisposing Factors

1 Cigarette smoking—amount, frequency and duration of smoking have positive relationship to cancer of the lung.
2 Industrial exposure to asbestos, arsenic, chromium, nickel, iron, radioactive substances, isopropyl oil, coal tar fumes, petroleum oil mists.

Preventive Measures

1 Maintain close watch of patients who are smokers—disease is insidious and exists before producing symptoms.
2 Encourage patients to abstain from cigarette smoking.
3 Recognize the presence of the tumour before symptoms appear.
   a. Continuous surveillance of smokers, especially those over 40.
   b. Chest x-rays at prescribed intervals.

Nursing Alert: Suspect cancer of the lung in patients who belong to a susceptible age group and who have repeated unresolved respiratory infections.

Clinical Manifestations

Usually occur late and are related to size and location of tumour, extent of spread and involvement of other structures.

1 Cough—especially a new type or changing cough.
2 Haemoptysis.
3 Thoracic discomfort; chest pain.
4 Wheezing.
5 Repeated infections of upper respiratory tract.
6 General symptoms; weight loss, fatigue, anorexia.
7 Usual sites of metastases: regional nodes, liver, adrenals, brain, bones, kidneys.
8 Signs of superior vena cava obstruction.
9 Change of voice.

Diagnosis

1 X-rays of chest—including flurosocopy and tomography; lung cancers may be partly or completely hidden by other structures.

2 Bronchoscopy and biopsy; bronchial brushing.
3 Cytologic examination of sputum or saline washings from suspected bronchus.
4 Scalene node biopsy; mediastinoscopy.
5 Pulmonary function tests.
6 Adrenal function tests preoperatively—under the stress of surgery the patient requires increased secretion of adrenocorticoids. (If the adrenal glands have been affected by metastatic cancer the patient may develop acute adrenal insufficiency).
7 Cardiac evaluation.
8 Lung, brain, bone and liver scans if indicated.
9 Computed tomography.

NOTE: Support and encourage patient and relatives during the period of diagnosis and assessment, in a situation loaded with doubt and fear.

Treatment

Objective

To provide the maximum likelihood of cure.

There are three methods of treatment: surgery, radiation and chemotherapy, used separately or in combination.

1 Surgical removal of the lesion and regional lymph nodes.
    Operation may be a segmental resection, lobectomy or pneumonectomy with removal of adjacent lymph nodes, depending on patient's clinical status and stage of the disease.
2 Radical megavoltage radiation therapy (cobalt or linear accelerator).
3 Treatment of inoperable cancer of the lung.
    a. Palliative radiotherapy to decrease tumour size and relieve pressure on vital structures.
    High dose irradiation used for small cell (oat cell) carcinoma.
    b. Systemic chemotherapy (combined therapy with two or more agents)—for symptomatic control of metastatic disease.

Nursing Managment

1 Prepare patient for surgical intervention if he is a candidate for operation (see p. 348).
2 Support and encourage patient receiving palliative treatment.
3 Treat underlying bronchitis or pulmonary infections.
    a. Bronchial drainage and removal of secretions.
    b. Bronchodilators and water vapour therapy.
    c. Antibiotic agents for infection.
4 Give supplementary nutrition and encourage extra periods of rest.
5 Observe for central nervous system disturbances due to metastasis to brain, and for pain in back, pelvis or extremities from bone metastasis.

6   See Volume 1, Chapter 7 for nursing management of the patient with cancer.
7   See Volume 1, Chapter 7 for nursing management of the dying patient.

Chest Trauma

Chest trauma is an injury to the chest caused by any form of violence.

1   Chest injuries are potentially life-threatening because of (1) immediate disturbances of cardiorespiratory physiology and haemorrhage; and (2) later developments of infection, damaged lung and thoracic cage.
2   Patients with chest trauma may have injuries to multiple organ systems.
3   Patient should be examined for intra-abdominal injuries, which must be treated
aggressively.

Altered Physiology

1   In penetrating injuries, some air escapes into the pleural space. (Negative
intrapleural pressure is replaced by atmospheric pressure).
2   A loss of negative pressure within the pleural cavity may cause collapse of the
lung.
3   The change of pressure interferes with expansion of the uninvolved lung, and
there is shifting back and forth of the collapsed lung and mediastinum.
4   This shifting interferes with filling of the right side of the heart, lessening cardiac
output and causing cardiopulmonary collapse.

Emergency Management

The order of priority is determined by the clinical status of the patient.

Objective

To restore normal cardiorespiratory function as quickly as possible.
    This is accomplished by maintaining the airway, restoring the chest wall integrity,
and re-expanding the lung.

1   Assess patient's condition, physiological state.
    a. Examiner's ear is placed close to patient's mouth and nose, allowing him to
    listen at the airway, watch uncovered chest movements and monitor pulse—this
    provides a rough estimate of the adequancy of ventilation.
    b. Check neck for position of trachea, subcutaneous emphysema and distended
    neck veins.
2   Establish and maintain an open airway.
    a. Aspirate secretions, vomitus and blood from nose and throat via:
    (1) Tracheal aspiration, if patient is unable to clear the tracheobronchial tree
    by coughing (p. 239).
    (2) Utilize endotracheal tube if patient is bleeding from nasopharynx or if
    trachea is injured (short-term use).
    (3) Employ bronchoscopic aspiration if necessary.
    (4) Prepare for tracheostomy if necessary.

(a) Tracheostomy helps to obtain clear, dry tracheobronchial tree, helps patient breathe with less effort, decreases amount of dead air space in the respiratory tree, and helps reduce paradoxical motion.

(b) The use of a cuffed tracheostomy tube permits a closed system for air exchange when connected to a ventilator.

b. Stabilize the chest wall.

c. Free the pleural cavity of blood and air.

d. Sucking chest wounds should be closed with an emergency dressing. The presence of lung injury and chest tube drainage must also be considered.

3   Control haemorrhage.

4   Treat for shock. (Shock may be due to blood loss, impairment of cardio-respiratory function.)

a. Use one or more intravenous infusion lines; obtain blood for baseline studies.

b. Restore blood volume to adequate levels—plasma, plasma expanders, electrolyte solutions.

c. Give infusion rapidly.

d. Monitor serial central venous pressure readings to prevent hypovolaemia and circulatory overload.

Types of Chest Injuries

Haemothorax

Blood in the pleural cavity from injury to the intrathoracic organs or to blood vessels of the chest wall.

1   Blood in the pleural cavity produces a compression of the lung and can displace mediastinal structures.

2   Patient may be asymptomatic; or he may be dyspnoeic, apprehensive or in shock.

3   Treatment.

a. Blood and air are aspirated via needle thoracentesis *or*

b. An intercostal catheter (thoracotomy tube) is inserted and drainage is instituted to accomplish more complete and continuous removal of blood—effects re-expansion of lung and permits monitoring of blood loss.

The chest catheter is sutured in position and connected to a water-seal drainage bottle (p. 358).

c. Prepare for immediate blood replacement and thoracotomy if bleeding continues.

Pneumothorax

Air in the pleural space occurring spontaneously from injury or disease. In patients with chest trauma it is usually the result of a laceration to the lung parenchyma, tracheobronchial tree or oesophagus.

Patient's clinical status depends on the rate of air leakage and size of wound and on previous respiratory condition.

1   *Spontaneous pneumothorax:*

a. May occur in healthy individuals; is usually due to rupture of a subpleural bleb of the lung.

b. Treatment is generally nonoperative if pneumothorax is not too extensive;

needle aspiration or chest tube drainage may be necessary to achieve re-expansion of collapsed lung.

c. Surgical intervention (thoracotomy) advised for patients with recurrent spontaneous pneumothorax. Intervention may be (1) pleurodesis (via thoracoscopy tube) or (2) pleural resection (via thoracotomy)

2 *Tension pneumothorax:*

a. A rapid flow of air or a small leak with valve action into the pleural space will produce *tension pneumothorax* (air in the pleural cavity producing displacement of the mediastinum to the uninvolved side, with resultant severe cardiorespiratory embarrassment).

b. If tension pneumothorax is present, the pleural space is temporarily decompressed with a syringe attached to a 16–18 gauge needle inserted into the second intercostal space.

c. Chest-tube drainage (closed thoracotomy) of pleural space to evacuate air. (Chest tube connected to underwater-seal suction.)

Sucking Wound of Chest

Air passing through hole in the chest wall causes lungs to collapse and mediastinum to shift. There is an audible passage of air during inspiration and expiration.

1 The negative intrapleural pressure is eliminated, creating a disturbance in ventilation; this may cause rapid death by asphyxia.

2 Treatment:

a. Close the chest wound immediately to restore adequate ventilation and respiration.

b. Instruct the patient to inhale and exhale forcefully against a closed glottis (Valsalva manoeuvre) as the pressure dressing (petrolatum gauze) is laid in place. (This manoeuvre helps to expand collapsed lung.)

c. If necessary, prepare patient for surgical intervention or for catheter drainage of the pleural space (see p. 358). Thoracotomy tube is inserted after the emergency treatment above.

d. Be alert for lung injury—a dressing without thoracotomy tube drainage could produce a tension pneumothorax.

e. If condition permits, place patient in semisitting position to permit greater ventilatory efficiency.

Fracture of Ribs and Sternum (most common chest injury)

1 Manifestations:

a. Localized tenderness or crepitus (crackling) over fracture site.

b. Chest pain referred to the fracture site.

c. Painful, shallow respirations (due to splinting of involved chest).

2 Pneumonitis is a complication of rib fracture if patient is not encouraged to deep-breathe periodically.

3 Intercostal nerve block of involved area is helpful in relieving pain at times.

4 Analgesics (usually non-narcotic) given to assist patient to cough and deep-breathe effectively.

5 Wrapping the chest with 15 cm (6 in) elastic bandage promotes comfort.

6 Strapping and tight binders are usually avoided since these restrict chest wall movements at the risk of retaining secretions and producing atelectasis.

Flail Chest

Loss of stability of chest wall, with subsequent respiratory impairment. This is usually the result of multiple rib fractures.

1 Pathophysiology:
   a. When this occurs, one portion of the chest has lost its bony connection to the rest of the rib cage.
   b. During respiration, the detached part of the chest will be pulled in on inspiration and blown out on expiration (paradoxical movement).
   c. Normal mechanics of breathing impaired to a degree that seriously jeopardizes ventilation.
2 Clinical manifestations:
   a. Pain, dyspnoea, cyanosis.
   b. Paradoxical (reverse of normal) movements of involved chest wall.
3 Treatment:
   Objective: to stabilize the paradoxically moving chest.
   a. Stabilize the flail portion of the chest with the hands; apply a pressure dressing and turn patient on his injured side, or place 10-lb sandbag at site of flail.
   b. Prepare for immediate endotracheal intubation or tracheostomy with continuous positive pressure mechanical ventilation—this 'floats out' the flail segment, improves alveolar ventilation, restores thoracic cage stability and intrathoracic volume and decreases the work of breathing.

Wet Lung Syndrome

Presence of fluid in the lungs (mucus, blood, serum) as a result of severe chest injury, contusion of pulmonary tissue, aspirative pneumonitis.

1 Manifestations:
   a. Constant loose cough, rattling, wheezing.
   b. Râles present on auscultation.
   c. Dyspnoea, tachycardia, cyanosis.
2 Objective of treatment: to improve tracheobronchial drainage
   a. Clear the airway; stabilize the chest wall with positive pressure ventilation (bag and mask) or endotracheal tube with oxygen.
   b. Give oxygen when cyanosis and dyspnoea are present.
      Encourage patient to cough.
      (1) Give manual support to the chest.
      (2) Give adequate analgesia to permit coughing.
      (3) Aspirate blood or air in pleural cavity (see thoracentesis, p. 248).
4 Give periodic IPPB to help clear tracheobronchial tree.
5 Administer bronchodilator drug if bronchospasm is present.
6 Prepare for tracheostomy with continuous ventilatory support if patient's respiratory efforts are exhausting him.

Cardiac Tamponade

Progressive collection of fluid or blood fills the pericardial space; interferes with diastolic filling of the ventricles.

1 Pathophysiology.

Pericardial tamponade follows penetrating injury to heart in which blood escapes into the pericardial sac; or may follow heart surgery.

2   Manifestations (depends on whether there is acute injury or chronic effusion):
   a. Faint heart sounds.
   b. Narrowed pulse pressure.
   c. Elevated venous pressure.
   d. High central venous pressure.
   e. Falling arterial blood pressure.
   f. Distended neck veins.
   g. Dyspnoea, cyanosis, shock.

3   Treatment:
   a. Pericardial aspiration (pericardiocentesis), aspiration or drainage of the pericardium; permits heart action to be resumed.
   (1) Repeated aspirations may be necessary.
   b. Open operation (thoracotomy) to control haemorrhage and to repair cardiac injury may be necessary.

Nursing Alert: In the patient with hypovolaemia the venous pressure may not rise, thus masking the signs of cardiac tamponade.

THORACIC SURGERY

The Challenge: Meticulous attention must be given to the preoperative and postoperative care of patients undergoing thoracic surgery. These operations are wide in scope; obstructive lung disease may be present, and the margin of safety is apt to be narrow.

Preoperative Care

Objectives

To determine if patient can survive planned procedure.
To ensure optimal condition of patient for surgery.

Determine the Preoperative Status of the Patient, his Physical Assets and Liabilities

1   Assist the patient undergoing diagnostic studies.
   a. History and physical examination.
   b. Chest x-rays (see p. 239).
   c. Pulmonary function studies (p. 245)—to ascertain if patient will have adequately functioning lung tissue postoperatively.
   d. Special diagnostic studies as required.
   e. Baseline studies to ascertain any unsuspected abnormalities and to serve as a baseline reference during the postoperative period.
   (1) ECG—to disclose presence of arteriosclerotic heart disease or conduction defect.
   (2) Blood urea nitrogen, serum creatinine—to obtain a 'rough' measurement of renal function.
   (3) Blood sugar or glucose tolerance—to detect unrecognized diabetes.

(4) Blood electrolytes, serum protein studies and blood volume determinations as indicated.

(5) Arterial blood gas studies.

2 Nursing assessment of the patient.

a. What signs and symptoms are present (cough, expectoration, haemoptysis, chest pain)?

b. What is his smoking history (amount and duration)? How much is he presently smoking?

c. What is the patient's cardiopulmonary tolerance, while bathing, eating, walking, etc.?

d. What is the 'physiological age' of the patient (general appearance, mental alertness, behaviour, degree of nutrition)?

e. What other medical conditions exist?

f. What is his breathing pattern?

g. How much exertion is required to produce dyspnoea?

h. What are his personal preferences and dislikes?

Improve Alveolar Ventilation

1 Encourage the patient to stop smoking since this increases bronchial irritation.

2 Employ all measures to minimize pulmonary secretions.

a. Measure sputum daily in patients with large volume of secretions to determine if volume of secretion is decreasing.

b. Instruct the patient to cough against a closed glottis to increase intrapulmonary pressure.

c. Humidify the air to loosen secretions.

d. Administer bronchodilators for bronchospasm.

e. Give antibiotics for infection.

f. Give expectorants, enzymes and mucolytic agents as directed.

g. Employ IPPB therapy to improve pulmonary ventilation (see p. 281).

h. Carry out postural drainage positioning on patients with bronchiectasis, etc. (see p. 252).

i. Teach diaphragmatic breathing preoperatively (see p. 256).

j. Set up a schedule of breathing exercises that encourage the use of abdominal muscles (see p. 256).

Evaluate Cardiovascular and Pulmonary Status so that Complications may be Anticipated and Prevented

1 Study the results of diagnostic tests to learn of existing deviations from normal.

2 Observe the patient and his reactions to various activities of daily living.

3 Give cardiac drugs to patients with congestive heart failure.

4 Correct anaemia, dehydration and hypoproteinaemia—intravenous infusions, tube feedings, blood transfusions as indicated.

Prepare the Patient and his Family for the Surgical and Postoperative Experience by Offering Reassurance, Explanations and Skilful Preoperative Nursing Care

1 Orient the patient to events in the postoperative period.

a. Cough and breathing routine.

b. Presence of chest tube and drainage bottles.

    c. Oxygen therapy; ventilator therapy.
    d. Measures used to control discomfort.
    e. Leg exercises and range of motion exercises for affected shoulder.
2 Encourage expression of psychological and safety needs.
3 See that consent form has been explained and signed.

Participate in Preoperative Preparations as Indicated

1 Shaving of incision area.
2 Antiseptic skin cleansing.
3 Restriction of oral intake.
4 Special medications.
5 Placement of needed tubes as prescribed (intravenous infusion lines, indwelling catheter, nasogastric tube).

Postoperative Care

Objective

To restore normal cardiopulmonary function as quickly as possible.

1 Maintain an open airway.
    a. Look and listen at the patient's open mouth as he breathes for evidences of obstruction, and listen to his chest (auscultation) with a stethoscope.
    b. Monitor the arterial blood gases—a progressive fall in PO_2 is an indication for the use of the ventilator; an elevated PCO_2 also usually signifies need for ventilator support (except in patients with chronic obstructive airway disease).
    c. Patient may have endoctracheal tube and be assisted by a ventilator until he demonstrates that he can support adequate respiration—initiating ventilator therapy at appropriate time may reverse the trend towards respiratory failure.
    d. Aspirate all secretions with suctioning until patient is able to raise secretions effectively—endotracheal secretions are present in excessive amounts in post-thoracotomy patients because of trauma to the tracheobronchial tree during operation; diminished lung ventilation and diminished cough reflex.
      (1) Excessive secretions will produce airway obstruction; air in the alveoli distal to the obstruction will become absorbed and the lung will collapse.
      (2) Carry out tracheal aspiration on 'wet' comatose patient to prevent atelectasis.
2 *Technique for tracheal suctioning if patient cannot clear râles or refuses to cough.* Sterile technique should be used. This procedure should be learned under expert clinical supervision.
    a. Place the patient in a sitting or semi-Fowler's position. Attach the sterile catheter to a 'Y' or 'T' tube that has been connected to a suction device.
    b. Preoxygenate the patient several minutes before each suctioning procedure.
    c. Give patient a gauze square; instruct him to pull his tongue outward; this tilts the epiglottis forwards (or have someone else do this).
    d. Pass the catheter (lubricated with water-soluble gel) through the nostril to the pharynx.
    e. Check the position of the tip of the catheter; it should be in the lower pharynx.
    f. Instruct the patient to take a deep breath—this action serves to open the

epiglottis and also encourages the catheter to move in the direction of the negative pressure generated by inspiration.

g. Advance the catheter into the trachea only during inspiration.

h. Apply suction *intermittently* by closing the open end of the 'Y' (or 'T') catheter with the finger and slowly rotating between the thumb and forefinger.

i. Suctioning must *never* be prolonged more than 5–10 s since cardiac arrest may ensue in patients with borderline oxygenation.

j. While the catheter is being withdrawn apply gentle suction to clear the tracheal walls of secretions.

k. Ventilate the patient with oxygen for about 2–5 min prior to a second passage of the catheter (if this is necessary). Check the pulse rate.

Nursing Alert: Look for changes in colour and consistency of aspirated sputum. Colourless, fluid sputum is not unusual; opacification or colouring of sputum may mean dehydration or infection.

3 Maintain continuing nursing surveillance of the patient.

a. Take blood pressure, pulse and respiration every 15 min or more frequently as indicated; repeat, allowing longer intervals according to the patient's clinical status.

b. Evaluate *character* of respirations and patient's colour—depth of respiration is an important criterion in evaluating whether lungs are being adequately expanded.

c. Monitor heart rate and rhythm via auscultation and ECG, since arrhythmias are more frequently seen after thoracic surgery.

(1) Arrhythmias can occur any time, but frequently begin between second and sixth postoperative day.

(2) Rate of occurrence of arrhythmias increases with age of patient.

d. Maintain an arterial line to facilitate frequent monitoring of blood gases, serum electrolytes, haemoglobin, haematocrit and arterial pressure.

e. Monitor the central venous pressure for prompt recognition of hypotension and for assessing effective blood volume.

4 Maintain surveillance and careful management of the chest drainage system (p. 358). Understand the system being used.

a. Chest drainage employed following surgery/trauma that invades pleura and collapses lung (with exception of pneumonectomy*).

b. Chest tube(s) inserted at time of surgery to prevent fluid and air from accumulating in pleural or mediastinal space and to assist in re-expansion of remaining lung tissue.

c. Check amount and character of drainage immediately postoperatively and at necessary intervals thereafter—drainage should progressively decrease after first 12 hours. The drainage is usually bloody immediately after surgery but becomes serous in 24 hours or so.

d. Persistence of bloody drainage indicates bleeding. Prepare for blood replacement and possible reoperation to achieve haemostasis.

* A patient with a pneumonectomy usually does not have water-seal chest drainage since it is desirable that the pleural space fill with an effusion which eventually obliterates this space. Some surgeons do use a 'modified' water-seal system. The instructions on clamping and briefly unclamping the tube must be scrupulously observed.

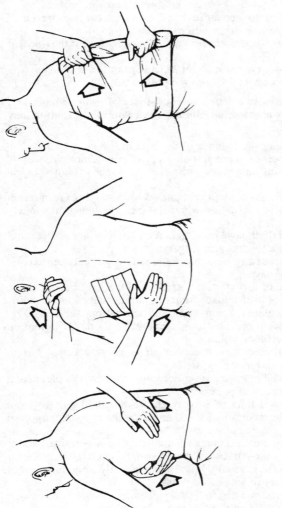

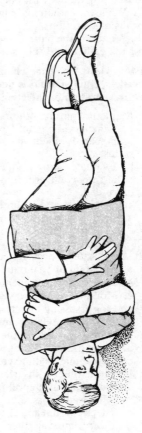

Figure 3.21.   Promotion of an effective cough.

5   Give humidified oxygen in immediate postoperative period to assure maximum oxygenation—respirations are still depressed and residual secretions in the peripheral respiratory passages may partially block gas exchange. Monitoring by means of arterial blood gas analysis may be necessary.

   a. Assess for respiratory distress and a feeling of tightness in the chest.

   b. Watch for restlessness—often the first sign of hypoxia.

6   Encourage and promote an effective cough routine (Fig. 3.21); a persistent and ineffective cough exhausts the patient, and retained secretion lead to atelectasis and pneumonia.

   a. Sit patient on side of bed with feet supported on a chair if his condition permits.

   b. Support the chest firmly over the operated side and against opposite chest to lessen incisional pain.

   c. Instruct the patient to take a deep breath (to increase cough pressure), to pull in his abdominal muscles and to cough vigorously.

   d. Assist the patient to cough at least every hour during the first 24 hours and when necessary thereafter.

     (1) If audible râles continue, it may be necessary to utilize chest percussion with cough routine until lungs are clear of râles (p. 254).

     (2) If coughing and/or tracheal aspiration (suctioning) fail to clear râles, bronchoscopic removal of secretions may be necessary.

7   Listen to both lungs (anterior and posterior) with a stethoscope to determine if there are any changes in breath sounds since diminished breath sounds may indicate collapsed or hypoventilated alveoli.

   a. Are breath sounds normal, indicating free flow of air in and out of the lungs?

   b. Are breath sounds distant? Wheezing? Râles present?

8   Give aerosol therapy to reduce viscosity of secretions and avoid excessive drying of tracheobronchial secretions.

9   Administer IPPB treatments as directed to improve ventilation.

10 Use blow bottles or inspiratory spirometer as ordered.

11 Provide intelligent pain relief—pain limits chest excursions, thereby decreasing ventilation.

   a. Severity of pain varies with type of incision and with patient's reaction to and ability to cope with pain. Usually a posterior-lateral skin incision is the most painful.

   b. Give narcotics (usually in frequent small doses) for pain relief, to permit patient to breathe more deeply and cough more effectively; place on oral analgesic (codeine) as soon as possible.

   c. Avoid depressing respiratory and vascular systems with too much narcotic; patient should not be so somnolent that he does not cough.

   d. Position in bed properly.

   e. Support chest tubes to avoid pull on chest wall.

   f. Assist patient having intercostal nerve block for pain control.

12 Monitor hourly urine output from indwelling catheter since urine volume reflects cardiac output and organ perfusion.

   a. Patient should excrete at least 30 ml (1 oz) of urine hourly.

   b. Decreasing urinary output is frequently due to hypovolaemia and hypo-hydration.

    c. Urine specific gravity helps assess state of hydration.

13   Administer blood and parenteral fluids at a slower rate after thoracic surgery—pulmonary oedema due to transfusion/infusion overload is an ever-present threat; following pneumonectomy the pulmonary vascular system has been greatly reduced.

14   Maintain care in positioning the postoperative thoracotomy patient.

    a. Position patient flat in bed at intervals unless this produces dyspnoea.

    b. Position patient in semi-Fowler's position to permit residual air to rise to upper portion of pleural space and be removed via the upper chest catheter.

    c. Patients with limited respiratory reserve may not be able to turn on unoperated side as this may limit ventilation of the operated side.

    d. Vary the position from horizontal to semierect; remaining in one position tends to promote the retention of secretions in the dependent portion of the lungs.

    e. Sit patient upright to cough.

15   Watch for evidences of acute gastric distension (not uncommon following thoracic surgery).

    a. Insert nasogastric tube for decompression.

    b. Keep nasogastric tube functioning to avoid vomiting and tracheobronchial aspiration.

16   Anticipate and forestall complications.

    a. Pulmonary insufficiency.   **e.** Cardiac arrhythmias.

    b. Haemorrhage.   **f.** Renal failure.

    c. Respiratory acidosis.   **g.** Gastric distension.

    d. Pneumonitis; atelectasis.

17   Restore normal range of motion and function of shoulder and trunk.

    a. Encourage breathing exercises to mobilize thorax (p. 254)

    b. Encourage skeletal exercises to promote abduction and mobilization of the shoulder.

    c. Ambulate as soon as pulmonary and circulatory systems are compensated.

Discharge Planning and Health Teaching

1   There will be some intercostal pain for a period of time which can be relieved by local heat and oral analgesia.

2   Weakness and fatigability are common during the first 3 weeks following a thoracotomy.

3   Range of motion exercises for the arm and shoulder on the affected side should be carried out several times daily to avoid ankylosis of the shoulder ('frozen shoulder').

Water-Seal Chest Drainage

Following pneumonectomy, the space in the thorax gradually fills with (a) a small amount of blood from the mediastinum and the chest wall and (b) with inflammatory exudate from the raw surfaces. During and after the exudate, oxygen in the space is gradually absorbed, resulting in a negative pressure. This causes a transudate to collect, which will gradually obliterate the space.

If this process does not proceed normally, mediastinal shift may occur: (a) towards the side of the operation—this may occur if there is a leakage of air from the space into the subcutaneous tissues, or from the drainage tube, thus causing negative pressure and (b) away from the side of the operation—this may occur if an effusion builds up rapidly, causing a positive pressure in the space. This complication is most likely within the first 48 hours. Mediastinal shift can be observed clinically by the position of the trachea which will deviate at its lower end.

Further complications include (a) bronchospasm, (b) atelectasis or pneumonitis of remaining lung, (c) bronchopleural fistula and (d) empyema.

Pathophysiology

1   Water-seal chest drainage is a system designed to drain the so-called pleural space and mediastinal space. The anatomy and physiology of the chest and the effects of pathology on the pleural space must be considered in this treatment modality.

2   The pleural space is essential to thoracic drainage. The pleura is a thin sheet of tissue covering the undersurfaces of the ribs, diaphragm and the structures of the mediastinum; it continues as a covering over the entire surface of both lungs, thus forming a pleural space, named parietal pleura and visceral pleura.

3   Actually, the pleural space is really a potential space since the two pleural surfaces are touching each other. With injury, disease, or surgery this space becomes more evident.

4   The pleural space normally always has a 'negative' pressure because the lungs are elastic and tend to pull away from the chest wall.

5   Pressures in the pleural space are approximately 8 mm H_2O during inspiration and 2 mm H_2O during expiration. During forced inspiration (as against a closed glottis) a negative pressure in the range of 54 mm H_2O can be measured, whereas during forced expiration (coughing) a positive pressure develops to about 68 mm H_2O.

6   An opening in the chest, from any cause, produces a loss of negative pressure, and the lung collapses. Collections of fluid or materials in the chest also cause collapse of the lung because these substances take up space. Air and collections of other substances are detrimental to cardiorespiratory function.

7   Three types of pathologic materials collect in the pleural space.
   a. Solids, such as fibrin or clotted blood.
   b. Liquids—serous fluids, blood, pus, chyle or gastric juice.
   c. Gas—as air from the lung, tracheobronchial tree or oesophagus.

8   A chest drainage system must be capable of removing whatever collects in the pleural space a little faster than it accumulates, so that a normal pleural space and normal cardiorespiratory function are restored and maintained.

Principles of Chest Drainage

Chest drainage can be categorized into three types of mechanical systems (Fig. 3.22).

The Single Bottle Water-seal System

1   The end of the drainage tube from the patient's chest is covered by a layer of water, which permits drainage and prevents lung collapse by sealing out the atmosphere.

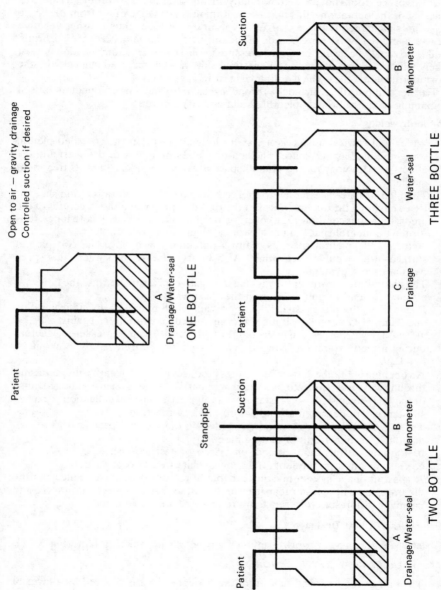

Figure 3.22. Systems of chest drainage. (Drawing courtesy: Edward R. Munnell, M.D.)

2   Functionally, drainage depends on gravity, the mechanics of respiration and, if desired, suction by the addition of *controlled* vacuum.

    a. The tube from the patient extends approximately 2.5 cm (1 in) below the level of the water in the container (Fig. 3.22).

    b. There is a vent for the escape of any air that might be leaking from the lung.

    c. The water level fluctuates as the patient breathes; it goes up when the patient inhales and goes down when the patient exhales.

    d. At the end of the drainage tube, bubbling may or may not be visible. Bubbling would mean either persistent leakage of air from the lung or other tissues or a leak in the system.

The Two-bottle System

1   Consists of the same water-seal chamber plus a manometer bottle.

2   Drainage is similar to that of the single unit, but suction may be added. This is controlled by the depth of immersion of a standpipe into the second vessel containing sufficient fluid to establish the degree of vacuum desired (Fig. 3.22).

3   Effective drainage depends on gravity and on the amount of suction added, as controlled by the manometer bottle.

    a. When vacuum is added to the system from a vacuum source, such as wall suction, water is added to the manometer bottle to determine the amount of vacuum applied to pleural space.

    b. The sterile solution added on some manufactured devices or covering the standpipe of Bottle B is measured at approximately 20 cm (7.6 in).

The Three-bottle System

1   Similar in all respects to the previous two except that the initial chamber collects the drainage (Bottle C) so the fluid in the water-seal chamber stays constant as drainage accumulates (Fig. 3.22). (This has an advantage since in the other two systems as the chest drainage collects in the water-seal bottle, the resistance of flow from the pleural space is increased; when this fluid in the water-seal bottle equals the amount of fluid in the manometer bottle, any effective suction is cancelled.)

2   In the three-bottle system (as in the other two), drainage depends on gravity and the amount of suction added, as controlled by the manometer.

3   The mechanical suction motor or wall suction creates and maintains a negative pressure throughout the entire closed drainage system.

4   The manometer bottle regulates the amount of vacuum in the system. This bottle contains three tubes (Fig. 3.22).

    a. A short tube above the water level comes from the water-seal bottle.

    b. Another short tube leads to the vacuum or suction motor or wall suction.

    c. The third tube is a long tube (standpipe) which extends below the water level in the bottle and which is open to the atmosphere outside the bottle. This is the tube that regulates the amount of vacuum in the system. This is regulated by the depth to which this tube is submerged in the water—the usual depth is 20 cm (7.6 in).

5   When the vacuum in the system becomes greater than the depth to which the tube is submerged under water, outside air is sucked into the system. This results in constant bubbling in the pressure-regulator bottle (manometer bottle), which indicates that the system is functioning properly.

NOTE: When the motor is off or the wall vacuum is turned off, the drainage system should be open to the atmosphere so that intrapleural air can escape from the system. This can be done by detaching the tubing from the suction motor to provide a vent.

GUIDELINES: Managing the Patient with Water-Seal Chest Drainage

Purposes

1   To remove solids, liquids and gas from the pleural space or thoracic cavity and the mediastinal space. (Solids may be fibrin or clotted blood; liquids are serous fluid, blood, pus and occasionally other fluids; gas is air from the lung, tracheobronchial tree or oesophagus).
2   To bring about re-expansion of the lung and restore normal cardiorespiratory function after surgery, trauma or medical conditions (not normally used after pneumonectomy).

Equipment

Closed chest drainage system
Holder for drainage system (if needed)
Vacuum motor

Two plastic-coated clamps or haemostats—taped to patient's bed.

Procedure

Nursing Action	Reason
1 Attach the drainage tube from the pleural cavity to the tubing that leads to a long tube with end submerged in sterile normal saline.	1 Water-seal drainage provides for the escape of air and fluid into a drainage bottle. The water acts as a seal and keeps the air from being drawn back into the pleural space.
2 Tape the places where the tubing is connected, if needed. Some connectors will hold without taping.	2 Taping the connecting points of the tubing will make certain that the tubing remains airtight to re-establish negative (intrapleural) pressure.
a. The tube should be approximately 2.5 cm (1 in) below the water level.	**a.** If the tube is submerged too deep below the water level, a higher intrapleural pressure is required to expel air.
b. The short tube is left open to the atmosphere.	**b.** Venting the short glass tube lets air escape from the bottle.

Nursing Action	Reason
3 Mark the original fluid level with tape on the outside of the drainage bottle. Mark hourly/daily increments (date and time) at the drainage level.	3 This marking will show the amount of fluid loss and how fast fluid is collecting in the drainage bottle. It serves as a basis for blood replacement, if the fluid is blood. Grossly bloody drainage will appear in the bottle in the immediate postoperative period and if excessive may require reoperation. Drainage usually declines progressively after the first 24 hours.
4 Fasten the tubing to the drawsheet with rubber bands and safety pins so that flow by gravity will occur. The tubing should *not* loop or interfere with the movements of the patient.	4 Kinking, looping or pressure on the drainage tubing can produce back pressure, thus possibly forcing drainage back into the pleural space or impeding drainage from the pleural space.
5 Allow the patient to assume a position of comfort. Encourage good body alignment. When the patient is in a lateral position, place a rolled towel under the tubing to protect it from the weight of the patient's body. Encourage the patient to change his position frequently.	5 The patient's position should be changed frequently to promote drainage and the body kept in good alignment to prevent postural deformity and contractures. Proper positioning helps breathing and promotes better air exchange. Pain medication may be indicated to enhance comfort and deep breathing.
6 Put the arm and shoulder on the affected side through range-of-motion exercises several times daily. Some pain medication may be necessary.	6 Exercise helps to avoid ankylosis of the shoulder and assists in lessening postoperative pain and discomfort.
7 'Milk' the tubing in the direction of the drainage bottle hourly.	7 'Milking' the tubes prevents them from becoming plugged with clots and fibrin. Constant attention to maintaining the patency of the tube will facilitate prompt expansion of the lung and minimize complications.
8 Make sure there is fluctuation ('swinging') of the fluid level in the long glass tube (Fig. 3.22, Bottle A).	8 Fluctuation of the water level in the tube shows that there is effective communication between the pleural cavity and the drainage bottle, provides a valuable indication of the patency of the drainage system, and is a gauge of intrapleural pressure.

Nursing Action	Reason

9 Fluctuations of fluid in the tubing will stop when:
a. The lung has re-expanded.
b. The tubing is obstructed from blood clots or fibrin.
c. A dependent loop develops (see step 4).
d. Suction motor or wall suction is not operating properly.

10 Watch for leaks of air in the drainage system as indicated by constant bubbling in the water-seal bottle.
a. Clamp the tubing (*momentarily*) close to the chest to look for air leak only if ordered by the doctor.
b. Report excessive bubbling in the water-seal chamber immediately.

10 Leaking and trapping of air in the pleural space can result in tension pneumothorax.
   If the leak is in the patient and the tube is clamped for more than a few seconds, air may back up in the pleural cavity and extend the patient's pneumothorax.

11 Observe and report immediately signs of rapid, shallow breathing, cyanosis, pressure in the chest, subcutaneous emphysema or symptoms of haemorrhage.

11 Many clinical conditions may cause these signs and symptoms, including tension pneumothorax, mediastinal shift, haemorrhage, severe incisional pain, pulmonary embolus and cardiac tamponade. Surgical intervention may be necessary.

12 Encourage the patient to breathe deeply and cough at frequent intervals. If there are signs of incisional pain, adequate pain medication is indicated.

12 Deep breathing and coughing assist in raising the intrapleural pressure thus emptying accumulation in the pleural space and removing secretions from the tracheobronchial tree with resultant expansion of the lung and prevention of atelectasis.

13 Stabilize the drainage bottle on the floor or in a special holder.
   Caution visitors and personnel against handling equipment or displacing the drainage bottle.

13 If any part of the apparatus is damaged, the closed system of drainage will be destroyed and the patient will be endangered by atmospheric pressure in the pleural space and resultant collapse of the lung. The drainage system must be kept airtight to re-establish negative intrapleural pressure.

14 If the patient has to be transported to another area, place the drainage bottle below the chest level (as close to the floor as possible) if he is lying on a stretcher. Clamps should be attached to the patient's gown while he is transported.

14 The drainage apparatus must be kept at a level lower than the patient's chest to prevent backflow of fluid into the pleural space.

The patient may be mobilized while the tube is still in place, particularly in the case of a pneumothorax. A special bag or container should be provided to hold the underwater-seal bottle, so that the patient can carry this while walking. Care must be taken that the patient understands that the bottle must always be below chest level.

Nursing Action	Reason
15 When two nurses work together to remove the tube: **a.** Ask the patient to perform the Valsalva manoeuvre (forcible exhalation against a closed glottis, holding one's breath). **b.** One nurse clamps the tube and cuts the stitch holding the tube in place. **c.** The second nurse holds the ends of the purse string suture round the wound, ready to tighten it as the tube is removed. She has a pad of three or four pieces of sterile gauze to place over the wound immediately.	15 The chest tube is removed as directed when the lung is re-expanded (usually 24 hours to several days). During removal of the tube, the chief priorities are prevention of entrance of air into the pleural cavity as the tube is withdrawn and prevention of infection.

APPENDIX

Physiology of Gas Exchange—Concept of Partial Pressure

Gases are exchanged through a thin membrane by diffusion, i.e., the gas of high pressure passes through the membrane to the lower pressure, in order to equalize the pressure on either side of the membrane.

There are two areas in the body where this gaseous exchange occurs.

1   The exchange of gases between the alveoli and the capillary network which closely surrounds them. This exchange is known as external respiration.
2   The exchange of gases between the capillaries and the tissue cells in every part of the body. This is known as internal respiration.

In atmospheric air, which is a mixture of gases, and which at sea level exerts a total pressure equal to 760 mmHg (101.3 kPa), each of the gases exerts a pressure or tension in proportion to its percentage of the whole. (As well as the gases, there is a variable amount of water vapour. Due to the specialized structure of the lining of the air passages, air is saturated with water vapour by the time it has reached the lungs.)

The presssure, or tension exerted by the individual gases in a mixture is known as the partial pressure.

The composition of air is approximately:

nitrogen, 79%; oxygen, 21%; carbon dioxide, 0.04%.

To estimate the partial pressure of these gases, it is necessary to calculate their proportion of the total air pressure. For example, nitrogen, 79% of 760=600.

Therefore the partial pressure of nitrogen P_{N_2} is 600 mmHg. In order to convert this to S.I. units, divide by 7.5, which gives 80 kPa.

The partial pressure of oxygen is 21% of 760=159·6. Therefore P_{C_2} 159·6 mmHg = 21.3 kPa.

External Respiration

The Composition of alveolar air is:

Nitrogen, 80%:	573 mmHg	= 76.7 kPa
Oxygen, 14%:	100 mmHg	= 13.0 kPa
Carbon dioxide, 5.5–6%:	40 mmHg	= 5.3 kPa
Water vapour:	47 mmHg	= 6.3 kPa

The blood arriving at the capillary network surrounding the alveoli has the following composition:

$$P_{O_2} = 40 \text{ mmHg} = 5.3 \text{ kPa}; \qquad P_{CO_2} = 46 \text{ mmHg} = 6.1 \text{ kPa}.$$

Therefore, it is obvious that by diffusion, oxygen will pass from the alveoli into the capillaries, and carbon dioxide will pass from its higher pressure in the capillaries to the lower pressure in the alveoli. Due to this exchange, the blood leaving the lungs contains P_{O_2} 100 mmHg = 13 kPa, P_{CO_2} 40 mmHg = 5·3 kPa, that is, in equilibrium with the alveolar air.

Internal Respiration

The blood in the capillaries arriving at the tissues has a higher pressure of oxygen than the tissue fluid, and a lower pressure of carbon dioxide, so that oxygen diffuses out of the capillaries and carbon dioxide passes back into them.

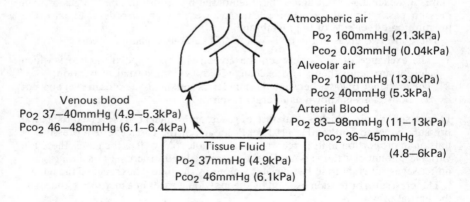

Atmospheric air
Po2 160mmHg (21.3kPa)
Pco2 0.03mmHg (0.04kPa)
Alveolar air
Po2 100mmHg (13.0kPa)
Pco2 40mmHg (5.3kPa)
Arterial Blood
Po2 83–98mmHg (11–13kPa)
Pco2 36–45mmHg
(4.8–6kPa)

Venous blood
Po2 37–40mmHg (4.9–5.3kPa)
Pco2 46–48mmHg (6.1–6.4kPa)

Tissue Fluid
Po2 37mmHg (4.9kPa)
Pco2 46mmHg (6.1kPa)

Pulmonary Ventilation

The amount of air which is taken in with each breath under resting conditions, is about 400 ml. This is known as the tidal volume. In order to establish the pulmonary ventilation, the tidal volume is multiplied by the number of breaths per minute. The usual range of pulmonary ventilation is from about 400 ml × 15 breaths = 600 ml to 400 ml × 20 breaths = 800 ml, i.e. 6–8 l/min. This can be considerably increased during vigorous exercise to 50 l/min. Not all the air which is taken in with a breath reaches the alveoli. Out of 400 ml which is taken in, about 150 ml remains in the air passages, where no gaseous exchange occurs. This area is known as the dead space.

It is sometimes necessary to know the alveolar ventilation, which is calculated by respiratory rate × (tidal volume − dead space).

$$\text{Alveolar volume} = 15 \times (400 - 150) = 3750 \text{ ml/min.}$$

Carriage of Oxygen

Oxygen is carried by the haemoglobin contained in the red blood cells. 1 g of haemoglobin has the ability to combine with 1.34 ml of oxygen. Thus, a person with 15 g haemoglobin/100 ml blood would, theoretically, be able to carry 1.34 × 15 = 20 ml oxygen/100 ml blood. This is known as the oxygen capacity.

At a tension of 100 mmHg (13.0 kPa), the oxygen capacity is very close to this amount i.e., 95–97% of the oxygen capacity, where there is 19 ml oxygen/100 ml blood.

When internal respiration takes place under resting conditions, about 5 ml oxygen per 100 ml blood are given up. During exercise, more oxygen is given up, increasing to 15 ml oxygen/100 ml blood. This can be shown on a graph and is known as the oxygen dissociation curve.

During vigorous exercise, there is an increase in temperature and hydrogen ion production, this decrease in the pH of the blood has the effect of moving the curve to the right, i.e. proportionately more oxygen is extracted (figure 3.23).

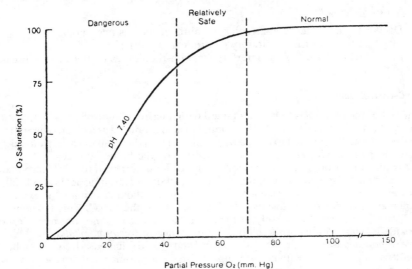

Figure 3.23. Oxygen–haemoglobin dissociation curve showing levels of pH that are normal, relatively safe and dangerous.

Hypoxia. This is a situation in which there is lack of oxygen in the body.
Hypoxaemia. This is an oxygen deficiency in the blood.

$$\text{Normal } PaO_2 = 83\text{--}98 \text{ mmHg } (11\text{--}13 \text{ kPa})$$

Causes of hypoxaemia.

1 Most common cause is diseases which affect the alveolar membrane so that diffusion of gases is impaired, although perfusion of the lungs is normal. This can occur, for example, in pneumonia and emphysema.
2 A low partial pressure of oxygen in the inspired air, e.g., at high altitudes.
3 Some of the blood by-passing the pulmonary circulation, as in ventricular septal defects.
4 Decrease in the amount of haemoglobin available for the carriage of oxygen e.g., in anaemia, and also in carbon monoxide poisoning (carbon monoxide has a very great affinity for haemoglobin, so that only a small amount of inspired carbon monoxide may decrease the available haemoglobin for the carriage of oxygen by half).

Hypoxia will occur for these reasons, plus a sluggish circulation which occurs in cardiac failure or shock. In this case, the amount of oxygen passing into the blood and the amount of haemoglobin are both normal, but the circulation is inadequate to supply the needs of the tissues.

Hypercapnia

This is retention of carbon dioxide in the blood, i.e. the P_{CO_2} is above 45 mmHg (60 kPa) at rest.

Causes of hypercapnia

1 Diseases which affect the alveolar membrane, such as pneumonia.
2 Interference with the respiratory centre, e.g., by drugs.
3 Mechanical difficulties, or interference with the nerves or the neuromuscular junction.

Acid-base Balance

The pH of the blood has to be maintained within narrow limits of 7.35–7.45, and a balance has to be made between the amount of acid produced as a result of metabolic processes, and the amount excreted by (a) the lungs in the form of carbon dioxide + water (carbonic acid) and (b) actively excreted by the kidney tubules.

In order for carbonic acid to be carried in the blood, it is buffered by bicarbonate, and in order for this to happen, the normal bicarbonate/carbonic acid ratio is 20:1. However, if respiration is inadequate, and carbon dioxide cannot be excreted, hypercapnia will result, causing a drop in the pH of the blood. This is known as *respiratory acidosis*. Conversely, if hyperventilation occurs, and too much carbon dioxide is 'washed out' of the blood, the pH will rise (*respiratory alkalosis*).

Metabolic acidosis occurs when the production of acid is increased, e.g., in diabetes mellitus, or when kidney function is impaired, e.g., in chronic renal disease and renal failure.

Metabolic alkalosis occurs when acid is lost from the body, e.g., from prolonged vomiting, or nasogastric suction, or when there is increased ingestion of alkali, which may occur by self-medication of patients with indigestion by taking antacid drugs containing sodium bicarbonate.

The respiratory system is able to compensate for a change in the pH level by altering the rate and depth of respirations.

FURTHER READING

Books

Belcher, J R and Sturridge, M F (1972) Thoracic Surgical Management, Baillière Tindall

Belinkoff, S (1976) Introduction to Respiratory Care, Little Brown

Chilman, A and Thomas, B (1981) Understanding Nursing Care, Churchill Livingstone

Clarke, D B and Barnes, A D (1975) Intensive Care for Nurses, Blackwell Scientific

Cole, R B (1971) Essentials of Respiratory Disease, Pitman Medical

Emergy, E R J et al. (1978) Principles of Intensive Care, Hodder & Stoughton Unibooks

Feldman, S A and Crawley, B E (1977) Tracheostomy and Artificial Ventilation, Edward Arnold

Flenley, D C (1981) Respiratory Medicine, Baillière Tindall

Gibson, J (1975) Modern Medicine for Nurses, Blackwell Scientific

Goodfield, R and Spalding J M K (1979) A Nurse's Guide to Artificial Ventilation, Edward Arnold

Green, J H (1980) Introduction to Human Physiology, Oxford University Press

Lewis, E P (1972) Nursing in Respiratory Disease, American Journal of Nursing Company

MacLeod, J (1981) Davidson's Principles and Practise of Medicine, Churchill Livingstone

Meredith Davis, B (1979) Community Health, Preventative Medicine and Social Services, Baillière Tindall

Partridge, M (1981) Chronic Bronchitis, Update Books

Rickard, M P et al. (1975) Intensive Care of the Heart and Lungs, Blackwell Scientific

Stringer, L W (1976) Emergency Treatment of Acute Respiratory Diseases, Robert J. Brady

Wilson, F (1981) Tracheostomy for Nurses, Edward Arnold

Articles

Ashworth, P (1979) Breathing, Nursing, 6: 251–252

Ashworth, P (1979) Psychological aspects of respiratory care nursing, Nursing, 7: 295–300

Bailey, R (1979) Drugs and the respiratory system, Nursing, 7: 315–318

Brown, S E (1979) Respiratory physiotherapy and the nurse, Nursing, 7: 257–259

Cody, T J and Bennett, A (1978) Technology in nursing—respiratory function, Nursing Times, Series 1–11

Dickens, B (1979) David—a case for ventilation, Nursing, 7: 319

Evans, C C (1979) Pneumonia, Nursing, 7: 320–323

Fairbrother, C (1979) I can't breathe nurse, Nursing, 7: 319

Harrington, V E (1979) Philip, an asthmatic child, Nursing, 6: 273–277

Howe, P (1979) The respiratory effects of surgery, Nursing, 7: 324–327

Jackson, H (1979) Patients with chest injuries and their nursing care, Nursing, 7: 303–309

Legg, S (1979) Breathlessness—what happens?, Nursing, 6: 253–256

Levi, T (1979) Breathing equipment, Nursing, 6: 260–263 and 7: 336–339

Skeates, S (1978) Intensive care. 5. Acute respiratory failure, Nursing Times, 74: 445–447

Watson, S (1979) Chronic bronchitis—a case study, Nursing, 6: 286–291

Williams, R F (1980) Infection of respiratory tract and lungs, Nursing Times, 76: 286–291

Chapter 4

DISORDERS OF THE DIGESTIVE SYSTEM

2. Gastronintestinal Conditions

1. Conditions of the Mouth, Neck and Oesophagus

MOUTH CONDITIONS

Nursing Objectives for Effective Mouth Care

Psychosocial Significance

1 Enhance the person's attractiveness by maintaining clean and well-cared-for teeth and gums.
2 Promote the individual's comfort and general well-being.

Nursing Management

1 Reduce bacterial count and prevent tissue infection when food is removed and mouth is rinsed.
2 Prevent dental caries when plaque is removed periodically by the dentist.
3 Emphasize importance of regular periodic dental examination to maintain good mouth health.

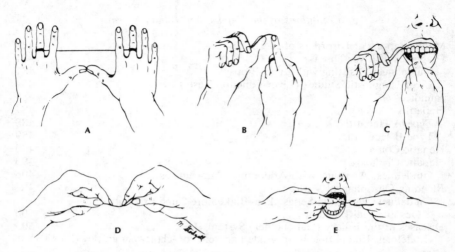

Figure 4.1.   Flossing technique. a. Wrap floss on middle fingers. b. Thumb to the outside for upper teeth. Flossing between upper back teeth. d. Holding floss for lower teeth. e. Flossing between lower back teeth. (From: Effective Oral Hygiene. Developed by USAF School of Aerospace Medicine, Brooks Air Force Base, TX. Published by the American Academy of Periodontology, Chicago.)

4   Maintain healthy mouth structures by tooth brushing, flossing between teeth (Fig. 4.1) and massaging gums.
5   Promote proper nutrition, since dentition and mouth tissue tone are directly affected.
6   Encourage topical application of fluoride as well as fluoridation of water, since this chemical significantly reduces dental caries.
7   Recognize that fatigue, emotional upsets and injury lower resistance of dental tissue to infection.
8   Examine soft tissues of the mouth frequently for evidences of irritation, unusual growths, discoloration, encrustation and leucoplakia, since abnormal manifestations may herald malignancy and early detection may achieve early correction.
9   Participate in community dental health programmes to promote prevention, early detection and correction of dental problems.

CAUSES OF TRAUMA TO ORAL STRUCTURES

Mechanical: Stiff-bristled toothbrush, ill-fitting dentures, carious or broken teeth, grinding of teeth, cheek and lower lip biting
Thermal: Smoking, hot liquids, hot foods
Chemical: Sucking hard sweets, using full-strength antiseptic mouthwashes, chewing or smoking tobacco, drinking alcoholic beverages, chewing Aspergum, sucking mouth lozenges, using breath sweeteners, drinking citrus juices.

Bacterial   Poor oral and nutritional attention that permits food to collect
Irradiation: Exposure to sun, ultraviolet rays, radium and x-rays.

Diagnosis

Oral Cell Smear for Cytologic Examination

1 Examine the patient's mouth carefully (see Assessment of Mouth).
2 Grasp the tongue with a 4″ × 4″ gauze square and gently move the tongue to expose the questionable area.
3 Using a moistened tongue depressor, scrape the area or lesion.
4 If a hyperkeratotic lesion is present, scrape off surface keratin so that deeper epithelial cells are available for a specimen (these are usually involved in early malignant change).
5 Smear cells on a glass slide, immerse carefully in alcohol and send to laboratory.

Lesions of the Lips

Actinic Cheilitis

Heat-ray or sun-induced inflammation of the lip.

1 Often results from overexposure to sun radiation.
2 May lead to squamous-cell carcinoma.
3 *Manifestations:*
    White hyperkeratosis, fissuring, erythema.
4 *Treatment:*
    a. Lips may be protected with sunscreen ointment.
    b. Cryosurgery or electrosurgery may be required.

Contact Dermatitis

Skin irritation produced by allergen.

1 Allergens from cosmetics, lipsticks, ointments, toothpaste or chewing gum may be causative factors.
2 *Manifestations:*
    Itching of lips, erythema, vesiculation or burning may develop.
3 *Treatment:*
    a. Eliminate irritant or suspected contactant.
    b. Apply corticosteroid ointment.
    c. Use hypoallergenic cosmetics.

Lesions of the Mouth

Herpes Simplex

A viral infection commonly producing herpes labialis—cold sore, canker, fever blister.

1   *Manifestations:*
   a. Small vesicles may erupt on lips (and/or tongue, cheeks and pharynx).
   b. Vessels then erupt to form sore shallow ulcers.
   c. This infection often appears in association with other febrile infections (meningococcus meningitis, malaria, and *Streptococcus pneumoniae* infections).
2   *Treatment:*
   a. Does not respond to chemotherapeutic agents that are available.
   b. Some relief is obtained from ointments containing benzocaine or lignocaine (note that there is the potential for allergic sensitization when used over long periods).
   c. Antihistamine such as diphenhydramine (Benadryl) is helpful before meals; this is normally applied as an aqueous rinse with crushed ice.

Gingivitis

Inflammation of gums.

1   This is the most common infection of oral tissues.
2   *Manifestations:*
   a. Inflammation and slight swelling of superficial gingivae and interdental papillae.
   b. With continued neglect, this may advance to chronic degenerative gingivitis and eventually to periodontal disease.
3   *Treatment:*
   a. Conscientious mouth hygiene.
   b. Periodic professional dental cleaning.

Necrotizing Gingivitis

'Trench mouth,' Vincent's gingivitis.

1   This is a pseudomembranous ulceration affecting gums, mouth mucosa, tonsils and pharynx.
2   *Aetiology:*
   a. Thought to be a combination of a spirochete and a fusiform bacillus.
   b. May be due to poor oral hygiene, low tissue resistance and infection from complex micro-organisms.
3   *Manifestations:*
   a. Painful bleeding gums, mild fever, swelling of lymph nodes of neck.
   b. If infection spreads to tonsils and pharynx, swallowing and talking may be painful.
4   *Nursing objectives in treatment:*
   a. Encourage mouth irrigations using dilute hydrogen peroxide or 2% sodium perborate (to combat anaerobic spirochetes) to treat infection, to control bad breath and to produce comfort.
   b. Administer antibiotics as prescribed to curb infection.
   c. Offer soft foods and liquids to reduce gum trauma.
   d. Instruct patient to avoid highly seasoned foods, alcoholic beverages and smoking, all of which irritate infected oral tissues.
   e. Teach patient the importance of regular eating habits and sufficient rest.

Conditions of the Salivary Glands

Parotitis

Inflammation of the salivary gland.

1 Occurs in elderly, acutely ill and debilitated persons when salivary glands fail to secrete sufficiently because of dehydration.
2 Causative organism is usually *Staphylococcus*.
3 *Manifestations:*
   a. Condition appears suddenly and fever exacerbates.
   b. Gland swells and is tender with pain felt in the ear.
   c. Swallowing becomes increasingly difficult.
   d. Swelling increases rapidly; overlying skin becomes red and shiny.
4 *Preventive nursing measures:*
   a. Encourage dental attention (if necessary) before surgery.
   b. Maintain adequate nutritional and fluid intake as well as good oral hygiene.
   c. Postoperatively, allow patient to chew gum or suck hard sweets, which may prevent obstruction of salivary gland ducts.
5 *Treatment:*
   a. Apply ice bag over affected gland for comfort and to control swelling.
   b. Administer antibiotics to treat infection.
   c. Recognize that a suppurating gland may require incision and drainage.

Salivary Calculus (Sialolithiasis)

1 Salivary stones may form in the submaxillary gland following glandular infection or ductal stricture due to trauma or inflammation.
2 Salivary stones are usually mostly calcium oxalate.
   a. Stones found in the gland are irregularly lobulated.
   b. Stones found in the duct are small and oval in shape.
3 *Diagnosis:*
   Sialogram—x-ray with radiopaque dye.
4 *Manifestations:*
   a. None unless there is an infection.
   b. If calculus obstructs gland, the following conditions may occur:
      (1) Sudden, local pain, which is suddenly relieved by a gush of saliva.
      (2) Gland is swollen and tender.
      (3) Stone may be palpable.
      (4) Stone is visible with x-ray studies.
5 *Treatment:*
   a. Surgical extraction of stone.
   b. Gland may have to be removed if condition occurs repeatedly.

Maxillofacial Fractures

Fractures of the maxillofacial area usually include injury to the soft tissues and may occur as a result of a fall or if patient has been hit by a fist or a flying object.

Immediate Assessment and Management

1 Determine whether there is obstruction to the airway.
   a. Remove any obstruction from pharynx, such as broken teeth, dentures, blood clots or broken bits of bone.
   b. Prepare for emergency tracheostomy if airway is obstructed.
2 Control haemorrhage by direct pressure on vessels supplying the area.
   Prepare for fluid replacement.
3 Note extent and involvement of other parts of the head and body.
4 Ascertain localization of pain to determine nerve injury.
5 Administer analgesics to relieve pain and anxiety but not to depress respirations.
6 Reassure patient that he is being given the best possible care.

Mandibular Fractures

Clinical Manifestations

1 Malocclusion, asymmetry, abnormal mobility and crepitus (grating sound with movement).
2 Tissue injury; note extent and involvement.

Preoperative Medical and Nursing Intervention

1 Determine priorities for repair.
   a. Irrigate laceration with copious amounts of normal physiological saline.
   b. Prepare for debridement and suturing of lacerations.
   c. Apply sterile pressure dressings to control swelling, to prevent tension on stitches and to maintain as clean an area as possible to minimize or prevent infection.
   d. Administer tetanus prophylaxis as prescribed.
   e. Give antibiotics as prescribed.
2 Prepare patient for x-rays to determine method of reducing and immobilizing fractures.
3 Reduce mandibular fractures first; maxillary fractures follow in positioning.
   Lower jaw is held tightly against upper jaw by cross-wires or rubber bands placed around arch bars wired to the teeth (intermaxillary fixation).

Postoperative Nursing Care

1 Immediately position patient on his side with head slightly elevated to facilitate breathing and for ease of suctioning.
2 Note wire cutter or scissors taped to bandages or in some other obvious place.
   a. These cutters or scissors are to cut wires or rubber bands in the event the patient vomits; this will prevent aspiration.
   b. After the patient emerges from anaesthesia, scissors or cutters must still be kept nearby for emergency use.
3 Suction drainage and stomach contents as required to lessen danger of aspiration.
   a. Connect nasogastric suction to low-pressure suction.
   b. Administer antiemetic medications as prescribed, if vomiting is anticipated.
   c. Insert small catheter into nasopharyngeal area for suctioning if a nasogastric catheter has not been inserted during surgery.

d. Aspirate oral cavity; this is facilitated by inserting a tongue blade to move cheek away from teeth.

e. Insert oral catheter behind third molar (or where a tooth may be missing) to aspirate within the oropharynx.

4 Modify care as patient emerges from anaesthesia.

a. Remind patient that his jaw is wired but that he can breathe and swallow.

b. Provide a means of communication such as a 'magic slate' (or chalk and chalkboard) or signal system.

c. Elevate the head of the bed for comfort and to facilitate breathing.

d. Continue to administer parenteral intravenous fluids as prescribed until nourishment can be taken by mouth.

e. Administer medications to control pain and restlessness as well as to prevent nausea and infection.

5 Promote a climate to prevent complications and to promote recovery.

a. Apply lubricant to the lips to prevent drying and cracking.

b. Provide frequent and careful attention to the mouth.

(1) Irrigate the mouth with tap water or normal saline after each feeding; use a syringe or irrigating set under low pressure.

(2) Swab the area between teeth and cheek by using a tongue depressor to retract the cheek. Provide light with a torch.

6 Maintain adequate nutritional levels to promote healing.

a. Provide privacy for the patient to eat, since he might be sensitive to his appearance and to the noisy sounds he makes as he tries to eat and drink.

b. Provide a straw if the patient can manage it; the patient may suck soft foods from a spoon.

c. Serve food attractively and arrange as pleasant an environment as possible (music, television, view from window) to encourage nutritional intake.

7 Set up a plan of instruction so that patient will be able to manage at home even with the jaw wired.

a. Encourage exercise and proper diet to promote general good health, tissue healing and to prevent constipation.

b. Develop a plan that is convenient for him to follow in maintaining mouth cleanliness.

c. Work with his family, if required, in determining interesting pursuits to counterbalance any worries he might have about appearance, cost of treatment and other problems.

d. Remind him of follow-up visits to his doctor.

e. Prepare him for possible reconstructive or orthodontic work if this is required.

Premalignant Mouth Lesions

Leucoplakia Buccalis ('Smoker's patch')

1 This condition is characterized by the appearance of one or more small, often crinkled pearly patches on the mucous membrane of tongue or mouth.

2 It is due to the keratinization of the mucosa and sclerosis of the underlying tissues.

3   *Manifestations and treatment:*
  a. If there are no symptoms other than appearance, emphasize importance of careful oral hygiene:
    (1) Recommend dental care and gingival treatment.
    (2) Advise patient to avoid alcohol, tobacco, coffee and tea.
    (3) Suggest mouth rinses of half-strength milk of magnesia after meals and at bedtime.
    (4) Encourage increased vitamin intake, particularly of vitamin C.
  b. If in addition to appearance of white patches there is pain, induration and ulceration, do the following:
    (1) Suggest biopsy to rule out cancer.
    (2) Follow above regime (3a).

Cancer of the Lip

Incidence

1   Cancer of the vermilion border of the lip is the most frequent (20–30%) of all mouth cancers.
2   Most lip cancer is of squamous-cell type.
3   More men than women are affected.
4   This cancer usually occurs in the age group 50–70.
5   The lower lip is most often the site; occasionally the upper lip is involved, and in this location more women than men are affected.

Predisposing Factors and Clinical Manifestations

1   Chronic irritation from actinic rays of sun accounts for most lip cancer; irritation from warm pipe stems may also be a factor.
2   The condition presents first as a well-differentiated small lesion that is infiltrating or ulcerating in character.
3   It continues to grow and may involve entire lip, progressing from there to the soft tissues of the chin.
4   Often it appears as a painless, indurated ulcer with raised edges.
5   Later it progresses to chronic labial fissures, particularly in the midline of the lower lip; repeatedly this fissure heals and breaks down.

Treatment

Objective

To remove malignancy with best cosmetic result.

1   Small lesions are excised liberally. The lip is reconstructed by approximating the layers of the mucous membrane, the subcutaneous tissues and the skin.
2   More extensive resection involves excising half of the lip or the entire lip.
3   If lesion involves more than one-third of lip, best treatment may be radiotherapy.
4   If lymph nodes are involved, a radical neck dissection is indicated.

Nursing Management

For Small Excision

1 Observe appearance of lip for uncontrolled bleeding that forms a haematoma. If untreated, the following may occur:
   a. Undue pressure on mucous membrane results in sloughing.
   b. Cosmetic results are poor.
2 Avoid trauma to incision when the patient eats.
   a. Keep a small dressing over lip.
   b. Feed patient liquids and blenderized foods through straw or nasal tube.
3 Observe for possible secondary infection.

For More Extensive Resection (excision of half or entire lip)

1 Preoperative nursing management:
   Provide meticulous oral hygiene (particularly in presence of infected teeth, gingivitis and a generally poor mouth condition)—to avert infection in the incision line, thereby interfering with proper healing.
2 Postoperative nursing management:
   a. Observe incision to detect signs of inflammation or infection.
   b. Aspirate oral secretions frequently to keep mouth clean and to avoid crusting of secretions around sutures.
   c. Note any swelling around incision which might indicate onset of infection or slow bleeding.
   d. Prevent the patient from exerting undue strain on operated lip when eating, talking, smiling, laughing or using other facial expressions.
   e. Feed patient preferably via a nasogastric tube to prevent strain on suture line.
   f. Offer sips of water, crushed ice or tea to keep oral mucous membrane moist and free of drying secretions.
   g. Liberalize light liquid nourishment by mouth about the fifth day.
   h. Permit soft or semisolid foods after 10 days.
3 Health teaching: instructions for the patient.
   a. Cigarette smoking should be terminated.
   b. A sunscreening ointment should be applied to the lips when they are exposed to wind and sun.

Cancer of the Tongue

Anterior Tongue

Incidence

1 Occurs usually in males in the 40–80-year age group.
2 Strongly associated with history of heavy alcohol intake, smoking and practising poor mouth hygiene.

Manifestations

1 A small ulcer (or thickening) on the anterior undersurface of lateral aspects of tongue that has not healed in 3 weeks.

2 Pain or soreness of tongue on eating hot or highly seasoned foods.
3 Limitation of motion of tongue.
4 Spread of growth to neighbouring structures leads to:
   a. Excessive salivation, blood-tinged sputum.
   b. Slurred speech, trismus (contraction of mastication muscles).
   c. Pain on swallowing liquids.
5 If untreated:
   a. Inability to swallow.   **d.** Cervical lymph node metastasis.
   b. Earache, face-ache and toothache.   **e.** Haemorrhage.
   c. Inability to eat or sleep.   **f.** General debilitation.

Objectives of Treatment

1 To remove the malignancy and salvage as much of the tongue as possible.
   a. When the lesion is small, particularly at the tip of the tongue, surgical excision is done because it is effective and produces minimal impairment of function.
   b. For more extensive lesions, irradiation, such as with interstitial implantation of radium needles, is used.
   c. If radiation is not effective, surgical excision may be indicated.
   d. Cervical lymphadenectomy may be done prophylactically, since a high percentage of tongue cancers tend to metastasize.
2 To develop other lines of communication if patient is going to be unable to speak either for a short or a long period of time.
   a. Practise methods of communicating that the patient understands and can become adept at, such as use of 'magic slate', hand signals, eye blink code and flash cards (words or pictures).
   b. Include the family in using the most effective means of communication.

Postoperative Medical and Nursing Management

See below, Cancer of the Mouth.

Posterior Tongue

Manifestations

Symptoms are less obvious:

1 Slight dysphagia, sore throat.
2 Salivation.
3 Blood-tinged sputum.

Poor Prognosis

1 It is a difficult site for effective radiation
2 Total glossectomy is very mutilating.

Postoperative Medical and Nursing Management

See Cancer of the Mouth, below and Advanced Cancer Nursing Care.

Cancer of the Mouth

Incidence

1 Males are afflicted three times more often than females.
2 Evidence suggests that the risk of cancer in the heavy smoker and drinker may be as much as 15 times greater than in those who neither smoke nor drink.

Clinical Manifestations

For precancerous mouth lesions—(leucoplakia buccalis, keratosis labialis)

1 Pearly patches—one or two small thin, often crinkled areas on mucous membranes of the tongue, mouth or both, due to:
   a. Keratinization of mucosa.
   b. Sclerosis of underlying tissue.
2 Later, most of tongue and mouth may become covered.
   a. Creamy white, thick fissured mucous membrane.
   b. Sometimes desquamates, leaving a beefy-red base.

For Cancerous Lesions

1 White patchy area, sore spot or ulcer on lips, gums or mouth which fails to heal.
2 Swelling, numbness or loss of feeling in the part.
3 An asymmetric, firm nodal enlargement or mass.
4 Erythroplakia—red plaques or well-defined velvety red patches, often with the tiny areas of ulceration.

Preventive Measures

1 Eliminate causes of chronic irritation.
2 Practise good oral hygiene.
3 Obtain proper dental care—remove or repair jagged, carious and infected teeth.
4 Reduce or eliminate smoking and chewing tobacco; also eliminate pipe smoking if it irritates the lip.
5 Restrict or eliminate ingestion of highly spiced foods and reduce alcohol consumption.
6 If syphilis is suspected, seek treatment.

Diagnosis

1 X-rays of head and neck to determine involvement.
2 Cytologic examination of sputum.
3 Biopsy of suspected tissue.

Treatment

1 Selection of treatment depends upon size of lesion and how extensively surrounding tissues are involved.
2 Small lesions can be removed by wide excision or can be treated with radiotherapy or interstitial irradiation.

3 Large lesions may be excised widely or treated by external irradiation followed by radical neck dissection (see p. 382).

4 Inoperable cancer.

a. Radiation therapy can be quite palliative, providing it has not been given previously.

b. Extensive surgical removal may be feasible but is done only with patient's full understanding that cure is not achievable.

c. Intra-arterial chemotherapy has been done, but only with limited success. A brief regression in tumour size may be achieved.

d. Thalamotomy may be a useful palliative procedure for the patient with advanced malignancy and severe pain.

Nursing Management

Preoperative Care

1 Promote optimum physical condition and psychological adjustment.

a. Assess patient's reaction to his condition.

(1) Evaluate his apprehension and offer emotional support.

(2) Correct any misinformation.

(3) Determine therapeutic plan of care for patient's rehabilitation.

b. Maintain a good nutritional level.

2 Provide optimum mouth care.

a. Proper care of teeth because they are essential to mastication.

(1) Stress regular dental care.

(2) Promote good nutrition.

b. Mouth cleanliness to reduce incidence of infectious disease such as mumps and surgical parotitis.

(1) Brush teeth frequently.

(2) Use oxygen-releasing and antibiotic mouth-rinsing solutions.

(3) Apply lanolin to dry and cracking lips.

(4) Remove dentures and clean them frequently.

c. Adequate fluid intake, particularly in debilitated patients who are prone to mouth infections.

d. Stimulation of flow of saliva.

(1) Offer chewing gum.

(2) Encourage patient to suck lemon sweets, a fresh lemon or orange slices.

(3) Administer antibiotics as prescribed to assist in control of infection.

3 Care for mouth lesions and control mouth odours.

a. Feeding problems may be handled in the following way:

(1) Use straws, teaspoon, feeders, etc.

(2) Provide food that is soft, liquid and nonirritating—not too hot or cold or highly seasoned.

(3) Serve small, frequent meals attractively.

b. Excessive salivation and mouth odours may be handled as follows:

(1) Insert gauze wick in corner of mouth; place basin conveniently to catch drippings.

(2) Use small rubber catheter and suction.

(3) Encourage use of mouthwashes, particularly oxidizing agents such as hydrogen peroxide half strength.

(4) Use power spray, if available.

4   Prepare for postoperative communication, since patient may not be able to talk for a few days after surgery.

Practise lip reading, hand signals, 'magic slate', eye blink codes and flash cards (words or pictures).

5   Provide regular preoperative care.

Postoperative Care

1   Maintain a patent airway.

a. Recognize that the patient may have an airway, endotracheal tube, or tracheostomy to facilitate air exchange.

b. Observe patient closely for signs of respiratory embarrassment such as changes in vital signs, dyspnoea and restlessness.

c. Place patient in prone position, or in supine position with head turned to side, or laterally; position should facilitate drainage and prevent aspiration.

d. Suction as required; precautions are necessary to avoid injury to suture line and sensitive tissues.

e. When the patient is out of anaesthesia, elevate head of bed for comfort, to facilitate deep breathing and coughing up of secretions and to lessen oedema.

2   Check pressure dressings that are used to control oedema.

a. Note whether dressings are hindering respirations.

b. Observe surrounding tissues to determine whether dressings are constricting blood circulation.

c. If portable suction is used, pressure dressings may not be applied.

3   Control pain so that respirations are not depressed.

Employ nursing measures to make the patient comfortable so that narcotics for pain relief are not used unless absolutely required.

4   Maintain nutritional and electrolytic levels.

Following intravenous therapy, administer tube feedings by nasogastric tube or gastrostomy (see p. 423).

5   Keep mouth clean for comfort and to assist in healing process.

a. Mouth irrigations, using normal saline, diluted hydrogen peroxide, sodium bicarbonate or alkaline mouthwashes.

b. Gentle lavaging, using a catheter between cheek and teeth to loosen mucus.

c. Power spray to clean inaccessible spaces.

d. Vaporizer to provide moisture to traumatized tissue and discourage crusting.

6   Encourage speech rehabilitation and social adjustment.

a. Recognize that face and neck surgery can be disfiguring and the patient often is embarrassed, withdrawn and depressed.

b. Supply pad and pencil, 'magic slate', signal system (eye blinks or hand), so that patient can express his needs and thoughts. Note that if the patient usually wears glasses to read and write, he may not be able to put his glasses on because of dressings, skin flaps, etc.

c. Allow patient to have his meals in privacy if he desires.

d. Encourage his family and friends to visit so that he is aware others care for him.

e. Assist him in caring for his personal appearance.

f. Observe closely for indications of his needs which may be communicated in other ways.

g. Refer him to a speech therapist if the services of this specialist are indicated.

h. Be consistent with emotional support.

7   Provide an environment conducive to the patient's recovery.

a. Maintain proper humidification and aeration of room.

b. Prevent odours by removing soiled dressings; use effective and pleasant deodorizers.

c. Inform patient that his general throat discomfort is due to endotracheal anaesthesia and will improve in a few days.

8   Prepare patient for convalescence and extended care at home.

a. Provide detailed instructions to the patient or a member of his family.

b. If suctioning is required, instruct as to method, type of equipment and where it can be obtained.

c. Emphasize adequate nutrition—proper consistency, proper seasoning and right temperature. Suggest commercial baby foods or the use of a blender if available.

d. Repeat the details of good mouth care and cleanliness of dressings.

e. Review signs of obstruction, haemorrhage, infection and depression and what to do about them if they are evident.

RADICAL NECK DISSECTION FOR MALIGNANCY

Objective

To remove all lymph-node-bearing tissue on the involved side of the neck.

Scope of Surgery

Removal of all tissue under the skin from the ramus of the jaw down to the clavicle; from midline back to the angle of the jaw. This includes: sternocleidomastoid muscle, other smaller muscles, jugular vein in the neck.

Concomitant Surgery

Tracheostomy.

Nursing Management

Preoperative Care

Preoperative care including diagnosis—see specific related condition, such as Cancer of Mouth,, p. 379, Cancer of the oesophagus, p. 396, etc

Postoperative Care

Postoperative nursing objectives are based on the following patient concerns:

1   His ability to breathe normally.

a. Place him in upright position.

b. Observe for signs of respiratory embarrassment, such as dyspnoea, cyanosis, and oedema.

2   His ability to avoid haemorrhage and infection.
   a. Evaluate vital signs which may suggest haemorrhage or infection onset.
   b. Note condition of dressings to detect early signs of haemorrhage.
3   His ability to swallow.
   a. Observe for throat irritation: oedema, clearing of throat.
   b. Note how he accepts liquids: refusal may mean difficulty in swallowing, which in turn may be indicative of superior laryngeal nerve damage.
   c. Encourage his intake of fluids in order to 'thin' secretions.
   d. Encourage coughing to remove secretions.
   e. Allow patient to assume sitting position to bring up secretions (the nurse should support his neck with her hands).
   f. Suction secretions if patient is unable to bring them up himself.
4   His wound healing.
   a. Reinforce pressure dressings from time to time to assist in obliterating dead spaces and providing immobilization.
   b. Observe dressings for evidence of haemorrhage and constriction which may affect respiration.
   c. If suction drainage (Redivac) is used, approximately 80–120 ml of serosanguineous secretions are drawn off during the first postoperative day; this diminishes with each day.
   d. Apply aeroplast or other antiseptic plastic sprays to protect the wound.
5   His ability to communicate.
   a. Inform the patient that temporary hoarseness can be expected with extensive neck surgery and tracheostomy.
   b. Encourage him to write messages for first few days; if writing is a problem, it may be due to denervation of the trapezius muscle.
   c. Recognize that for this patient to nod 'Yes' or 'No' may be difficult because of the neck dissection.
   d. Manipulate his environment so that he is able to reach his call bell or other required articles without straining.
6   His appearance.
   a. Respect his desire for privacy during treatments, dressing change and feedings.
   b. Inform his visitors of his appearance before they see him so that their expressions do not cause him to be upset.
   c. Provide frequent aeration of the room and utilize deodorants to prevent unpleasant odours.
   d. Observe for lower facial paralysis, since this may indicate facial nerve injury.
   e. Watch for shoulder dysfunction which may follow resection of spinal accessory nerves.
      (1) Utilize postoperative muscle exercises and muscle re-education (see below).
      (2) Work with the patient to obtain good functional range of motion.
   f. Consult with the surgeon and patient in decisions on future cosmetic surgery or in use of a prosthetic device.
7   His prognosis.
   a. Encourage the patient to verbalize his concerns and feelings.
   b. Consult the doctor to determine the nature and extent of explanation and

prognosis he has given to the patient.

c. Encourage the patient to seek confirmation of his personal philosophy and religious beliefs if this would provide answers for him.

d. Accentuate the positive.

e. Encourage the patient to participate in his plan of care.

f. Recognize that a great effort has to be made in behaviour modification to change a lifestyle which included alcohol consumption and cigarette smoking. It is difficult to do.

8   His family.

a. Collaborate with the doctor in informing the family of the nature and extent of the patient's disease and surgery.

b. Help them to understand that without surgery, the patient's condition would be worse.

c. Prepare them for the patient's postoperative appearance; how this will be done depends on the strengths and weaknesses of the family and the individual circumstances.

d. If there is difficulty with a spouse or person close to the patient in accepting his appearance, refer the person to the doctor, social worker, psychiatrist or whatever resource seems advisable.

Rehabilitation Exercises Following Head and Neck Surgery

Exercises are recommended when the neck incision is sufficiently healed.

Objective

To regain maximum shoulder function as well as head and neck motion following surgery.

1   Perform exercises morning and evening. At first, exercises are done only once; then the number is increased by one each day until each exercise is done ten times.

2   Following each exercise the patient is instructed to relax.

3   For neck:

a. Gently rotate head to each side as far as possible.

b. Tilt head to the right side as far as possible; repeat for left side.

c. Drop chin to chest and then raise chin as high as possible.

4   For shoulder:

a. Standing beside bed, place hand from unoperated side on bed for support.

b. Gradually swing arm on operated side up and back as far as is comfortable for patient.

c. Each day work toward finishing a complete circle.

Haemorrhage as a Major Complication Following Mouth Surgery and Radical Neck Dissection

Principal Causes of Sudden Haemorrhage Following Surgery

1   Loose ligature around a large vessel.

2   Sudden distension of tied off blood vessel followed by rupture.

3   Slipping of ligature that may occur in violent coughing spasm.

4   Rupture of a vessel due to trauma incident during surgery.
5   Rupture of a vessel weakened by erosion, tumour or slough.
6   Sloughing associated with secondary infection.

Treatment

Immediate Treatment for Sudden Haemorrhage

1   Pressure over the common carotid and internal jugular vessels in the neck may be life saving.
2   Have someone notify the surgeon immediately.
3   Treat patient for shock.

Definitive Treatment

1   Surgical intervention to repair vessel defect.
2   Correct fluid and blood loss with proper replacement.
3   Initiate postoperative monitoring programme until vital signs remain consistently normal.

CONDITIONS OF THE OESOPHAGUS

Nursing Assessment

During the taking of the nursing history, ask the following questions:

1   What problems or discomfort do you have when you eat? Do you have pain? Where? Is there food sticking in your throat or chest? Are you nauseated? How long does the discomfort last? Is it daily or intermittent?
2   How is your appetite? Are there any signs of anorexia (loss of appetite)?
3   Do you have to restrict the kinds of food you eat as determined by size or consistency (meat for example), as determined by seasoning, or as determined by spiciness or acidity (citrus fruits)? Do you have to limit food because of temperature (hot or cold)?
4   Do you experience any nausea, heartburn, dysphagia, regurgitation, reflux or vomiting?
5   Does the position of your body (bending, stooping, lying down) affect the problem? Do you lie flat when sleeping or do you have the head of the bed elevated? Does assuming a particular position help or make the problem worse?
6   Do you have any gas formation? Early satiety? Belching?
7   How has your weight been (stable, increasing or decreasing)?
8   What relieves the discomfort?
9   Do you find food or saliva on your pillow in the morning on awakening?
10   How are your teeth? Do you have difficulty chewing?

Upper Gastrointestinal Radiography

See p. 410.

Oesophageal Endoscopy

This is the direct visualization of the entire mucosa of the oesophagus to detect inflammation, ulceration, masses (tumours) or varices, and to obtain specimens for cytologic studies or biopsy.

Nursing Management and Patient Instruction

1   Give the patient nothing by mouth for 6 hours prior to the test. This is done to decrease the possibility of aspiration and to be sure the oesophagus is clear of particles that would block visibility.
2   Explain the procedure to the patient before it is done, and explain the steps during the examination.
3   Administer diazepam (Valium) or pethidine if prescribed for relaxation.
4   Spray the throat with local anaesthetic to dull the effects of passing the oesophagoscope and to reduce vomiting.
5   If the oesophagus is dilated (fluid-filled oesophagus was seen on x-ray) first pass nasogastric tube and then evacuate and irrigate oesophagus.

Nursing Alert: For *all* **endoscopies, bouginage and pneumatic dilatation procedures, have the following ready: oropharyngeal suction and emergency cardiopulmonary resuscitation equipment.**

6   If a rigid scope is used, position the patient on his back. During insertion of oesophagoscope, his neck is hyperextended and his head is supported.
7   With the flexible oesophagofibrescope, scope is passed with patient sitting, then examination is completed with patient lying on left side.

Following Endoscopy

1   Withhold fluid and foods until the patient's swallowing reflex has returned (about 2 hours). Test the patient's swallowing with sips of water before foods or fluids are given.
2   Offer anaesthetic lozenges or normal saline gargles for throat discomfort.
3   Observe the patient for 24 hours for symptoms such as bleeding, dysphagia, fever and neck pain (cervical area) that are suggestive of perforation. Check also for substernal or epigastric pain (thoracic area); shoulder pain, dyspnoea, abdominal pain (diaphragmatic area), and subcutaneous emphysema.

Oesophageal Biopsy and Exfoliative Cytology

1   Biopsy of tissue may be taken during oesophagoscopy; prepare tissue for laboratory examination.
2   Cytology.
   a. Usually an overnight fast is required (no food or fluids).
   b. A No. 12 or No. 16 French nasogastric tube is passed to the cardio-oesophageal junction (45 cm).
   c. Residual contents are aspirated.
   d. Physiological saline (50 ml) or Ringer's lactate solution are forcefully instilled with a syringe and are immediately aspirated below the cardia; this procedure is repeated at various levels of the oesophagus (5-cm intervals from 45 to 25 cm from incisor teeth).
   e. Aspirated contents are collected in separate containers surrounded by ice; when all specimens are collected, take them *immediately* to laboratory for analysis (must be centrifuged and pallet spread on slide as soon as possible after aspiration).

Oesophageal Trauma

Oesophageal trauma is injury to the oesophagus caused by external or internal insult.

1 Externally—stab or bullet wounds, crush injuries, etc.
2 Internally—swallowed foreign bodies, i.e., metal objects, fishbones, dentures, poison (e.g., acid burn).

Treatment and Nursing Management

Objectives

To institute emergency life-saving treatment.
To restore continuity of oesophagus
To facilitate healing and prevent infection and constriction.

1 Assess condition of patient to determine his physiological needs.
2 Maintain open airway. Often, difficulty in respiration is due to oedema of throat or a collection of mucus in pharynx.
3 Control haemorrhage if present.
4 Treat for pain and shock. (Shock may be due to haemorrhage, impairment of cardiorespiratory function).
5 Provide high fluid intake; may require parenteral therapy.
6 For external wound:
   a. Initiate emergency first-aid wound care and prepare for surgery.
   b. Maintain feeding through a nasogastric tube.
7 For internal chemical damage, give specific antidote. If lysol or other caustic or organic solvent is swallowed, do NOT try to induce vomiting.
   a. A gastrostomy may be performed, either as a temporary or a permanent means of feeding the patient (see p. 422).
   b. Resulting strictures may be relieved by dilating the narrow oesophagus with bougies.
   c. Reconstructive surgery may be necessary to create a new passageway for food between pharynx and stomach.
8 For swallowed foreign bodies.
   a. When foreign body is made of metal, such as safety pins, needles, nails, and other similar objects, it is not considered safe to allow object to make its way through gastrointestinal tract.
   b. Usually these can be removed with the aid of an oesophagoscope. A large-bore, rigid oesophagoscope is best.
   c. A skilled operator is required; magnets can be used on end of retrieving instrument passed through oesophagoscope.

Oesophagitis

Oesophagitis is an acute or chronic inflammation of the oesophagus. Severity of symptoms may be unrelated to the degree of inflammation seen at endoscopy.

Clinical Manifestations

Sudden or gradual in onset.

1   Hot burning pain (heartburn) behind xiphoid or sternum→spreading to throat, jaw, arms and back.
2   Pain with belching, regurgitation of acidic or bitter fluid.
3   Symptoms aggravated by recumbency.
4   Symptoms may be precipitated by increases in intra-abdominal pressure such as when patient bends over, lifts heavy objects, or has to strain to pass stool or urine (constipation or prostatism).
5   Dysphagia—worse at onset of meal. Food 'sticking' in throat or chest—produced by spasm, oedema or narrow lumen. While swallowing bolus of food, patient may require 'washing down' of food with liquids.
6   Pain on drinking citrus liquids, alcohol or hot or cold fluids. Coffee often aggravates the pain.
7   Bleeding—acute or chronic; melaena or haematemesis also occurs.
8   Relief may be obtained by taking water, milk, antacids or by standing rather than lying.

Causative Factors

1   Fungal—*Candida.*
2   Chemical—ammonia, aerosols, lysol.
3   Physical—alcohol, excessively hot liquids.
4   Trauma—swallowing foreign body.
5   Reflux oesophagitis due to incompetent lower oesophageal sphincter; condition appears to have no relationship to hiatal hernia.
6   Malignancy associated with achalasia.
7   Prolonged nasogastric intubation.
8   Following gastric or duodenal surgery.
9   Repeated vomiting (common in alcoholics).
10 Bending, stooping, coughing, and straining at stool.

Diagnosis

For all oesophageal disorders.

1   Oesophagograms.
2   Oesophagoscopy (see p. 385) with cytology and biopsy may differentiate oesophagitis from carcinoma.

Medical and Nursing Therapy

Objectives

To reduce gastric acidity and prevent regurgitation.
To treat the basic problem.

1   Institute a feeding regime similar to that for peptic ulcer (see p. 415).
    a. Frequent feedings progressing to five meals—bland, low residue—no bedtime feedings.

Nursing Alert: Milk actually is contraindicated for ulcer or oesophagitis due to high calcium content which stimulates gastric acid secretion.

   b. Avoid foods high in residue, very hot foods, spices, alcohol, tobacco and coffee (even decaffeinated).
   c. Avoid salicylates, phenylbutazone (Butazolidin) and anticholinergics.
   d. Do not give food within 2 hours of retiring.
   e. Chew food well and eat slowly.
2 Administer antacids, especially at bedtime.
3 Place 15–20 cm (6–8 in) bed blocks at head of bed.
4 Provide adequate mouth and dental care.
5 Administer cholinergic agents.
6 Promote a relaxing environment during mealtime.
7 For strictures, dilation therapy may be initiated; this is done initially several times weekly, then on a monthly basis.
8 Surgery is indicated when conservative measures fail.
   a. Fundoplication (Belsey or Nissen procedure) for reflux to throat—severe stricture
   b. Combined with vagotomy—pyloroplasty if associated with gastroduodenal ulcer.
   c. Stricture may need to be resected and an oesophagogastrostomy may be required.

Nursing Alert: Anticholinergics are contraindicated because they may further impair competence of lower oesophageal sphincter.

Achalasia

Achalasia refers to a benign spasm of the lower oesophageal sphincter often with marked dilatation of the oesophagus. It is a neuromuscular disorder due to absent or defective nerves (of the myenteric plexus) going to the involuntary muscles in the oesophagus.

Clinical Manifestations

1 Difficulty in swallowing both liquids *and* solids, substernal pressure, fullness and regurgitation, often heartburn appears.
2 Secondary pulmonary complications due to spillover of oesophageal contents (aspiration pneumonia).
3 Loss of peristaltic activity and failure of oesophageal sphincter to relax during swallowing process (detected by x-ray or manometry) may occur.
4 Emotional upsets, sudden shock or dietary indiscretion may aggravate this disorder.
5 Weight loss is eventually noticed inasmuch as the patient has a decreased intake in order to avoid discomfort; eventually this can lead to emaciation.
6 Increased risk of oesophageal carcinoma (8–10%). The patient may also have carcinoma at cardia invading oesophagus, simulating achalasia.

Diagnosis

1   Cine film of oesophagus with barium; this reveals weak or absent peristaltic waves and failure of sphincter relaxation.
2   Oesophagoscopy with cytologic studies and biopsy.
3   Oesophageal manometry with perfused open-tip catheters.
4   Nursing assessment:
   a. Determine what the patient can and cannot swallow.
   b. Note location and kind of pain.
   c. Determine how relief is obtained.
   d. Ascertain what aggravates the problem.

Treatment and Nursing Management

Objective

To enlarge the passageway so that contents pass more readily from oesophagus to stomach.

1   Pneumatic bag dilatation.
2   Surgical oesophagomyotomy.

Nursing Management—Medical Therapy or Minor Surgical Therapy

1   Direct patient to eat slowly, chew food thoroughly and arch his back while swallowing to provide relief.
2   Suggest that the patient sleep with his head elevated to avoid reflux or aspiration.
3   Provide a bland diet and tell patient to avoid alcohol as well as spicy, very hot and very cold foods in order to minimize symptoms.
4   Administer pharmacologic agents such as Bethanecol (urecholine) to increase lower oesophageal sphincter tone.

Nursing Alert: Anticholinergic drugs are contraindicated for achalasia because they further decrease oesophageal peristalsis.

5   If pharmacotherapy fails, pneumatic dilatation is tried (see Guidelines: Pneumatic Dilatation, p. 393).

Nursing Management—Major Surgical Therapy

Used only if pneumatic dilatation fails.

1   Oesophagomyotomy—a division of muscular fibres enclosing the narrowed oesophagus that permits mucosa to pouch out through the divided area in muscle layers.
2   Cardiomyotomy—when above operation is extended to include cardiac end of stomach.
3   Incisional approach determines nature of postoperative care; thus, an incision through chest implies nursing care similar to a thoracotomy.

Diffuse Spasm of Oesophagus

Diffuse oesophageal spasm is a motor disorder of the oesophagus.

Clinical Manifestations

One or more of the following:

1 Pain on swallowing.
2 Dysphagia.
3 Chest or back pain.

Clinical Features

1 Diffuse spasm may be associated with achalasia, obstruction of the cardia by tumour, precipitation by reflux acid.
2 It is common in old age.
3 It may be an early stage of achalasia.

Treatment

Conservative

1 Administer sedatives for pain.
2 Avoid food and beverages that precipitate symptoms.
3 Eliminate source of tension as a precipitating factor producing stress during mealtime.
4 Administer nitroglycerine or long-acting nitrites if reflux is not a factor.

Later, if necessary

Utilize pneumatic dilatation if manometric studies reveal increased lower oesophageal sphincter pressure (providing gastro-oesophageal reflux is not part of the problem).

GUIDELINES: Oesophageal Dilatation (Bougienage)

Purpose

To dilate the cardio-oesophageal sphincter so that food may pass from the oesophagus into the stomach.

Equipment

Water-soluble lubricant
Bougies—flexible, woven silk-tipped or rubber, of various sizes
Dilators of the doctor's preference.

Procedure

Preparatory Phase

1 Explain the procedure to the patient and indicate why it is necessary for him to fast and drink no fluids for 12 hours beforehand.
2 Administer sedative or narcotic as prescribed to allay apprehension and assist him in relaxation.
3 Have the patient in a sitting position in a chair or in bed.

4   Place a drape bib-fasion around his chest and over shoulders to protect his clothing.
5   Provide him with a vomit bowl.

Nursing Action	**Reason**

Performance Phase

1 Spray the patient's throat with a local anaesthetic (gargle may be preferred).	1 The spray or gargle will desensitize local tissues.
2 Lubricate bougie with water soluble lubricant (some bougies are weighted with mercury).	2 Lubrication reduces friction between the mucous membrane and tube.
3 Assist the doctor as he passes the tube and first dilator. Support the patient's head and encourage him to swallow.	3 The more relaxed the patient, the easier the bougie will descend to the cardiac sphincter.
4 Larger bougies are passed progressively until pain occurs. (For achalasia, a pneumatic or hydrostatic balloon is used with fluoroscopy).	4 Sizes are increased to progressively dilate the structure. By increasing the pressure of the balloon, under fluoroscopy the sphincter may be gradually dilated.

NOTE: If bougies do not pass the stricture, it will be necessary to pass a guide wire through the stricture via oesophagoscope. The scope is then removed and metallic olive dilators are passed down the guide wire, progressively increasing the size.

Follow-up Phase

1 Have the patient rest in bed following procedure. **a.** Check pulse and temperature at least hourly for 6 hours.	1 Observe for 24 hours for evidence of oesophageal perforation. **a.** Elevated pulse and temperature plus chest pain and evidence of subcutaneous emphysema may indicate presence of air in the mediastinum.
b. Be attentive to complaints of chest pain. **c.** Observe upper chest for signs of subcutaneous emphysema. Should any of the above occur, notify the medical officer.	It may be necessary to have x-ray verification.
2 Follow-up barium swallow may be required 2–4 hours later to determine success of dilatation. If test results are clear, oral fluid intake may then be resumed.	2 At this time it can also be determined whether or not perforation has occurred.
3 After 24 hours of no untoward signs or symptoms, continue to instruct patient as follows:	

Nursing Action	Reason
a. Chew foods thoroughly; mix foods with liquids.	**a.** Saliva and liquids will facilitate passage of food.
b. Utilize those positions which are most conducive to the patient's comfort.	**b.** Sitting and elevated head positions allow gravity to assist with passage of food.

GUIDELINES: Pneumatic Dilatation

Pneumatic dilatation is the introduction of a pneumatic dilator under fluroscopic control to dilate a cardio-oesophageal sphincter (tightened by spasm) utilizing measured pressure control.

Procedure

Preparatory Phase

1 Explain procedure to patient; tell him some discomfort may be experienced but that he will be given medication to help combat this.
2 Intake is limited to fluids for 3 days prior to dilatation.
   a. Give nothing by mouth after midnight prior to treatment.
   b. Medications are prescribed prior to treatment, usually pethidine, atropine and perhaps diazepam (Valium).
   c. The throat is sprayed with a local anaesthetic, which may also be given in the form of a gargle (viscous lignocaine can be swallowed).
3 Procedure is done with fluoroscope control (x-ray department)

Medical Action	Reason
1 Place patient in sitting position and pass a nasogastric tube.	1 This is to aspirate secretions and contents of oesophagus.
2 Remove tube following aspiration.	
3 Pass pneumatic dilator and position to straddle cardio-oesophageal junction.	3 Done under fluoroscopic control.
4 Inflate balloon to 100 mmHg.	4 Keep at this pressure for 1 min still under fluroscopic control.
5 Note slight constriction of sphincter.	5 The constriction should be positioned in centre of balloon.
6 Inflate balloon to 200 mmHg.	6 Keep the balloon inflated for 2 min; nurse to observe patient's response and provide support.
7 Inflate balloon to 300 mmHg.	7 Patient may experience moderate to moderately severe pain.
8 Release pressure and remove dilator.	8 A small amount of blood on balloon is frequently seen when it is deflated and removed.

(Procedure may be repeated over several days—gradually increasing pressure in balloon).

Nursing Action	Reason

Follow-up Procedure

1 Continue to keep patient fasting.

2 Monitor vital signs every 30 min for 2 hours.

3 Continue to monitor vital signs every 4 hours.

4 Observe patient for vital sign changes and complaints of severe pain. Should changes or complaints occur, notify medical officer and give patient nothing by mouth.

5 Be prepared for medical officer to order blood grouping and cross-matching, and chest x-ray.

1 This is done until patient's condition is stabilized.

2 When vital signs are stable, full fluids may be given.

3 Monitor signs for an additional 16 hours.

4 These may be indicative of bleeding or perforation; reassure patient.

5 These tests may be required to assist in assessing cardiovascular conditions.

Oesophageal Diverticulum

An *oesophageal diverticulum* is an outpouching of the wall, usually in the cervical posterior side.

Types

1 Pharyngo-oesophageal (pulsion)—also called Zenker's diverticulum; upper end of oesophagus through cricopharyngeal muscle.
2 Midoesophageal (traction)—near tracheal bifurcation.
3 Epiphrenic (traction-pulsion)—lower third of oesophagus.

Clinical Manifestations

Pharyngo-oesophageal

1 Difficulty in swallowing, fullness in neck, a feeling that food stops before it reaches the stomach, and regurgitation of undigested food.
2 Belching, gurgling or nocturnal coughing brought about by diverticulum becoming filled with food or liquid, which is regurgitated and may irritate the trachea.
3 Halitosis and foul taste in mouth caused by decomposing of food in pouch (diverticulum).
4 Weight loss.

Midoesophageal

Generally no symptoms.

Epiphrenic

1 At times associated with achalasia or diffuse oesophageal spasm (see p. 390).

2   No symptoms at first, but condition eventually may cause dysphagia, pain and pulmonary complications.

Diagnosis

1   X-rays using barium should be taken.
2   Oesophagoscopy is risky, because of danger of perforation of diverticulum, which may lead to mediastinitis.

Treatment

Pharyngo-oesophageal

Surgical intervention, usually with a vertical incision; however, some surgeons prefer a transverse cervical incision.

1   Caution taken to avoid injury to common carotid artery and internal jugular vein.
2   Sac is dissected free and then excised flush with oesophageal wall.
3   If transthoracic approach is used, nursing management is similar to that described for chest operations.
4   Nasogastric tube inserted.

Midoesophageal

Therapy is usually not required because of absence of symptoms and rarely does it cause complications.

Epiphrenic

Underlying primary condition must be treated.

Nursing Management

1   Institute nasogastric feedings utilizing fluids.
    a. Irrigate tube carefully with water following each feeding.
    b. Record kind and amount.
2   Observe wound for evidence of leakage from oesophagus—may lead to fistula formation.
3   If patient is tolerating liquid diet well, consider offering a bland diet.

Oesophageal Varices

See pp. 498–503.

Oesophageal Perforation

Oesophageal perforation is an acute surgical emergency in which the oesophagus is punctured by a swallowed foreign body (e.g., dental prosthesis, open safety pin), by gunshot, which results in trauma, or by an oesophagoscope or stiff tube.

Clinical Manifestations

1 Chest pain, usually substernal—may be mild or severe.
2 Temperature elevation occurring within 24 hours.
3 Abdominal pain and tenderness, and epigastric muscle spasm.
4 Subcutaneous emphysema and crepitus of neck, face and chest wall—noted in cervical and thoracic oesophageal perforations.

Diagnosis

1 History of recent oesophageal trauma.
2 Chest film to look for air in mediastinum.
3 Oesophagogram.

Surgical Treatment and Nursing Measures

1 Utilize emergency resuscitative procedures.
2 Prepare for surgical intervention (may not be needed if diagnosed and treated early).
3 Administer parenteral fluids and antibiotic agents as prescribed.
4 Pass nasogastric suction tubing to minimize pleural or mediastinal contamination. Give nothing by mouth.

NOTE: For Spontaneous Oesophageal Perforation, See Fig. 4.2, which shows clinical manifestations, operative findings and treatment.

Cancer of the Oesophagus

Incidence

1 Benign tumours and sarcomas of oesophagus are unusual, except for leiomyomas.
2 About 80% of cancers of the oesophagus involve men.
3 Middle third of oesophagus is most involved.
4 Proximity of lesion to vital body structures, e.g., heart and lungs; lymph-node-spread is easy and rapid.
5 Before significant symptoms occur, the tumour may already have invaded surrounding structures.

Causes

Causative factors have not been proven; the condition is associated with achalasia.

1 Chronic trauma—frequent use of alcohol, tobacco, spicy foods, hot Oriental tea.
2 Poor mouth hygiene.

Clinical Manifestations

1 Progressively increasing difficulty in swallowing (dysphagia). At first, only solid foods give trouble; then, as growth progresses and obstruction becomes more complete, even liquids pass with difficulty into the stomach.
2 Pain on swallowing.

3 Possible haemorrhage—usually only occult bleeding.
4 Progressive loss of weight and strength due to starvation.
5 Later symptoms—substernal pain, hiccup, respiratory difficulty, foul breath, regurgitation of food and saliva.

Diagnosis

1 Oesophagogram.
2 Oesophagoscopy.

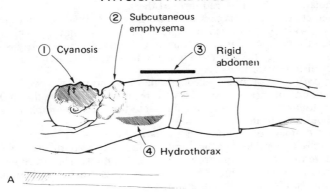

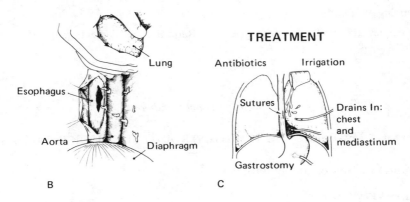

Figure 4.2. Oesophageal perforation. a. Characteristic physical findings with spontaneous rupture of the oesophagus. Emergency operation to close perforation and to drain mediastinum is indicated. (Adapted from: Sawyers, J L (1972) Oesophageal perforation and mediastinitis, AORN J, 15: 42).

3   Bronchoscopy—usually performed with lesions in the upper two-thirds of the oesophagus in order to determine tracheal involvement and whether the lesion can be removed.
4   Cytologic examination and tissue biopsy.
5   Mediastinoscopy to determine involvement of nodes and other mediastinal structures.

Treatment

1   Lesions in middle and upper third, particularly, are often not suitable for excision.
   a. Irradiation is the preferred form of therapy.
   b. Some clinics report success with insertion of a prosthetic tube through the mouth to bridge the involved area and to facilitate swallowing. This insertion is done after dilatation of tumour-bearing portions of the oesophagus.
2   Lesions of middle and lower oesophagus are excised if there is no evidence of local or distant metastases.
   a. The portion of oesophagus containing the tumour is removed.
   b. Continuity of gastrointestinal tract is restored by bringing the stomach (or a tube in stomach or a segment of colon) into the chest and implanting proximal end of oesophagus into it.
   c. Chest drainage of pleural cavity is carried out.
3   If growth is inoperable, a gastrostomy (p. 422) may be performed as a palliative procedure to permit administration of food and fluids. This procedure does not appear to prolong life, since gastrostomy patients cannot swallow saliva either and are miserable from this problem.

NOTE: Some clinics prefer to treat patients with carcinoma of the oesophagus by radiation therapy followed by resection.

Nursing Management

Principles are similar to those given for Radical Neck Dissection (p. 382) and Thoracic Surgery (p. 348).

2. Gastrointestinal Conditions

MAJOR MANIFESTATIONS OF GASTROINTESTINAL DISTURBANCE

Anorexia, Nausea and Vomiting

Normal Physiology

Appetite

A desire for food, or an agreeable attitude toward ingesting food, often specific kinds of food.

1   The frontal and parietal areas of the cerebrum, but especially the hypothalamus, are known to be associated with appetite.
2   Desire for food is acutely associated with increased rates of gastric hydrochloric acid secretion, with gastric hyperaemia, and hypermotility.

Hunger

A strong sensation or urge to eat following a period of fasting.

1   Hunger is temporarily associated with rhythmic contractions of the stomach.
2   The precise mechanisms by which hunger is produced is unknown; it is related to a low blood-sugar level.

Satiety

A condition following consumption of sufficient food to meet present requirements; a feeling that one has had enough to eat.

Anorexia

Lack of appetite for food; lack of interest in all food.

1   Associated with a disinterest in consumption of even those foods which ordinarily one has great interest in and liking for.
2   Associated with decreased secretion of gastric hydrochloric acid.
3   Possible causes:
    a. Unpleasant or upsetting experiences.
    b. Apprehension, fear and anxiety.
    c. Excitment, both pleasurable and desirable.
    d. Systemic and local diseases, such as hepatic failure and uraemia.

Nausea

A most unpleasant sensation usually associated with a distinct revulsion towards the ingestion of food; it may or may not precede vomiting.

1   Very often, anorexia is succeeded by nausea and vomiting. However, either of these states may occur without the others.
2   Associated with decreased motor activity of the stomach, pallor of gastric mucosa and contraction of proximal duodenum.
3   Frequently associated with evidence of diffuse autonomic discharge: profuse watery salivation, sudden drenching perspiration, tachycardia.
4   Difficult to describe by many patients:
    a. Vague unpleasantness in epigastrium.
    b. Distressing feelings in the throat.
    c. Vague unpleasantness spread diffusely in abdomen (must be distinguished from mild visceral abdominal pain).

Vomiting

Sudden forceful expulsion of stomach contents through the mouth.

1   Vomiting centre is located in the medulla.
2   May or may not be preceded by nausea and retching.

3   Exaggerated and often extreme vasomotor activities may immediately precede and accompany the vomiting act; watery salivation, sweating, pulse rate change, vasoconstriction and pallor.
4   Tachycardia prior to vomiting becomes bradycardia during process.
5   Incited by neuromuscular 'reverse peristalsis' or mechanical obstruction.

Nursing Management

1   Observe the preliminary symptoms.
    a. Patient is often lightheaded, weak and dizzy.
    b. Irregularity of respiration before and during vomiting.
    c. Blood pressure may fall before and then fluctuate during vomiting.
2   Observe character and quantity of expectorated material.
    a. Yellowish or greenish colour—may contain bile, which indicates pylorus is open.
    b. Faecal components—may indicate intestinal obstruction or infarction.
    c. Bright red (arterial) blood—may indicate haemorrhage from peptic ulcer. Dark red (venous) blood—may suggest haemorrhage from oesophageal or gastric varices.
    d. 'Coffee-grounds'—may indicate digested blood from slowly bleeding gastric or duodenal lesion.
    e. Undigested food—may indicate gastric tumour or ulcer obstruction.
    f. If taste is 'bitter'—suggestive of bile.
    If taste is 'sour' or 'acid'—may indicate gastric contents.
    g. Odourless.
    h. Sour-smelling.
    i. Liquid.
    j. Containing mucus or pus.
3   Be aware of progression of events when there is a diminution of intake and output—weight loss, dehydration, fluid and electrolyte imbalance:
    a. Skin becomes dry and loses elasticity.
    b. Poor mouth hygiene leading to halitosis.
4   Recognize progression of events which might lead to shock, tachycardia, hypotension, oliguria.

Disturbances Associated with Anorexia, Nausea and Vomiting

Psychic and Neurologic Factors

1   Life situations that evoke subjective manifestations of fear, frustration, depression and anxiety may be associated with these symptoms.
2   *Anorexia* is commonly a manifestation of a depressed state which can lead to a profound impairment of food intake and possibly anorexia nervosa.
3   *Nausea and vomiting.*
    a. Occurring on a psychic basis.
        (1) Frequently occurs during or shortly after meals.
        (2) Often unaccompanied by nausea and retching.
        (3) Frequently does not empty stomach.
        (4) After vomiting, patient may desire to continue to eat.
        (5) No recurrence of vomiting occurs.

b. Projectile type associated with increasing intracranial pressure.
(1) Commonly not preceded by nausea.
(2) May indicate meningitis, internal hydrocephalus, space-occupying lesion, cerebellar lesions.
c. Accompanying migraine headache.
(1) Hypoxaemia affecting the vomiting centre.
(2) Vascular changes.
(3) Associated visual disturbances.
d. Caused by unusual stimulation of labyrinth of the ear.
Associated with vertigo.
e. Associated with systemic diseases, e.g. liver failure, uraemia.
f. Associated with gastritis (alcohol, viruses, bacteria or poisons).
g. Associated with pyloric or intestinal obstruction.
h. Associated with cholecystitis, pancreatitis or peptic ulcer.

Drugs and Toxic Agents

1   Pathophysiologic effect.
a. Medullary chemoreceptor zone may be stimulated.
b. Direct effect on gastrointestinal organs brought about by mercury.
c. Stimulation of hypothalamus nuclei brought about by alcohol, morphine, histamine, epinephrine.
2   Mucosal damage of upper gastrointestinal tract caused by mercury, ammonium chloride, copper sulphate, aminophylline, alcohol, acetylsalicylic acid (aspirin).

Intra-abdominal Disorders

1   Mechanical obstruction in gastrointestinal tract (see p. 462).
2   Intra-abdominal inflammatory disorders—pancreatitis, peptic ulcer.

Nausea and Vomiting of Pregnancy

Other Factors

1   Febrile illness.
2   Uraemia.
3   Motion sickness.
4   Ménière's disease.
5   Hepatocellular disease.

Nursing Management

1   Observe and assess status of patient when he experiences anorexia, nausea and vomiting.
Note the effect of these symptoms on the patient generally:
a. Food and fluid intake.
b. Balance between intake and output.
c. Effect on body weight, indicating malnutrition.
d. Character and amount of vomitus—measure and record.
e. Effect on patient's activity—malaise or apathy.
f. Changes in patient's skin colour and elasticity and in mucous membranes.
g. Note other fluid losses—perspiration, faeces, urine fluid and electrolyte balance which may result in dehydration.

2   Improve psychological desire for food in order to overcome anorexia, nausea and vomiting.
   a. Determine patient's eating habits, cultural preferences, etc.
   b. Include patient's family in soliciting information.
   c. Encourage adequate rest before, during and after his meal; allay anxiety.
   d. Prepare patient for his meals by being certain he has had good oral hygiene, is comfortable and has clean bedding and clothing.
   e. Promote physical comfort of patient so that he may enjoy his food and not be distracted by discomfort during or after his meal.
   f. Protect his environment from noise, foul odours, confusion, too many visitors, etc.
   g. Serve food with attractive appearance and in appropriate quantity.
   h. Be sure that food is served at proper temperature.
3   If patient is nauseated but does not vomit:
   a. Reduce environmental stimuli.

Visual	other 'sick' patients	Sensory	colostomy cauterization
	soiled dressings		bedpan
Olfactory	drainage bottle	Auditory	noise

   b. Encourage rest and deep breathing.
   c. Cater to patient's preferences in food.
   d. Limit size of servings.
   e. Remove meal tray as soon as he is finished.
   f. If he does vomit, carefully observe vomitus and remove promptly; clean area and patient if necessary and offer mouthwash.
4   Provide opportunity for patient to express his feelings.
   a. Keep channels of communication open.
   b. Provide time to allow patient to talk.
5   Correlate administration of medication with needs of the patient.
   a. If patient has pain, analgesics may be administered.
   b. If patient is tired and exhausted, sedatives may be ordered.
   c. If patient appears tense and worried, tranquillizers may be indicated.
   d. Specific antiemetic agents.
6   If secondary to intestinal obstruction, nasogastric suction or the insertion of a Miller–Abbott tube is indicated.

Constipation and Diarrhoea

Constipation

Constipation is a decrease in the frequency, volume or ease of stool passage.
   Obstipation is absence of intestinal output (no stool).

1   Constipation is usually caused by altered routine in dietary and activity patterns; by drugs such as morphine, codeine and atropine; by mechanical obstruction or surgery; by psychological factors resulting from restricted use of toilet facilities; and by old age. It may also occur as a result of chronic, strong-laxative abuse.
2   Manifestations of constipation include changes in colour, consistency and ease of expulsion of stools, which may be darker, harder and difficult or painful to pass.

Diarrhoea

Diarrhoea is an increase in frequency, fluidity and/or volume of stools.

Nursing Assessment

1 Determine whether onset was sudden or gradual.
2 Find out how long the patient has had diarrhoea—days?—weeks?—months?
3 Describe the character, consistency and appearance of stools. Note that colour changes are produced by presence of abnormal constituents.
   a. 'Tarry' stools—may indicate digested blood that usually originates in upper gastrointestinal tract.
   b. Bloody stools—may indicate haemorrhage, usually from lower gastrointestinal tract.
   c. Blood streaking in stool surface or on toilet paper—may indicate haemorrhoid or fissure.
   d. Pale, pasty (clay-coloured) stools—indicate totally obstructed biliary tract
   e. Foamy, foul smelling stools—indicates malabsorption or malabsorption syndrome.
   f. Other colour changes due to food or medication ingested indicates dietary excesses or effect of medication.
4 Learn whether the bouts of diarrhoea are in the day time only, after meals, or occur either day or night.
5 Determine whether diarrhoea is associated with cramping or abdominal pain, fever, chills, nausea, weakness, travel exposure, etc.
6 Is pain in rectum or anus experienced at the time stools are passed?—may be indicative of tumour, inflammation, haemorrhoids or anal fissure.

Nursing Alert: Alteration in bowel habits (such as constipation, then diarrhoea, then constipation, then diarrhoea) may mean partial obstruction.

Nursing Management

Constipation and Diarrhoea

1 Disturbances in elimination produce psychological discomfort; conversely, psychological deviation can produce elimination disturbances.
2 Assist patient in overcoming correctable problems by:
   a. Affording privacy.
   b. Helping patient approach as near-normal position during evacuation as possible.
   c. Providing comfort measures such as warmed bedpan.
   d. Providing sufficient time and a schedule as close to the patient's own as possible.

Constipation

1 Correct dietary habits to include adequate fluids, fresh fruits, roughage.
2 Suggest a small glass of prune juice or lemon juice in warm water each morning.
3 Encourage a regular time for evacuation each day.
4 Suggest a bulk-forming laxative such as methylcellulose (Celevac) that does not irritate the bowel.

1–2 heaping teaspoonfuls in a glass of water, once or twice daily, followed by a second glass of water.

Diarrhoea

1   Consider hospitalization if diarrhoea continues unresolved and there is significant dehydration.
2   Perform rectal examination to check for faecal impaction (common in the elderly, in mental patients and in patients with neurologic disorders). If found, manually disempact (see p. 478). Then give enemas.
3   Remove such causative factors as stress and food until cause is determined.
4   Administer prescribed medication.
    a. Mixture of kaolin and morphine—acts as an absorbent to bind gas and bacteria.
    b. Diphenoxylate (Lomotil)—decreases intestinal motility by acting on gastrointestinal smooth muscle (contraindicated when aetiologic agent is *Shigella* or invasive bowel disease).
    c. Opiates—act to decrease bowel motility.
5   Prepare for fluid therapy administration if dehydration is suspected.

Health Teaching

1   Have required bathroom facilities readily available.
2   Pay particular attention to proper hand and body hygiene, since diarrhoea may be infectious.
3   Use talcum powder or emollients to prevent skin excoriation.
4   Provide dry and clean bed linen and clothing.

DIAGNOSTIC STUDIES FOR GASTRODUODENAL CONDITIONS

GUIDELINES: Nasogastric Intubation—Levin Tube (Short Tube)

Purposes

1   To remove fluid and gas from the gastrointestinal tract (decompression).
2   To determine the amount of pressure and motor activity in the gastrointestinal tract (diagnostic studies).
3   To treat patients with mechanical obstruction and bleeding within the upper gastrointestinal tract.
4   To administer medications and feeding (nasogastric) directly into the gastrointestinal tract.
5   To obtain a specimen of gastric contents for laboratory studies.

Equipment

Nasogastric tube—usually Levin (rubber or plastic, 12 to 18 Fr.)—preferably disposable (plastic tubes are less irritating than rubber) or double-lumen sump tube
Water-soluble lubricant
Clamp for tubing
Towel and vomit bowl
Glass of water and straw, or preferably ice chips.

Procedure

Preparatory Phase

1   Explain procedure to patient and tell him how mouth breathing, panting and swallowing can help in passing the tube.
2   Have patient in a sitting position with neck flexed; place a towel across his chest.
3   Determine with the patient what signs he might use, such as raising his index finger, to indicate 'wait a few moments' because of retching or discomfort.
4   Remove dentures.
5   Mark distance tube is to be passed by measuring as indicated in Fig. 4.3. This will ensure the passage of the tubing into the stomach.

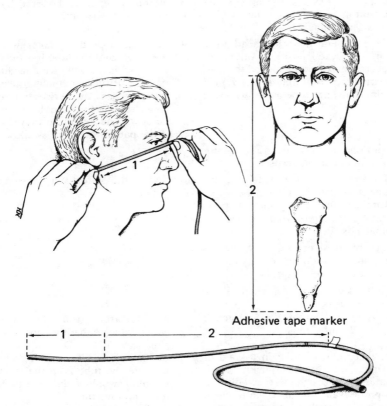

Adhesive tape marker

Figure 4.3.   To measure the distance a Levin tube is to be passed in a patient (to ensure that it enters the stomach): (1) measure the distance on the tube from the patient's tragus (ear lobe) to bridge of nose, plus (2) the distance from the bridge of nose to the bottom of the xiphoid process. Mark this distance with a piece of adhesive tape. Note that the Levin tube usually has circular markings on the tubing—when it is in the patient's stomach, it is between the second and third circular markings.

Nursing Action	**Reason**

Performance Phase

1 Lubricate tube for about 15–20 cm (6–8 in) with thin coat of water-soluble jelly.

1 Lubrication reduces friction between mucous membrane and tube.

2 Lift head before inserting tube into nostril and gently pass it into the posterior nasopharynx aiming downwards and backwards.

2 Passage of tube is facilitated by following the natural contours of the body.

3 When tube reaches the pharynx, the patient may retch; allow him to rest for a few moments.

3 Vomiting reflex is triggered by the presence of the tube.

4 Have patient hold his head in a partially flexed position; offer him several sips of water sucked through a straw or permit him to suck on ice chips. Advance tube as he swallows.

4 Flexed head position makes swallowing easier and the tube less likely to enter trachea. Swallowing facilitates passage of tube. Actually, once the tube passes the cricopharyngeal sphincter into the oesophagus, it can be slowly and steadily advanced even if the patient does not swallow.

5 Continue to advance tube gently each time patient swallows.

6 If obstruction appears to prevent tube from passing, do *not* use force. Rotating tube gently may help. If unsuccessful, remove tube and try other nostril.

6 Avoid discomfort and trauma to patient.

7 If there are signs of distress such as gasping, coughing or cyanosis, immediately remove tube.

8 To check whether the Levin tube is in the stomach:
a. Aspirate contents of stomach with a 20-ml syringe.

a. Aspirated stomach contents would indicate that the tube is in the stomach.

b. Place end of tube in a glass of water, but remove quickly, since patient may cough unexpectedly and aspirate water, if tube is in trachea.
c. Place a stethoscope over epigastrium; inject 5 ml of air into Levin tube.

b. Paroxysms of coughing would indicate the tube is in the trachea; bubbling would indicate tube is in lung; remove tube.
c. Air can be detected by a whooshing sound entering stomach rather than the bronchus.

9 Adjust tubing after these tests to proper position in the stomach.

Nursing Action	Reason

Follow-up Phase

1 Anchor tube with hypoallergenic tape.
   a. Prevent patient's vision from being disturbed.
   b. Prevent tubing from rubbing against nasal mucosa.

   b. To make the patient as comfortable as possible.

2 Anchor the tubing to the patient's gown.

   2 To permit mobility of patient.

3 Clamp the tube until the purpose for inserting the tube is about to take place.

Nursing Alert: All enteric tubes must be irrigated at regular intervals with small volumes of fluid to ensure patency.

4 Administer oral hygiene frequently. Cleanse tubing at nostril. Utilize a decongestant spray, if necessary.

   4 To promote patient comfort.

5 Apply cream to lips and nostril to prevent encrustation.

   5 To keep tissue soft.

6 If tube is to be in place for prolonged periods (beyond 12 hours), keep head of patient elevated at least 30°.

   6 To minimize gastro-oesophageal reflux.

Before Removing Nasogastric Tubing

1 Be certain that gastric drainage is not excessive in volume nor from the small bowel.
2 Ensure, by auscultation, that audible peristalsis is present.
3 Determine whether the patient is passing flatus so that abdomen is not distended.

Nursing Alert: Recognize the potential for complications when intubation is prolonged—nasal erosion, sinusitis, oesophagitis and gastric ulceration. Pulmonary complications may occur postoperatively in patients with nasogastric intubation because of interference with coughing and clearing of the pharynx.

GUIDELINES: Gastric Analysis (Aspiration of Stomach Contents via Nasogastric Tube)

Purpose

1 To determine secretory activity of the gastric mucosa because of diagnostic significance.
2 To study the secretory component, hydrochloric acid.
3 To analyse gastric contents in patients suspected of having pyloric or intestinal obstruction.
4 To remove poisons.

Equipment

Rubber or plastic tube, 12–18 Fr. depending upon patient's size
Tube clamp
Syringe, 50 ml or low-pressure intermittent suction apparatus
Water-soluble lubricant
Bowl of chipped ice for rubber tubing
Specimen containers

Procedure

Nursing Action	Reason

Preparatory Phase

1	Direct patient to fast (and take no fluids) for 8–10 hours preceding analysis.	1	An accurate sampling of stomach contents is ensured.
2	Withhold anticholinergics for 48 hours.	2	To permit normal emptying of the stomach and remove suppressive effect on gastric secretion.
3	Explain procedure to patient; cover his upper body with a drape to protect his clothing and provide a vomit bowl.	3	Patient's understanding of how to breathe through his mouth and occasional swallowing will assist in passing the tube.
4	Instruct patient to sit in a back-supporting chair leaning forward from the waist.	4	Gravity and this anatomic position will facilitate tubes passing into oesophagus. If neck is hyper-extended, tube is more likely to enter trachea.
5	Establish with the patient a signal system to indicate when he wishes to rest a few minutes.	5	Greater patient co-operation is obtained.
6	If dentures or bridges are present, they should be removed.	6	Dislodging of dentures could occur with risk of asphyxiation

Performance Phase

Pass the nasogastric tube (see Guidelines, p. 404).

1	Verify that the tube is in the stomach (for absolute assurance of tube position, fluoroscopic verification is required). Tip at least 50 cm down from nose. When syringing air in and out, gurgling over stomach is audible with stethoscope.	1	Blue litmus turns pink in the presence of acid.
2	Place patient semirecumbent in left lateral position.		
3	Aspirate fasting stomach contents completely; then measure and record. If abnormal, notify doctor before proceeding.	3	Normal: clear and watery; often contains green or yellow bile. Abnormal: see Nursing Alert.

Nursing Action	Reason
4 When tubing is properly positioned in the stomach allow patient to rest for 20–30 min and continuously aspirate contents. This procedure allows patient to attain a basal state and to adjust to the tube in his throat.	4 Production of hydrochloric acid may be inhibited by the irritation of the tubing and by anxiety.

Nursing Alert: In gastric analysis note the following:
1 **Residual of 100 ml or more, including undigested food particles may be indicative of gastric stasis or pyloric obstruction.**
2 **Faecal odour—suggests neoplasm or gastric fistula, intestinal obstruction.**
3 **Blood—indicates ulcerating lesion.**
   Streaks of blood—suggests trauma from tubing.

Types of Analyses

Basal Analysis

A test to determine nature of secretions in the absence of stimuli.

1 Give no food or fluids from midnight on.
2 Obtain specimens as follows:
   First specimen—label 'residual'.
   Second specimen (30 min later)—label as to amount and time of collection.
   Then four additional specimens must be collected at 15-min intervals—label as to amount and time of collection.
   Continuous or frequent aspiration is required (manually or with suction apparatus) to avoid losses through pylorus.

Stimulation Analysis (betazole hydrochloride or pentagastrin)

Usually performed following basal study.

1 This is a test of gastric secretion following injection of a stimulant.
   a. Collect fasting specimen of gastric contents.
   b. Administer betazole hydrochloride (Histalog) or pentagastrin.
   c. Collect specimens every 15 min for 90 min or longer if doctor desires.
2 Significance.
   a. In presence of gastric ulcer visualized radiologically or endoscopically, the absence of any acid after stimulation (pH never falls below 6.0) suggests that ulcer is malignant and that surgical treatment is indicated.

NOTE: In absence of an ulcer, achlorhydria does *not* have the same significance (present in 40% of adults over age 60 without ulcer or cancer).

   b. In presence of a duodenal ulcer, basal output is greater than 20 mEq/hour peak or maximal acid output greater than 50 mEq/hour. A basal/maximal ratio greater than 0.6 should strongly suggest Zollinger–Ellison syndrome.
   c. Otherwise, acid outputs, either basally or after stimulation, are of no diagnostic significance in peptic ulcer disease.

Hypoglycaemic Analysis (Hollander test)

A test that shows the vagal stimulation of parietal cells following a blood sugar drop to a hypoglycaemia level of less than 50 mg/100 ml. (Hypoglycaemia stimulates the secretory activity of the vagus nerve: if the nerve is divided, secretion will not occur. This test may be done postsurgically to determine effectiveness of vagotomy.)

1   Collect fasting specimen of gastric contents; label 'residual'.
2   Collect specimens every 15 min for 1 hour; label 'basal secretion'.
3   Administer prescribed insulin intravenously (calculated according to body weight).
4   Collect gastric specimens every 15 min for next 2 hours. Concomitantly, collect blood specimens every 14 min for determination of blood sugar.
      Measure, note characteristics and record.

Nursing Alert: Observe patient for signs of hypoglycaemia; weakness, vertigo, tremors, perspiration, convulsions, unconsciousness. Have 50% glucose ready for intravenous administration if blood glucose level drops too low.

Radiography

X-rays of the Gastrointestinal Tract (Upper Gastrointestinal Series)

1   The entire gastrointestinal tract can be delineated by x-rays following the introduction of barium sulphate as the contrast medium. This procedure may be combined with cineradiography.
2   Barium is a tasteless, odourless, completely insoluble powder:
      a. It can be ingested in an aqueous suspension for upper gastrointestinal tract study (upper gastrointestinal series); micronization of particles as well as chocolate or strawberry flavouring makes it more palatable.
      b. Effervescent fluids may also be administered to obtain air-contrast studies.
      c. Follow serially through small bowel over next 4–6 hours.
3   The fasting patient is required to swallow barium under direct fluoroscopic examination.
      a. Oesophagus.
         (1) Patency, calibre and motility noted—may indicate anatomic and functional derangement.
         (2) Abnormally enlarged right atrium noted—indicates impingement on oesophagus.
         (3) Oesophageal varices noted—usually indicates liver cirrhosis.

Nursing Alert: If patient stands when drinking barium, transit time may be too rapid through the oesophagus; if this is a problem, consider supine position with the head somewhat elevated.

   b. Stomach.
      (1) Motility and thickness of gastric wall noted.
      (2) Spasms, ulcerations, malignant infiltrates and anatomic abnormalities noted.
      (3) Pressure from outside of stomach detected.
      (4) Patency of pyloric valve observed.
   c. Small intestine.
      Barium swallow or a continuous infusion of a thin barium sulphate suspension

via duodenal tube may be done to visualize jejunum and ileum (small bowel enema).
4   During fluoroscopic examination, x-rays or cine films are taken for permanent records.

Nursing Management and Patient Instruction

1   The patient is to receive nothing by mouth after midnight prior to the test.
2   During this interim, the patient is to receive no purgative, however mild, and no other medication unless specifically ordered.
3   The patient remains in a fasting state until the last x-ray is taken.
4   Barium from prior barium enema must be fully evacuated before gastrointestinal series or it will interfere with visualization of stomach and upper intestine. Cleansing enema is of particular value here.

Nursing Alert: There is a risk of aspiration of barium in patient with an obstructed oesophagus

Upper Gastrointestinal Fibreoscopy (Fibre Optic Endoscopy)

Upper gastrointestinal fibreoscopy is the direct visualisation of the gastric mucosa through a lighted endoscope (gastroscope). Fibrescopes are flexible scopes equipped with a fibreoptic lens through which coloured photographs or motion pictures can be taken. This type of scope may be inserted with less discomfort to the patient, causes fewer perforations than the straight endoscope, and has thus completely replaced the older instrument.

Nursing Management and Patient Instruction

1   Explain the following to the patient:
   a. What is about to happen.
   b. That he must fast before the examination to prevent aspiration of gastric contents and to permit complete visualization of the stomach.
   c. That dentures must be removed to facilitate passing the scope and to prevent injury.
   d. That a topical anaesthetic may be used for local comfort and to prevent retching.
   e. That a sedative or tranquillizer may be given to help him to relax.
   f. That air will be pumped into the stomach during the procedure to permit visualization of the stomach.
2   Following a gastric examination, do this:
   a. Check the swallowing reflex before offering foods or fluids.
      (1) Tickle the back of the patient's throat with a tongue depressor or cotton swab; usually 2–4 hours after the examination, the reflex functions return to normal.
      (2) If fluids are handled normally, patient may then be offered food.
   b. Check for signs of perforation: abdominal pain, subcutaneous emphysema, dyspnoea, cyanosis, back pain, temperature elevation, hydrothorax, rigid abdomen.
   d. Inform patient that he may pass gas by belching or passing flatus.

Gastric Biopsy

Obtaining a piece of gastric mucosa can be done through a gastroscope during endoscopy or fibreoscopy. Forceps extended through the scope may be used to bite tissue, or tissue may be obtained via suction as it pulls mucosa to excising blades within the scope. Tissue in one area may be representative of tissue in all sections of the stomach; however, by looking through the scope, the doctor is discriminating in selection of specific tissue.

Nursing management is similar to that for gastric endoscopy (see above).

GASTRODUODENAL CONDITIONS AND TREATMENT

Peptic Ulcer

A *peptic ulcer* is an excavation found in the mucosal wall of the oesophagus, the stomach, in the pylorus, or in the duodenum due to the erosion of a circumscribed area of its mucous membrane. Basically, the problem is too much secretion of hydrochloric acid in relation to the degree of protection afforded by both mucous secretion and the neutralization of gastric acid by duodenal, biliary and pancreatic fluid.

Predisposing Factors

1   Emotional stress: anxiety, anger, resentment.
2   Drinking coffee and cola beverages and smoking cigarettes are associated with increased risk of ulcer development.
3   Drugs (salicylates, reserpine, phenylbutazone, aminophylline and others) may be irritating to the mucous lining of the stomach, pylorus, and duodenum.
4   Genetic susceptibility.
5   A combination of the above factors.

Incidence

1   Duodenal ulcer is found most frequently in the 25–40 age group and in males four times more than females.
2   Gastric ulcer occurs most frequently in the 40–55 age group and in males 2.5 times more often than females.
3   Duodenal ulcers occur 10 times more frequently than gastric ulcers.
4   No significant racial or national difference.
5   Duodenal ulcer occurs more frequently in patients with type O blood.

Altered Physiology (duodenal ulcer)

1   Increased mass of gastric mucosa and more parietal and peptic cells.
2   Increased sensitivity to gastrin (peptide hormone secreted by gastric antrum stimulates gastric secretion).
3   Increased vagal stimulation, which in turn releases gastrin.
4   Increased release of gastrin in response to a meal.
5   More rapid gastric emptying.
6   Increased acid load to duodenum.

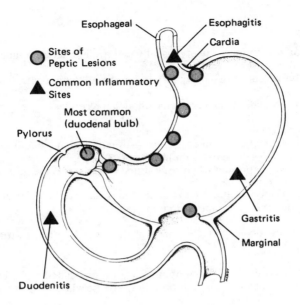

Figure 4.4. 'Peptic' lesions may occur in the oesophagus (oesophagitis), stomach (gastritis) or duodenum (duodenitis). Note peptic ulcer sites and common inflammatory sites.

Preventive Measures and Health Teaching

Instruct the patient as follows:

1   Establish regular eating habits.
2   Avoid foods such as alcohol and coffee that strongly stimulate gastric acid.
3   Bypass stress situations, because they stimulate gastric secretion and motility.
4   Avoid irritating drugs, such as aspirin, Alka-Seltzer and steroids. If it is necessary to administer these medications, have patient ingest milk and crackers between meals and at bedtime for buffering action.
5   Be aware of high-risk tendency if there is a family history of peptic ulcer.

Clinical Manifestations

Underlying Observations

1   Peptic ulcers are more apt to be in the duodenum than in the stomach (ratio of 10:1).
2   A peptic ulcer occurs only in the areas of gastrointestinal tract that are exposed to hydrochloric acid and pepsin (Fig. 4.4).
3   A small percentage of patients will have no symptoms and will first be diagnosed during a bleeding episode (more common in teenagers).

Pain

1   Types:
   a. Pain or discomfort—quality usually not well described—may be sharply localized in midepigastrium.
   b. Heartburn (substernal burning) is associated with peptic ulcer in many patients.
   c. Pain may radiate to the back if the duodenal ulcer has begun to penetrate the pancreas.
2   Time of occurrence:
   a. Pain is worst when stomach is empty—usual 30 min to 2 hours after meals; it may waken patient in early a.m. hours (12–3 a.m.).
   b. Pain is seldom present when patient first wakens, because gastric secretion is lowest at this time.
   c. Periodicity occurs in clusters—patient may have trouble for days to weeks, then experience long symptom-free intervals.
3   Relief:
   Obtained by food or antacids—if truly effective, this occurs within 5–10 min.

Nausea and Vomiting

Reflex vomiting occurs in 10–20% of patients; it is associated with ulcer pain, also seen with duodenal obstruction in chronic ulcer disease when it usually occurs with or just after evening meal.

Belching

Belching is due to increased air swallowing. (This is a nonspecific symptom and is most common in persons with *no* organic gastrointestinal disease).

Heartburn (Pyrosis)

This is burning sensation in lower oesophagus and just below the sternum.

Diagnosis

1   Observation, history and nursing assessment include the following:
   a. Determine location of pain, whether it is localized, whether it radiates, how long it lasts, and when it occurs.
   b. Find out if pain is relieved by food or alkalies.
   c. Learn if there is a history of tension, problem situations or anxiety.
   d. Determine whether the patient ingested drug irritants.
   e. Determine whether the patient smokes or consumes alcohol.
2   Fibreoptic panendoscopy, which permits visualization of entire stomach and proximal duodenum, is most accurate.
3   Upper gastrointestinal series (see p. 410).
4   Gastric secretory studies (p. 407) are of value mainly to check for possible Zollinger–Ellison syndrome.
5   Associated diseases.
   Associated occasionally with hyperparathyroidism, polycythaemia vera, alcoholism, chronic liver disease, chronic respiratory disease, uraemia.

Objectives of Treatment and Nursing Management

To Promote an Atmosphere Conducive to Physical and Mental Rest

1 Encourage bedrest to reduce physical activity and to separate patient from his usual environment.
2 Offer sedatives or tranquillizers to lessen the response to stimuli and to promote relaxation and sleep.
3 Provide frequent feedings, antacids and other medications given on time.
4 Inform visitors to avoid upsetting conversation.

To Relieve Pain and Discomfort, and to Promote Healing Through the Control of Gastric Acidity by Using Antacids and Antisecretory Medications

1 Administer antacid medications to neutralize hydrochloric acid and relieve pain.
2 Administer anticholinergic drugs to suppress gastric secretions and to delay gastric emptying. This is most useful at night.
3 Encourage hydration to minimize side-effects of anticholinergic medications.
4 Note that a new medication, cimetidine (Tagamet) (H_2 receptor blocker) appears promising in reducing acid production in the stomach wall, thus permitting the ulcer to heal.

To Reduce Motor and Secretory Activities of the Stomach by Means of a Therapeutic Diet

1 Eliminate foods which the patient says cause him pain or distress.
2 Offer regular milk since the fat in milk decreases secretion. (Skim milk is usually not given, because the calcium in milk increases secretion).
3 Give small servings to decrease distension and release of gastrin.
4 Provide frequent feedings to neutralize gastric secretions and to dilute stomach contents.
5 Advise patient to avoid coffee and other caffeinated beverages, and cola drinks.

To Assist the Patient in Understanding How Chronic and Long-lived His Problem is and the Very Real Part He Has in Controlling It

1 Emphasize the need to avoid anxiety-producing situations.
2 Alert him to the irritating nature to the gastric mucosa of certain drugs—especially aspirin and aspirin-containing drugs such as *Alka-Seltzer*.
3 Review the reasons for smaller meals and midmeal snacks.
4 Suggest that he cut down on smoking; suggest switching from coffee and cola to caffeine-free beverages.

Discharge Planning and Health Teaching

See above.

Complications

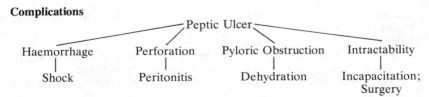

Haemorrhage

1   Experienced by 15–25% of patients with duodenal ulcer; accounts for 40% of deaths from peptic ulcer.
2   Manifestations:
   a. Giddiness, faintness, breathlessness with slight exertion.
   b. Tachycardia, sweating and coldness of extremities.
   c. Black, tarry stool (melaena). (Test for occult blood.)
   d. Vomiting of blood (haematemesis).
3   Medical and nursing intervention:
   a. Encourage bedrest and check vital signs frequently.
   b. Give medication for restlessness or pain, but be on alert for shock.
   c. Employ nasogastric suction to empty stomach of clots and to monitor rate of bleeding.
   d. Give whole blood and/or plasma to keep circulating blood volume at a safe level. (This is not needed if haematocrit is greater than 30 and vital signs are stable, with no drop in blood pressure or rise in pulse.)
   e. Note colour, consistency and volume of stools and vomitus.
   f. Provide treatment if patient goes into oligaemic shock.

Perforation

1   Clinical Manifestations:
   a. Severe upper abdominal pain, persisting and increasing in intensity and often spreading from upper to lower abdomen.
   b. Vomiting suddenly.
   c. Referring of pain to top of shoulders (phrenic nerve irritation).
   d. Abdomen—extremely tender and rigid.
   e. X-ray of abdomen: 50–75% free air visible.
   f. Shock.
   g. Patient lying still in bed, afraid to move; pain increased by patient's coughing or jostling the bed.
2   Surgical intervention:
   a. Repair fluid deficit.
   b. Close perforation; plication of ulcers is performed (see Postoperative Care, p. 420) if chronic symptoms preceded perforation.

Pyloric Obstruction

1   Aetiology:
   Area around pyloric sphincter becomes narrowed from spasm, oedema, or scar tissue formed when ulcer alternately heals and breaks down. Inflammation, muscle spasm or oedema may cause a temporary obstruction.
2   Major manifestations:
   Nausea, vomiting of retained food, constipation, weight loss, cramping, epigastric pain after meals.
3   Medical and nursing intervention:
   a. Gastric decompression and intravenous fluids.
   b. Later, test emptying with fluid load and then with solid bolus.
   c. Surgery may follow if clinical course is prolonged and obstruction is unrelieved.

Intractability

The failure of medical management to accomplish healing of the ulcer—usually a calloused posterior ulcer that penetrates into the pancreas.

1   Manifestations:
       Pain continues without adequate relief from milk or antacid.
2   Surgical intervention:
       a. Vagotomy and gastrojejunostomy or pyloroplasty—to abolish cephalic phase of secretion.
       b. Vagotomy and partial gastrectomy—to abolish cephalic and gastric phase of secretion.
       c. Gastric resection—to abolish acid-secreting parietal cells.

Surgical Treatment

Surgery is required in only about 15–20% of ulcer patients; operation is individualized, based on patient's age, ability to withstand procedure, preoperative nutritional status and particular indications.

Objectives

To relieve complications: (a) perforation (described above), (b) haemorrhage (described above), (c) pyloric obstruction (described above), (d) Intractability (described above).
To treat the tendency to ulcer formation.

Types of Gastric Operations

A comparison of these may be made for the following: M—mortality rate; UR—ulcer recurrence; PNR—poor nutritional result. (See Figs. 4.5–4.8 for the incidence of each of these occurrences.)

1   Gastrojejunostomy and vagotomy (Fig. 4.5)
       The jejunum is anastomosed to the stomach to provide a second outlet of gastric contents. The severed vagus nerve reduces secretions and movements of the stomach (90% good results).
2   Partial gastrectomy and vagotomy (Fig. 4.6).
       The resected portion includes a small cuff of duodenum, the pylorus and the antrum (about one-half of the stomach). The stump of the duodenum is closed by suture, and the side of the jejunum is anastomosed to the cut end of the stomach.
3   Vagotomy and pyloroplasty (Fig. 4.7).
       A longitudinal incision is made in the pylorus, and it is closed transversely to permit the muscle to relax and to establish an enlarged outlet. This compensates for the impaired gastric emptying produced by vagotomy.
4   Subtotal gastrectomy (Fig. 4.8).
       The resected portion includes a small cuff of the duodenum, the pylorus and from two-thirds to three-quarters of the stomach. The duodenum or side of the jejunum is anastomosed to the remaining portion of the stomach.

Nursing Management

See below, for management of the patient undergoing a gastric resection.

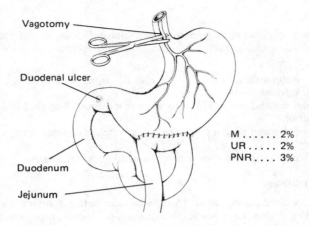

Figure 4.5.   Gastrojejunostomy and vagotomy.

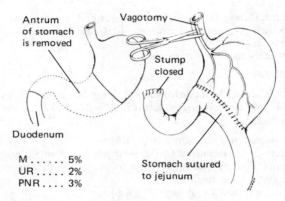

Figure 4.6.   Partial gastrectomy (polya type) and vagotomy.

Gastric Cancer

Clinical Manifestations

Early Manifestations

Most often, patient presents with same symptoms as gastric ulcer; later on evaluation, the lesion is found to be malignant.

1   Progressive loss of appetite.
2   Noticeable change in, or appearance of, gastrointestinal symptoms—gastric fullness (early satiety), dyspepsia of more than 4 weeks duration.
3   Blood (usually occult) in the stools.

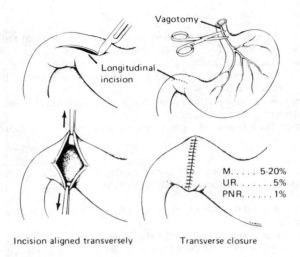

Figure 4.7. Vagotomy and pyloroplasty.

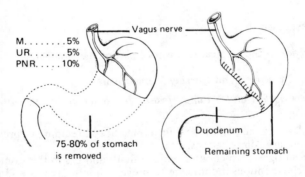

Figure 4.8. Subtotal gastrectomy. It is also possible to do the Billroth II procedure by suturing the gastric stump to the side of the jejunum.

4 Vomiting which may indicate pyloric obstruction of cardiac-orifice obstruction.
5 Occasionally, vomiting that has a coffee-ground appearance due to slow leaks of blood from ulceration of the cancer.

Later Manifestations

1 Pain is a late symptom often induced by eating and relieved by vomiting.
2 Weight loss, loss of strength, anaemia, metastasis (usually to liver), haemorrhage, obstruction.

Diagnosis

1   Patient's history—weight loss and loss of strength over several months.
2   Cytologic examination of gastric juice which may show cancer cells.
3   Palpable unusual abdominal mass.
4   Suspicion of metastasis by palpable lymph nodes—surface of liver, skin at umbilicus, supraclavicular nodes, etc.
5   Gastric analysis—absence of acid after maximal stimulation (Histalog, Pentagastrin) indicates ulcer is malignant.
6   X-ray studies, fluoroscopy and gastroscopy; also cytologic studies and biopsy.

Treatment

1   The only successful treatment of gastric cancer is surgical removal.
2   If tumour is localized to stomach and can be removed, chances are still poor that the patient can be cured.
3   If tumour has spread beyond the area that can be excised surgically, cure cannot be accomplished.
       Palliative surgery such as subtotal gastrectomy with or without gastroenterostomy may be performed to maintain continuity of the gastrointestinal tract. Surgery may be combined with chemotherapy to provide palliation and prolong life.

Gastric Resection

Gastric resection is the surgical removal of part of the stomach.

Objectives of Treatment and Nursing Management

To Promote Comfort and Wound Healing by Relieving the Patient of Pain and Discomfort

1   Frequently turn the patient and encourage deep breathing to prevent vascular and pulmonary complications.
2   Institute nasogastric suction to remove fluids and gas in the stomach.
3   Provide conscientious mouth care to prevent mouth dryness and ulceration.
4   Administer parenteral antibiotics to prevent infection.
5   See that patient has nothing by mouth until ordered (to promote gastric wound healing).

To Meet Nutritional Needs of the Patient

1   Give intravenous fluids to prevent shock and to provide adequate fluid and electrolytes.
2   Give fluids by mouth when audible bowel signs are present.
3   Increase fluids according to patient's tolerance.
4   Offer a diet with vitamin supplements when patient's condition permits.
5   Give protein-vitamin supplements to foster wound repair and tissue building.
6   Avoid high carbohydrate foods such as milk that may trigger 'dumping syndrome'.

To Anticipate Complications in Order to Prevent Them

1   Shock and haemorrhage.
   a. Assess status of blood pressure, pulse and respiration.
   b. Observe patient for evidence of apathy, apprehension, air hunger, pallor or clammy skin.
   c. Check the dressings and drainage bottle frequently for evidence of bleeding.
   d. Administer fluid and blood as ordered.
2   Cardiopulmonary complications.
   a. Encourage the patient to cough and take deep breaths to produce ventilatory exchange and enhance circulation.
   b. Assist the patient to turn and move, thereby mobilizing secretions.
   c. Promote ambulation as ordered to increase respiratory exchange.
3   Thrombosis and embolism.
   a. Initiate a plan of self-care activities to promote circulation.
   b. Encourage early ambulation to stimulate circulation.
   c. Prevent venous stasis by use of elastic stockings if indicated.
   d. Check for tight dressings that may restrict circulation.
   e. See also page 139.
4   'Dumping syndrome'.
   Instruct the patient as follows:
   a. Eat small, frequent meals rather than three large meals.
   b. Avoid meals high in sugars and salt.
   c. Reduce fluids with meals but take them between meals.
   d. Take anticholinergic medication before meals (if ordered) to lessen gastrointestinal activity.
   e. Relax when eating; eat slowly and regularly.
   f. Take a rest after meals.
5   Formation of a solid mass composed of vegetable matter.
   a. Avoid fibrous foods such as citrus fruits (skins and seeds) because they tend to form a solid mass.
      (1) Following a gastric resection, the remaining gastric tissue is not able to disintegrate and digest fibrous foods.
      (2) This undigested fibre congeals to form masses that become coated by mucous secretions of the stomach.
   b. Stress the importance of adequate mastication.

Discharge Planning and Health Teaching

Adjustment to self-care and return to the community.

1   Emphasize the importance of avoiding stress situations.
2   Review nutritional requirements and regime with patient.
3   Stress the importance of vitamin B_{12} supplements.
4   Encourage follow-up visits with the doctor.
5   Recommend annual blood studies and medical check-ups for any evidence of pernicious anaemia or other problems.
6   See above, 'Dumping syndrome'.

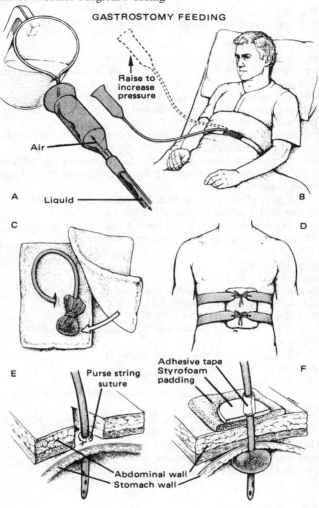

GASTROSTOMY FEEDING

Figure 4.9.   a. By tilting the receiving receptacle, feeding can be poured to allow air bubbles to escape. b. Liquid feeding is poured and permitted to flow into the stomach by gravity. Raising the funnel can increase pressure; lowering it can decrease pressure. At the end of the feeding flush tubing with water. c. Following the feeding, disconnect catheter and cover the outlet with a sterile gauze square; fasten with a rubber band. Coil tubing on dressing. d. A spigot may be used. e. A gastrostomy tube may be a rubber perforated tube; the stomach may be pulled upwards and fastened with sutures to prevent leakage. f. Another method is to use a Foley catheter as the gastrostomy tube. It is inflated with 5 ml of water or air and pulled snugly against the upper gastric wall. This tube is anchored in place with tape, which rests on a cushion of foam or padding. The nurse recognizes the extra precaution required in handling this latter type of gastrostomy.

Gastrostomy

A *gastrostomy* is an opening into the stomach performed for the purpose of administering food and fluids when a complete obstruction of the oesophagus exists. The obstruction may be due to scar-tissue contracture such as may result from a lysol burn or a carcinomatous growth. A gastrostomy may also be done occasionally in the unconscious or debilitated patient for prolonged nutrition (rare).

Preoperative Patient Care

1 Explain the nature of the problem to the patient and the recommended treatment; use simple line drawings for clarification.
2 Achieve adequate fluid, electrolyte and nutritional balance by administering the required foods and fluid.
3 Immediate preoperative care is similar to that described in Volume 1, Chapter 4, Care of the Surgical Patient.

Surgery

1 Frequently performed under local anaesthesia.
2 The anterior gastric wall is incised through a left rectus incision.
3 A tube is inserted and held in place in the stomach wall with several purse-string sutures. The tube may be a rubber tube or a Foley catheter inflated with 5–8 ml of water or air and pulled taut to the abdominal wall (Fig. 4.9).
4 The skin is closed close to the tube to prevent leakage.
5 The tube is clamped at all times except for feedings.

GUIDELINES: Assisting the Patient with Gastrostomy Feedings

Purpose

To provide a means of alimentation when the oral route is inaccesible.

Types of Feedings

1 Powdered feedings that are easily liquefied are commercially available.
2 Food blender is very useful in preparing a normal diet; physiological it is more acceptable, since fibre and residue content are retained and good bowel function is promoted.
3 Prepare a tray containing a funnel, tubing and adapter plus water at room temperature.
4 Pour feeding into a graduated container; warm to 37.8°C (100°F) in a basin of water.
5 Avoid using milk in excess.

Procedure

Preparatory Phase

1 Begin feeding the patient when peristalsis has returned.
2 Place patient in upright position unless contraindicated.

3 Place a half-sheet or bath towel over upper half of patient; fold top bedding down to cover the patient from the waist downward. This permits a space for gastrostomy tube exposure.

Nursing Action (Fig. 4.9)	**Reason**

Performance Phase

1 Connect funnel to tubing and connecting tube.	
2 Uncover opening of gastrostomy (or jejunostomy) tube and insert connecting tube.	2 Provides a receptable for feeding that will lead into gastrostomy tube.
3 Pour feeding into tilted funnel, unclamp tubing and allow fluid to flow into the stomach by gravity.	3 Tilting the funnel allows air bubbles to escape; when tubing is unclamped, air bubbles will not enter stomach.
4 Regulate flow by raising or lowering receptacle.	4 Raising increases pressure; lowering decreases pressure.

Nursing Alert: Force should not be used nor should feeding be given directly from the refrigerator; such action would cause abdominal discomfort to the patient.

Nursing Alert: If there appears to be an obstruction, stop feeding and report the problem.

5 After each feeding, the tube should be irrigated with water (room temperature) and clamped.	5 A water flush will prevent the tube from clogging and will assist in keeping it clean.
6 Apply a small dressing over the tube opening, using a rubber band to keep it in place (Fig. 4.9), or use a spigot.	6 This will keep the tube opening clean for the next feeding.
7 Twist a thin strip of adhesive around tube and attach firmly to abdomen, or coil the tubing on a dressing.	7 Prevents the tubing from being accidentally pulled out of the stomach.
8 Cover tubing with a dressing and apply a firm abdominal binder to hold in place.	8 Provides maximum mobility for the patient.

Patient Education

1 Since the tube should be changed every 2 or 3 days, the patient may be taught how to do it. (The tube should be clean but not necessarily sterile.)
2 The patient should learn how to feed himself. (He can learn what foods may be taken.)
3 Skin requires special care.
   a. It can be irritated by action of gastric juices that leak out.
   b. Daily dressing of wound averts skin maceration.
   c. Bland ointment, such as zinc oxide can be applied to area around the tube.
4 After several weeks, the tube may be removed and inserted only for feedings.

GUIDELINES: Total Parenteral Nutrition (TPN) (Hyperalimentation)

Total parenteral nutrition (TPN), formerly referred as 'parenteral hyperalimentation', is a means of providing body nutrients by way of the intravenous route when it is impossible or inadvisable to use the normal digestive routes.

Physiological Basis

1   The intravenous route has before not provided adequate nutrition; caloric and nitrogen deficiencies occurred.
2   Because of nutritional deficiencies, the process of *gluconeogenesis* takes place; this is the body's conversion of protein to carbohydrate.
3   Approximately 1500 calories/day are required by the average adult postoperative patient to prevent body protein from being utilized.
4   Body needs are increased when the patient has a hypermetabolic disease, a fever or injury; these needs may require up to 10 000 calories daily.
5   To meet the fluid volume necessary to provide so many additional calories would exceed fluid tolerance and lead to pulmonary oedema or congestive heart failure.
6   This process (TPN) provides desired calories in concentration directly into the intravenous system which rapidly dilutes incoming nutrients to satisfactory levels of body tolerance.
    a. Hypertonic glucose→fulfils caloric requirement→permits amino acids to be released for protein synthesis (not energy).
    b. Potassium→provides proper electrolyte balance→transports glucose and amino acids across cell membranes.
    c. Calcium, magnesium and sodium chloride→meet cell requirements as determined by serum electrolyte needs.
    d. Other trace elements whose function is not known may be deficient in TPN, since they are not included.

Clinical Indications

1   As a substitute for oral or nasogastric intubation when these are not effective, desirable or even hazardous. Use TPN under the following conditions:
    a. Chronic vomiting.
    b. Cancer, chemotherapy or radiotherapy.
    c. Cerebrovascular accident.
    d. Anorexia nervosa.
2   As a supplement for patients demonstrating large nitrogen losses, e.g., burn patients, those with metastatic cancer, and those who are receiving radiation and chemotherapy.
3   As a means of putting the gastrointestinal tract at rest.
    a. When there is evidence of gastrointestinal fistula.
    b. With severe and extensive inflammatory bowel disease.
    c. Following major intestinal resection.
    d. Instances of intestinal obstruction.

Equipment

Skin detergent germicide
Sterile drapes and gloves
20-ml syringe
No. 14 (5 cm) needle
16-gauge 20-cm radiopaque catheter
Connecting tubing and adapters

Intravenous 5% dextrose (500 ml)
3 × 3 dressings—adhesive for occlusive
  dressing
Suture material
Antibiotic ointment
Tincture of benzoin spray } if used

Procedure (Fig. 4.10).

Procedure as for subclavian vein catheterization.

Nursing Action	Reason
Preparatory Phase	
1 Explain the procedure to the patient and why it is important for him not to touch the area where the catheter is inserted.	1 To provide reassurance; to prevent dislodging and contaminating of catheter.
2 Tell the patient he will probably be ambulatory during the extended time of therapy.	2 In the absence of other conditions requiring bed rest, ambulation is possible.
3 Place patient in head-low position.	3 This position permits dilatation of neck and shoulder vessels, which makes catheter entry easier and prevents air embolus.
4 Suggest that the patient turns his face away from the area selected.	4 To prevent contamination of TPN site.
5 Support patient in proper position to permit hyperextension of shoulder.	5 This position can be facilitated by placing a rolled sheet or towel vertically along spinal column.
6 Shave area if necessary, remove surface oils with acetone or ether and prepare skin with a detergent-germicide.	6 To reduce probability of contamination to the barest minimum.
7 Instruct patient to be still during insertion of catheter.	7 To prevent the possibility of dislodging of catheter and perforation of subclavian vein.
Performance Phase (by doctor)	
1 Clean and drape area for catheter insertion (Fig. 4.10).	1 To prevent infection.
2 Inject local anaesthesia to skin and underlying tissues.	2 To promote comfort of patient and prevent patient movement.
3 Using a No. 14 (5 cm) needle with syringe, insert needle beneath the clavicle and into subclavian vein.	3 Subclavian vein is selected because it leads into the superior vena cava, which has a large volume of blood flow that provides rapid dilution of hypertonic solution.

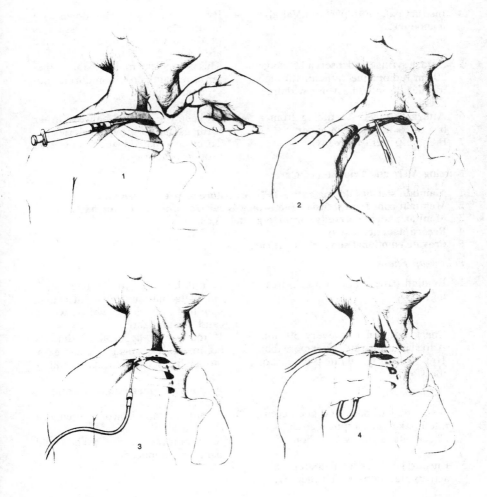

Figure 4.10.   Subclavian catheterization for intravenous feeding is achieved under controlled hospital conditions in these stages: (1) Syringe with Intracath needle inserted at clavicular curve parallel to patients chest, advanced under clavicle and over first rib until entire bevelled tip enters vein (demonstrated by aspirated blood). (2) Syringe detached, needle held by haemostat, catheter threated into superior vena cava. (3) Needle withdrawn, x-ray confirms correct catheter placement in middle portion of superior vena cava. (4) Catheter sutured to chest skin, attached to standard intravenous tubing, adhesive dressing applied, infusion started. Solutions may be delivered by gravity flow or propulsion pump. (From: Patient Care, 15 Jan 1975. Copyright 1975, Miller and Fink Corp., Darien, CT. All rights reserved.)

Nursing Action	Reason
4 Instruct patient to perform Valsalva manoeuvre.	4 By the patient's bearing down with mouth closed, positive pressure is produced when syringe and needle are replaced by catheter.
5 Detach syringe and insert a 16-gauge 20-cm radiopaque catheter through the needle into the vein; withdraw needle.	5 This permits the more flexible catheter to remain in position during subsequent feedings.
6 Attach Intracath to tubing from a bag of 5% dextrose in water.	6 To keep tube patent between other feedings and to provide calories.
7 Prepare patient for x-ray.	7 To ensure that tip of catheter is in proper location.

Nursing Alert and Priorities of Care:

1 **Maintain sterility during entire TPN procedure to prevent sepsis.**
2 **Maintain consistent infusion rate which is calculated on a 24-hour basis.**
3 **Monitor patient carefully—including vital signs.**
4 **Record data accurately.**
5 **Provide emotional support to patient.**

Follow-up Phase

1 Remind patient not to touch dressings.	1 Permit him to turn in bed or to ambulate, but caution patient against handling dressings which would cause contamination.
2 Check infusion rate every 30 min. Adjust infusion rate to not more than 10% of the original rate if too fast or too slow.	2 If too rapid→hypermolar diuresis occurs→excess sugar is excreted→ intractable seizures occur→coma→ death. If too slow→inadequate nutritional intake.
3 Weigh patient daily and keep accurate intake and output records.	3 Accurate comparison of daily change is noted.
4 Check vital signs every 4 hours.	4 Note temperature rise, which could signify a complication.
5 Encourage diversional therapy and activity during extended therapy.	

GUIDELINES: Duodenal Drainage

Purposes

1 To detect abnormal constituents of bile, pancreatic juice or duodenal fluid.
2 To assist in diagnosis of cholelithiasis (gallstones), choledocholithiasis (common duct stones), pancreatitis and pancreatic carcinoma.
3 To assist in diagnosing gallbladder problems when x-rays prove inadequate.
4 To assist in parasitologic studies, especially in detection of *Giardia intestinalis*.

Equipment

Duodenal tube (metal tip) with markings: 45, 60, 65, 70 and 90 cm (or rubber tubing with mercury weighted bag), or Abbot–Rawson tube with mercury-weighted tip.
Clamp for tubing
Towel and vomit bowl
30 g of magnesium sulphate in 50 ml of water
Glass of water; straw
Container for specimen
Optional: clear plastic tubing (7.5 cm) to use as a sleeve over rubber tubing; this can be slipped over tubing and kept near teeth to prevent biting of rubber tubing.

Procedure

Preparatory Phase

1 Explain procedure to patient and tell him how mouth-breathing and swallowing can help in passing the tube.
2 Have patient in a chair or upright position in bed with neck flexed; place a towel across his chest.
3 Determine with the patient what sign he might use, such as raising his index finger, to indicate 'wait a few moments' because of retching or discomfort.
4 Remove dentures.

Action

Performance Phase (by the doctor)	**Reason**
1 Ask patient to open his mouth and breathe through it.	1 Mouth breathing facilitates the relaxation process.
2 Place the tube's metal tip or the tubing with the mercury bag on the back of the tongue.	2 Proper positioning of the tip encourages and promotes swallowing.
3 Ask patient to close his mouth (without biting the tubing) and swallow.	
4 Permit patient to drink water through a straw as he swallows tubing until the 45-cm mark is reached. It is even better to have him suck on ice chips.	4 Water aids in lubricating and swallowing. However, avoid administering more than 100 ml in volume.
5 Instruct patient to sit in chair or on edge of bed and to lean forward with elbows on his knees. The tube is slowly advanced to the 60-cm mark.	5 These are all manoeuvres that have been found helpful in permitting the tube to pass through.
6 Next have the patient curl up on his *right* side with hips on a pillow and shoulders low. Advance tube to the 70-cm mark.	6 The tube tip should be in the second portion of the duodenum (Fig. 4.11). Check to see if bile can be aspirated and if the pH is greater than 7.0.

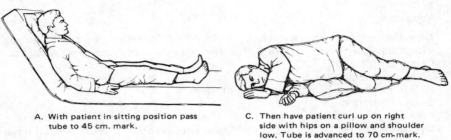

A. With patient in sitting position pass tube to 45 cm. mark.

C. Then have patient curl up on right side with hips on a pillow and shoulder low. Tube is advanced to 70 cm. mark.

45 cm.

60 cm.

70 cm.

90 cm.

B. Have patient sit up (this may be in bed or in a chair), leaning forward, sway back, with elbows on knees. Slowly advance tube to 60 cm. mark.

D. Turn patient on back for a few minutes.

E. Now turn patient to the right lateral position for collection of drainage. (Same as C)

Figure 4.11.   Positions to be assumed by the patient in passing a duodenal drainage tube. Note on the central diagram how the tubing is advanced by each position change.

Action	Reason
7 The patient is then rolled over on his back for 5 min.	
8 Drainage procedure may now take place with patient in right lateral position.	
Following are the ways of testing to see if tube is in duodenum:	
a. Aspirate gently—inspect fluid; instil 30 ml water.	a. Record colour, amount and consistency of bile as well as duration of flow (normal: clear, golden brown).
b. Instil 30 ml air rapidly and aspirate immediately; if as much as 5 ml can be recovered, the tip is probably in the stomach.	b. Usually no air can be recovered from the duodenum.
c. Use a stethoscope to locate tube's tip as air is slowly injected through tubing by syringe.	c. A bubbling sound is substantially louder than elsewhere. The spot should be small and well to the right of midline. If bubbling can be heard over an area as large as the hand, the tip is in the stomach.
d. To be absolutely sure of position of tube, check position fluoroscopically.	
9 Anchor tube by using plastic guard.	9 To prevent patient's biting rubber tube.
10 Collect specimens as directed by gravity drainage or by low-pressure intermittent suction with container on floor. If the tube is determined to be in the duodenum, an appropriate stimulant is injected and collection begins.	
a. Magnesium sulphate solution to stimulate relaxation of sphincter of Oddi and contraction of gallbladder.	a. If gallbladder function is to be evaluated.
b. Administer secretin or secretin-CCK to stimulate pancreatic secretion. Measure volume, bicarbonate concentration and amylase content.	b. If pancreatic function is to be evaluated.

Follow-up Phase

1 At conclusion of test, slowly withdraw tubing.	1 Rapid withdrawal may be injurious to mucous lining because of metal tip; teeth also may be injured by metal tip.

Action	Reason
2 As tube emerges from the patient's mouth, cover it immediately with a towel.	2 Covering the mouth will help prevent the urge to vomit.
3 Offer toothbrush and paste or mouthwash.	3 To freshen mouth.
4 Record test and patient's reaction.	

INTESTINAL CONDITIONS AND TREATMENT

Diagnostic Studies

Stool Specimen

1   The stool is examined for its amount, consistency and colour; a screening test for occult blood is also done. Normal colour varies from light to dark brown. Special tests may be made for faecal urobilinogen, fat, nitrogen, parasites, food residue and other substances.

2   Various foods affect stool colour.
   a. Meat protein—dark brown.
   b. Spinach—green.
   c. Beets—red.
   d. Cocoa—dark red or brown.
   e. Liquorice—black.

3   Various medications affect stool colour.
   a. Phenylbutazone (Butazolidin, Azolid)—black.
   b. Oxyphenbutazone (Tandearil, Oxalid)—black.
      Phenazopyridine (Pyridium)—orange-black.
   c. Aluminium hydroxide—grey-white.
   d. Pyrvinium pamoate (Povan)—red-orange.
   e. Bismuth compounds—black.
   f. Senna laxatives—yellow-green.
   g. Haematinics (iron salts)—black.
   h. Barium—white.

4   Haemoglobin and bleeding affect the stool in the following way:
   a. Considerable quantities of haemoglobin—occult blood (not visible to naked eye); use Haematest tablets for testing.
   b. Upper gastrointestinal bleeding—tarry black (melena).
   c. Lower gastrointestinal bleeding—bright red blood.
   d. Lower rectal or anal bleeding—blood streaking on surface of stool or on toilet paper.

5   Characteristic clinical entities related to characteristics of stool:
   a. Bulky, greasy, foamy, foul in odour, grey in colour with silvery sheen—steatorrhoea.
   b. Light grey 'clay-coloured' (due to absence of 'acholic' bile pigments)—biliary obstruction.
   c. Mucus or pus visible—chronic ulcerative colitis, shigellosis.
   d. Small, dry, rocky-hard masses—constipation, faecal obstruction.
   e. Marble-sized stool pellets—spastic colon syndrome.

Nursing Management

1   Use a spatula to place a small amount of stool in a disposable waxed container.
2   Save a sample of any faecal material if it is unusual in appearance—worms, blood or blood-streaked, unusual colour, much mucus.
3   Send specimen to be examined for parasites to the laboratory immediately so that the parasites may be observed under microscope while viable, fresh and warm.

Nasointestinal Intubation (Long Tube)

Purposes

1   To remove fluid and flatus from the intestinal tract (decompression).
2   To assess gastrointestinal bleeding.

Equipment (Choice Made by Doctor)

1   Type of Tube
       Single-lumen Tube:
          Harris, Cantor
          Distal end has a small rubber bag weighted with mercury; suction openings are proximal to bag.
          Some single-lumen tubes use air to inflate balloon or have a metal bulb at distal end.
       Double-lumen tube:
          1 Miller–Abbott
             a. One outlet is for drainage.
             b. The other outlet is for filling the small rubber bag near the distal end.
          2 Abbott–Rawson
             a. One lumen ends approximately 20 cm (8 in) beyond the other.
             b. The distal lumen has a small metal bulb or mercury weighted rubber bag.
2   Tube selection.
    a. Miller–Abbott tube is used in presence of mechanical bowel obstruction with hyperactive bowel sounds.
    b. Other tubes are used for adynamic ileus (absent bowel sounds).

Procedure

This is usually performed by the medical officer.

Preparatory and Performance Phases

Nursing Alert: All tubes and endoscopes should be routinely pretested for patency and function *before* **passage.**

1   Similar to passing of short nasogastric tube (p. 404).
    Exception: *Miller–Abbott*. Follow the procedures described below:
    a. Pretest the bag volume; the proper amount of air will fill the bag to just less than fully distended (slightly compressible). This also assures that the bag is not leaky.
    b. Place 1 ml mercury in the bag after it is in the stomach. This helps it to pass the pylorus.

c. After duodenum has been entered (position to be checked by x-ray), instil 20–50 ml air in bag according to its pretested volume; place other opening on suction.

Air-filled bag acts as bolus and is carried distally by peristaltic action, as suction evacuates retained air and fluid just ahead of bag.

Exception: *Abbott–Rawson tube*. Follow the procedures described below:

a. Pass the tubing (minus metal bulb) through the nostril.

b. When tubing is in the oropharynx, have patient open his mouth, then grasp tubing with clamp, and draw out in order to attach metal bulb.

c. Redirect metal bulb with tubing in oropharynx for the patient to swallow with small sips of water.

2   After the tubing enters the stomach, it has to pass by peristalsis and gravity into the small intestine; do not fasten tubing to face as with short nasogastric tube.

3   Change the patient's position from upright to a leaning forward position; this will assist in advancing the tubing to and through the pylorus; tilting to the right is helpful.

4   Upon x-ray confirmation that the tubing is past the pylorus, permit the patient to ambulate to facilitate tube passage.

(By passing the tube through the pylorus and into the duodenum under fibreoptic guidance, the entire procedure can be completed in less than 15 min with little patient discomfort.)

5   At specified time intervals, advance the tubing 5–10 cm (2–4 in).

6   Tubing may be taped to the face and suction may be applied when the tubing tip has reached its destination.

7   Measure drainage and record its characteristics every 8 hours.

Nursing Alert:

If drainage is clear and up to 3000 ml obtained/day, there is complete intestinal obstruction.

If drainage is yellow with a faecal odour, the patient may have a small intestinal obstruction.

Follow-up Phase

1   Similar to short nasogastric tube (p. 404).

Exception: In removing tubing, patient may feel tube resistance and become nauseated.

2   As tubing is drawn through posterior nasopharynx, have patient open his mouth so that balloon or bag can be grasped with a clamp in order that the balloon or bag can be removed. Withdraw the remaining tubing through nose.

3   If tubing has advanced beyond the ileocaecal valve, the doctor may release it so that it can pass through the gastrointestinal tract. After the distal tube has been retrieved at the rectum, the proximal end can be released at the nose. Peristalsis aids in passing the tubing.

Radiography of the Colon: Barium Enema

The fasting patient received a rectal instillation of a barium sulphate suspension which is viewed in the fluoroscope and then filmed. If patient is adequately prepared, fluoroscope will reveal:

1 Colon—contour of entire colon is visible.
2 Caecum and appendix—contour and motility observed.

NOTE: Air may be induced to give air contrast studies.

Nursing Management and Patient Instruction

1 Explain to the patient:
   a. What the x-ray procedure involves.
   b. That proper preparation provides a more accurate view of the tract.
   c. That it is important to retain the barium so that all surfaces of the tract are coated with opaque solution.
2 Two days before the examination, the patient may be given a minimal residue diet.
3 The day before the examination, some doctors restrict food intake to liquids; others advise liquids for the evening meal only.
4 The day before the examination, castor oil (60 ml (2 oz)) or magnesium citrate may be prescribed. (A 5- to 6-1 saline load by mouth may also be used to cleanse the colon.)
5 The evening before and on the morning of the examination, a cleansing enema may be given. Food and fluids are restricted for the examination.
6 The above preparation varies, but the objective remains the same: to have the large intestine as clear of faecal material as possible.

Nursing Alert: Use nursing judgement regarding the administration of laxatives or enemata in the presence of acute abdominal pain or obstruction.

7 Administer an oil-retention enema or laxative such as magnesium citrate following the barium enema to completely evacuate the barium.
8 Permit patient to eat following the examination, since he has been fasting and is undoubtedly hungry.

Visualization Measures

1 Two visualization measures are sigmoidoscopy and colonoscopy.
2 The details of these two procedures are presented in the following Guidelines.

GUIDELINES: Sigmoidoscopy

A *sigmoidoscopy* is the viewing of the lumen of the sigmoid and rectum by means of a sigmoidoscope, a tubular instrument that can be illuminated.

Equipment

Fletcher's disposable enema—used at least 1 hour before the sigmoidoscopy
Water-soluble lubricant
Sigmoidoscope—a two-part instrument (obturator and cannula)
              —a long, thin metal tube with light bulb at one end
Glass eyepiece to fit on scope during insufflation of air
Inflation bulb
Long applicator sticks (cotton)
Disposable gloves for preliminary digital examination

Procedure

Preparatory Phase

1   An hour before the sigmoidoscopy, a Fletcher's disposable enema may be administered by the nurse (or by the patient himself).
2   The enema is retained for 5 min before being evacuated.
3   Some doctor's request the patient to be on a light diet the evening before and the breakfast before the examination. Others prefer an aperient the evening prior to the examination.

Nursing Action	Reason
Performance Phase	
1 Have the patient assume knee–chest or Sims' lateral position.	1 The position used depends upon doctor's preference, patient condition and nature of examining table (or bed).

a. Knee–chest position
    (1) Knees are spread comfortably apart.
    (2) Thighs are perpendicular to table.
    (3) Feet are extended over the edge.
    (4) Head is turned sideways to right (head shares pillow with chest).
    (5) Left arm is flexed to side of chest.
    (6) Right arm may rest above head.
	a. This position permits the sigmoid to hang forwards, diminishing the angle at the rectosigmoid junction.

b. Sims' lateral position
    (1) Place patient on left side with left leg partially flexed at hip and knees; right leg should be fully flexed.
    (2) Pelvis to be perpendicular to table.
	b. Used for elderly, ill or arthritic patients or those who are reluctant to assume the knee–chest position.

2 Drape the patient so that only the perineum is visible.	2 A disposable large sheet with a circular opening is practical.
3 Check scope lights after connecting cord to battery.	
4 Doctor first examines anal and perianal region. Digital examination indicates the direction of the anal canal, its patency and the presence of any abnormality.	4 The purpose is to note inflammation, fistula, and ulceration. Digital examination also promotes anal relaxation and helps to lubricate orifice.

Nursing Action	Reason
5 Warm sigmoidoscope in tap water or sterilizer to slightly above body temperature; lubricate tip of scope.	5 A cold scope would cause discomfort and promote contraction rather than relaxation of perianal muscles. Water-soluble lubricant permits easier passage of scope.
6 Doctor spreads buttocks and anal margins with left hand and inserts instrument with right hand (or vice versa).	6 Keep instrument out of view of patient.
7 Nurse encourages relaxation and explains each step in advance.	7 Reassuring patient promotes relaxation.
8 Doctor may use a glass eyepiece over viewing end of scope; an insufflation bulb and tubing are attached. He may proceed to pump a small quantity of air into the bowel.	8 The purpose of inflating lower bowel with air is to expand the area viewed so that vision is not obstructed by mucosal folds.
9 The nurse should relay to the doctor expressions or complaints of pain by the patient.	9 Tenderness and pain may be experienced by the patient with a history of abdominal surgery; procedure may have to be terminated in order not to risk perforation.
10 As the scope advances, it may be necessary to attach suction to remove secretions, exudate, blood or excreta.	10 Connect tubing to suction equipment and turn to lowest degree at first.

Follow-up Phase

1 Upon withdrawal of scope, assist patient in gradually assuming a relaxed position.	1 Wipe the perineal area to prevent soilage of garments and to promote comfort.
2 If disposable scope is used, rinse scope and discard in proper receptacle. Reusable scopes are thoroughly cleaned in soap and water.	2 Sterilizable parts are sterilized before scope is stored.
3 Record the procedure and the reaction of the patient.	

GUIDELINES: Colonoscopy

Colonoscopy is the direct visual inspection of the large intestine by means of the colonoscope.

Purposes

1 As a diagnostic aid to view and assess the status of the large intestine (Fig. 4.12).

2   As an operative instrument to remove polyps, to obtain tissue for biopsy and to remove foreign bodies.

Equipment

Complete colonoscope, possibly with sidearm second observer scope
Water-soluble lubricant   Snares (for biopsy)
Suction apparatus   Drapes
Air-insufflating equipment   Fluoroscope

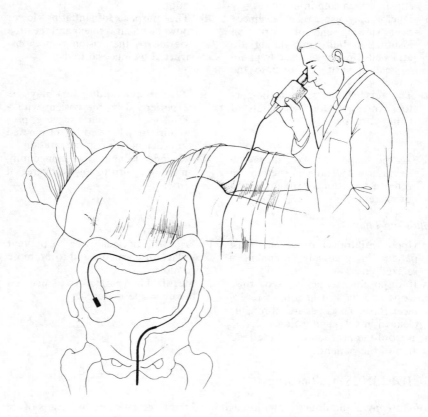

Figure 4.12.   Technique of colonoscopy. The patient is turned from one side to the other to take advantage of gravity as the scope is being advanced. Insert shows path of flexible scope from rectum through sigmoid colon and descending transverse, and ascending colon. If the doctor desires to check scope position with fluoroscopy, he should don a lead apron.

The Colonoscope

The colonoscope is an instrument consisting of a flexible 4-mm glass bundle (containing about 250 000 glass fibres).

1 There is a lens at both ends equipped to focus and magnify.
2 Light is transmitted from an external source by way of a fibreoptic bundle to the tip of the scope; an image is transmitted regardless of the looping or twisting of the flexible bundle.
3 Accessory channels provided for:
  a. Suction of fluid, blood and mucus.
  b. Insufflation of air or water.
  c. Biopsy.
4 There are two kinds of colonoscopes:
  a. To visualize left side of colon—105 cm.
  b. To visualize entire colon—165–185 cm.

Procedure

Preparatory Phase

1 Explain procedure to patient; his understanding and co-operation will promote his relaxation and facilitate his comfort during examination.
2 Limit the patient's intake to liquids for 24–48 hours prior to the procedure (as directed by the endoscopist).
3 Serve the patient citrate of magnesia or castor oil, as prescribed, in the evening for 2 days before the examination.
4 Give tap water or saline enemas approximately 3 hours prior to the colonoscopy until the returns are clear.
5 Administer sedative or analgesic as prescribed; sedation is desirable, but the patient must be sensitive to any pain during the examination so that his response can be relayed to the endoscopist.
6 Preferably, this procedure should be performed where fluoroscopy is available.

Nursing Action (as assistant)	Reason
Performance Phase (by endoscopist)	
1 Place patient in the left lateral position.	1 This position is assumed to follow the location of the sigmoid-rectum anatomically.
2 The lubricated scope is inserted and passed through the rectum.	2 This procedure is done under direct visualization; valvulae are prominent throughout the colon.
3 At apex of rectosigmoid area, there is a red 'blur-out'.	3 Blur-out occurs because the tip of the colonoscope touches the sigmoid colon wall.
4 The instrument is steadily inserted, rotated and flexed.	4 This will promote the sliding of the tip along the greater curvature of any loops in the sigmoid colon.

Nursing Action (as assistant)	Reason
5 If mucosa does not appear red, but seems to blanch or become white, the scope is withdrawn until red mucosa appears.	5 Whitening or blanching is indicative of compression of bowel wall with danger of perforation.
6 The endoscopist utilizes 'manoeuvres' to straighten difficult curves. A fluoroscope can also be used.	6 By various manoeuvres, such as 'alpha', 'hooking' or 'lifting', the endoscopist is able to continue with the insertion and examination of the walls of the colon. Fluoroscopy assists in monitoring position and direction.
7 Manoeuvres are resorted to at sharp turns such as the sigmoid-descending colon, the splenic flexure, the transverse colon and the hepatic flexure.	7 Occasional withdrawal, appearance of a triangular configuration, or a bluish colour are techniques and observations to assist in advancing the scope.
8 As the scope is advanced into the ascending colon, the nurse can position the patient on his back or on his right side.	8 This permits the manoeuvring of the colonoscope into the caecum. It takes about 20–45 min to reach this point in the examination.
9 Observation and close inspection is accomplished during insertion and withdrawal of scope.	

Polypectomy and Postcare

1   Prepare intestinal tract meticulously; if there is any faecal matter in the field near the polyp, the procedure will be postponed and bowel preparation will have to be repeated.
2   Skill is required to remove the optimum amount of polyp, to avoid burning the bowel wall and to prevent cutting the base too close to the bowel wall.
3   When the tissue has been cut by cauterization, the snare-cautery device is removed and the polyp tissue is withdrawn by suction.
4   Following polypectomy, the colonoscope may be reinserted, the inner bowel insufflated with air, and the operated area carefully examined for possible haemorrhage.
5   Postpolypectomy care depends upon size of the polyps removed and the general condition of the patient. Usually the ambulatory patient can be discharged with no medication and no dietary restriction.
6   For in-hospital patients, vital signs are checked for several hours, full liquid diet is given the day of surgery, and soft, low-residue diet is given for 2 weeks thereafter.
7   Follow-up by complete colonoscopic examination usually is scheduled for 6–8 weeks later.

Nursing Alert: If polypectomy is done through sigmoidscope or colonoscope, barium enema should not be done until 7–10 days thereafter because of risk of perforation at the polypectomy site.

Medical and Nursing Management of the Patient Undergoing Major Intestinal Surgery

Preoperative Objectives

To Ensure that the General Physical Condition of the Patient is the Best Possible

1 Administer parenteral therapy to correct fluid and electrolyte imbalance.
2 Correct nutritional deficiencies: protein supplements, between-meal feedings.
3 Provide blood replacement to overcome losses sustained by bleeding, infection and neoplasm.
4 Assist with diagnostic studies as they relate to the evaluation of the cardiopulmonary, hepatorenal bodily functions.
5 Give the patient psychological support as he encounters the stresses of accepting the diagnosis, surgery and possibly a colostomy.
6 Insert an indwelling urinary catheter immediately prior to the patient's going to the operating room.
7 Oversee general personal cleanliness to minimize skin and wound infection postoperatively.

To Reduce Bacteria in the Intestinal Tract to Prevent Postoperative Infection

1 Administer antibiotic agents to suppress aerobic colon microflora.
   Combinations of kanamycin or neomycin with tetracycline, erythromycin, lincomycin or metronidazole.

NOTE: Evidence that these are preferable to a good intestinal cleansing is lacking.

2 Reduce content of colon.
   a. Give low-residue diet and, when required, change to liquid diet.
   b. Offer laxatives as prescribed. Saline washout may be preferred.
   c. Administer enemas or colonic irrigations.
3 Decompress gastrointestinal tract by means of indwelling gastrointestinal tube to control distension and vomiting, if necessary.
   Miller–Abbott or Cantor tube.

Postoperative Objectives

To Meet Nutritional Needs by Administering Fluids, Electrolytes and Nutrients

1 Utilize intravenous catheter if intravenous therapy is to continue several days.
   Observe tissue for infiltration of fluid.
2 Maintain meticulous mouth hygiene while patient is on parenteral therapy.

To Promote Proper Functioning of Nasogastric Decompression and Patient Comfort

1 Observe and record quality and quantity of aspirated material.
2 Lubricate nostrils with water-soluble lubricant.
3 Humidify room to prevent dryness of mucous membranes.
4 Turn patient frequently to minimize discomfort.
5 Remove tube (when required) upon re-establishment of peristalsis (determined by auscultation, passage of flatus rectally).

To Alleviate Psychosocial Concern of Patient

1   Encourage patient to express concerns and questions. (See Colostomy and Ileostomy Management if these are pertinent, pp. 455 and 468).
2   Administer analgesics according to needs.
3   Promote restfulness with appropriate nursing measures prior to giving sedation or hypnotics.

To Prevent Complications by Recognizing Early Signs

1   Evaluate vital signs and recognize patterns of development that may suggest haemorrhage, infection, shock, obstruction, etc.
2   Stress preventive measures, each as turning frequently, maintaining fluid balance, encouraging coughing, emphasizing cleanliness and movement of legs.

To Prepare a Plan for Convalescence and Follow-up Care

1   Encourage ambulation and self-care activities.
2   Stimulate appetite by promoting those measures that will make patient want to eat what he should eat.
3   Help patient set goals toward which he can progress.
4   Emphasize the importance of follow-up visits to evaluate healing process, general physical and psychological adjustment.

Appendicitis

Acute appendicitis is an inflammation of the appendix due to an infection. It is almost always a surgical problem.

Incidence

1   Occurs most frequently in young adults but may occur in any age group.

Clinical Manifestations

1   Begins with a progressively severe abdominal pain, beginning in midabdomen (periumbilical) and moving to right lower quadrant after 6–12 hours.
2   An effective early assessment of the patient for acute appendicitis is to have him rise on his toes and then drop down on his heels with a thump or to have him cough. If he has an acute inflammation, he will feel localized pain in the inflamed area.
3   Within a few hours, the acute tenderness becomes localized in the right lower quadrant (McBurney's point).
4   Anorexia, slight or moderate temperature elevation, mild change in bowel habit (usually constipation), and perhaps nausea and vomiting occur.

NOTE: If these clinical manifestations occur in any person, encourage him to see a doctor immediately. There is a tendency in the ageing person to ignore aches and pains and to delay seeing a doctor. Consequently, mortality in such a person with a benign inflammatory bowel lesion is as high as 20%.

Diagnosis

1   Physical examination noting especially location and localization of pain, rebound tenderness, etc.
2   Blood studies with particular attention to white count; urinalysis.
    A white blood count reveals a moderate leucocytosis.
3   Careful history to rule out other possibilities.

Treatment and Nursing Management

Palliative Preoperative Care

1   Place patient in comfortable position to relieve abdominal pain and tension—usually upright position.
2   See that patient takes nothing by mouth—to decrease peristalsis and to allow stomach to empty preparatory to surgery. Note time and nature of last meal.
3   Place ice bag to right lower quadrant—NEVER HEAT because of the possibility of causing a rupture of appendix and peritonitis.
4   Do not administer aperients for the same reason as preceding precaution concerning heat.
5   Frequently evaluate vital signs—to assess progression of infection.
6   When diagnosis of acute appendicitis is made, administer chemotherapy and/or antibiotics.

NOTE: If there is evidence that perforation has occurred recently and a generalized peritonitis has developed, operative urgency is increased (see p. 444).

Operative

1   If diagnosis of acute appendicitis is established, a simple appendectomy is performed.
2   Because patient will obtain relief from pain, he usually accepts surgery very willingly, which affords a smooth recovery.
3   Anaesthetic may be general or spinal.
4   Incision may be McBurney, muscle-splitting or gridiron, or right rectus.

Postoperative Care

1   Without drainage
    a. Following recovery from anaesthetic, upright position is maintained, analgesic is given every 3 or 4 hours as needed, and fluids and food are given as tolerated.
    b. Enema given third postoperative day.
    c. Stitches removed between fifth and seventh day (usually in doctor's office).
2   With drainage.
    Treat same as for peritonitis (see p. 444).

Meckel's Diverticulum

Meckel's diverticulum is a congenital abnormality of the ileum consisting of a blind pouch resembling the appendix.

Incidence

A disease of 'two's'.

1   Such a diverticulum observed in about 2% of the population.
2   More common in men than women; 2:1.
3   Usually open into ileum about 61 cm (2 ft) proximal to ileocecal valve.
4   Two complications: Inflammation and bleeding.

Significance

1   Not infrequently the mucosal lining is composed of misplaced ectopic linings such as gastric or pancreatic and this tends to ulcerate and bleed (haemorrhage).
2   It may become inflamed leading to intestinal obstruction, perforation and peritonitis.

Clinical Manifestations

1   Abdominal pain which is umbilical in location.
2   Possibly passage of blood in stools—not bright red or tarry but rather dark crimson.

Treatment

Similar to that for an appendectomy (p. 443).

Peritonitis

Peritonitis is an inflammation of the peritoneal cavity.

Aetiology

Peritonitis indicates damage of peritoneum by trauma (blunt or penetrating) of inflammatory or neoplastic disease. The point of origin may be the gastrointestinal tract, the ovaries, the uterus or extraperitoneal organs (i.e., inflammation of the kidney).

Primary Peritonitis—(acute, diffuse)

1   Occurs primarily in young females; often due to pathogenic bacteria (strep-tococci, pneumococci, gonococci) introduced through fallopian tubes or through haematogenous spread.
2   In patients with nephrosis or cirrhosis, the offending organism is most often *Escherichia coli*.

Secondary peritonitis

1   Commonly seen in surgical patient; caused by appendicitis, peptic ulceration, biliary tract disease and colonic inflammation.
2   May occur following gunshot wound, stab wounds and motor vehicle accidents.

Postoperative

1   Theoretically preventable.

2   Noted following poor preoperative preparation—inadequate nutrition, fluid and blood replacement, and technical problems.
3   May occur in patients who are diabetic, or have malignancy or are taking steroids.

Altered Physiology

1   Any irritant such as blood, bile or pancreatic enzymes causes an exudation of plasmalike, protein-rich fluid—'internal burn'.
2   Secondary peritonitis often presents a mixed flora which include *E. coli* as well as the enterococci, *Clostridia, Klebsiella, Pseudomonas*, and *Bacteroides*.
3   If there is failure to seal the source of contamination, i.e., perforation along gastrointestinal tract, peritonitis will become progressively worse.
4   When damaged, the surface of the peritoneal cavity begins to exude a plasmalike fluid. This process can account for losses of as much as 5 l/day.
5   Paralytic ileus is usual, with fluid loss into dilated intestinal loops and stomach.
6   Individual is shocked because of fluid loss, abdominal distension with respiratory embarrassment; nutrients are not absorbed, leading to progressive rapid catabolism.

Clinical Features and Initial Physical Assessment

Dependent upon location and extension of inflammation.

1   Initially local type of abdominal pain tends to become constant, diffuse and more intense.
2   Abdomen becomes extremely tender and muscles become rigid; rebound tenderness and ileus may be present; patient lies very still, usually with legs drawn up.
3   Often nausea and vomiting occur; peristalsis diminishes; anorexia is present.
4   Elevation of temperature and pulse as well as leucocyte count.
5   Fever and thirst occur.
6   Percussion—resonance and tympany due to paralytic ileus; loss of liver dullness may indicate free air in abdomen.
7   Auscultation—decreased bowel sounds.

Diagnosis

1   Blood studies—to show leucocytosis (leucopenia, if severe).
2   Urinalysis—may indicate urinary tract problems as primary source.
3   Peritoneal aspiration—to demonstrate blood, pus, bile, bacteria (Gram stain), amylase.
4   X-ray of abdomen—may indicate free air in abdomen under diaphragm; of thorax—to rule out unexpected pneumonia.

Objectives of Treatment and Nursing Management

To Prevent the Cause of Peritonitis

1   Encourage the individual who has early signs and symptoms of appendicitis to see his doctor.

2　Instruct patient to avoid taking a laxative or applying heat to abdomen when abdominal pain of unknown cause is experienced.
3　Practise meticulous aseptic technique during abdominal surgery.

To Monitor the Patient so that the Eventual Goal of Normal Haemoglobin and Oxygenation, Urine Output of 30–50 ml/hour, and Normal Vital Signs are Realized

1　Monitor for central venous pressure.
2　Record urinary output hourly.
3　Note and record blood pressure every other hour.
4　Check vital signs frequently.
5　Obtain baseline and take frequent analyses of haematocrit, blood gases and electrolytes.

To Remove Cause of the Infection

1　If localized:
　a. If acutely inflamed appendix—an appendectomy is called for.
　b. If ruptured duodenal ulcer—ulcer closed or plicated.
　c. Resection of diseased bowel; decompression (gastrostomy, colostomy, ileostomy).
2　If not localized, patient is acutely ill and surgery is not performed until after distension as well as electrolyte and fluid problems are treated.

To Combat Infection and Promote Patient Comfort

1　Give nothing by mouth—to reduce peristalsis; ensure meticulous oral hygiene.
2　Provide fluids by vein to establish adequate fluid level and to promote adequate urinary output.
3　Record accurately intake and output including the measurement of vomitus.
4　Administer antibiotics as prescribed.
5　Observe and describe symptoms accurately: pain and tenderness have a tendency to shift and must be reported precisely.
6　Reassure the patient and establish his confidence, because he usually realizes the seriousness of his condition.

To Promote Recovery and Reduce the Possibility of Complications

1　Following recovery from anaesthetic, place patient in upright position to facilitate drainage.
2　Administer fluids by vein, since nothing is given by mouth initially.
3　Prevent nausea, vomiting and distension by use of nasogastric suction; institute proper nursing measures for nasal and oral comfort.
4　Reduce parenteral fluids and give oral food and fluids when the following occur:
　a. Temperature and pulse rate come down.
　b. Abdomen becomes soft.
　c. Peristaltic sounds return (determined by abdominal auscultation).
　d. Flatus is passed and patient has bowel movements.
5　Be alert for possibility of complications. Report immediately.
　a. Burst abdomen—"It feels as it something just gave way."
　b. Abscess formation—an area of abdomen is tender or painful and fever increases.

Abdominal Hernia

A *hernia* is a protrusion of viscus through the wall of the cavity in which it is normally contained. It is often called a 'rupture'.

Incidence

1 Occurs three times more frequently in men than women; may occur at any age.
2 Results from congenital or acquired weakness of the abdominal wall.
3 Tends to increase in size and occurrence with increase in intra-abdominal pressure brought about by coughing, straining or pressure from a nearby tumour.

Classification

According to Area

1 Inguinal.
   a. In male—due to weakness in abdominal wall where spermatic cord emerges; enters inguinal canal and then scrotum.
   b. In female—due to weakness in abdominal wall where round ligament is located; enters inguinal canal and then labia.
(1) Direct inguinal.	(2) Indirect inguinal.
Medial-to-deep epigastric artery.	Lateral-to-deep epigastric artery.
Majority are acquired.	Majority are congenital.
2 Femoral.
   a. Occurs most often in women.
   b. Located below Poupart's ligament (below groin).
3 Umbilical.
   a. Results from failure of umbilical orifice to close.
   b. Occurs most often in obese women and children and in patients with cirrhosis and ascites.
4 Ventral or incisional.
   a. Due to weakness in abdominal wall.
   b. May occur following impaired healing of incision because of drainage, infection, etc.

According to Severity

1 Reducible—the protruding mass can be replaced in abdomen.
2 Irreducible—the protruding mass cannot be moved back into abdomen.
3 Incarcerated—an irreducible hernia in which the intestinal flow is completely obstructed.
4 Strangulated—an irreducible hernia in which the blood and intestinal flow are completely obstructed.
   Symptoms—pain, vomiting, swelling of hernial sac, fever, lower abdominal signs of peritoneal irritation.

Treatment

Mechanical (reducible hernia only).

A *truss* is an appliance having a pad that is held snugly in the hernial oriface.

1 Does not cure a hernia—it prevents abdominal contents from entering hernial sac.
2 May be used in treatment of hernia in adults when, because of disease or age, it is inadvisable to perform surgery. In general, surgical treatment is preferred.

Surgical

Recommended to correct the hernia before a strangulation occurs which then becomes an emergency situation.

1 Hernial sac, is dissected free.
2 Contents of sac are replaced in abdominal cavity.
3 Neck of sac is ligated.
4 Muscle and fascial layers are sewed together firmly to prevent a recurrence. If this is not possible, synthetic mesh may be sutured over area.
5 Strangulated hernia requires resection of ischaemic bowel in addition to hernia repair.

Nursing Management

Preoperative

1 If hernia is strangulated, emergency conditions prevail. (See p. 462), Intestinal Obstruction.)
2 If surgery is elective, patient is usually in good physical condition.
3 Shave suprapubic region and anterior surface of upper thigh.
4 Observe for upper respiratory infection—if present, surgery will be postponed because coughing or sneezing postoperatively may break the sutures.

Postoperative

1 Ambulate patient in a day or two.
2 Take following measures for scrotal oedema or swelling.
   a. Bed rest.
   b. Ice pack, scrotal suspensory for support.
3 Observe for urinary retention.

Patient Instruction

Athletics and extremes of exertion are not permitted for 8–12 weeks postoperatively.

Ulcerative Colitis

Ulcerative Colitis is an inflammatory disease of the mucosa and less frequently, the submucosa, of the colon and rectum. Occasionally it involves the distal ileum as well.

Aetiology and Incidence

1 Unknown (idiopathic); however, there are several unproven possibilities:
   a. Emotional response alters blood supply to colon mucosa which eventually causes ulceration.
   b. Unidentifiable organisms cause pathology.
   c. A combination of causative factors: infection, stress, allergy, autoimmunity.
2 Most common in young adulthood and middle life; almost equal between sexes (slightly more in females); more prevalent among Jews; highest among third and fourth decades, familial incidence.

Clinical Manifestations

1 Bloody diarrhoea, tenesmus (painful straining), sense of urgency and cramping.
2 Multiple crypt abscesses of intestinal mucosa that may become necrotic and lead to ulceration.
3 There often is weight loss, fever, dehydration, hypokalaemia, anorexia, nausea and vomiting, iron-deficiency anaemia and cachexia.

Clinical Features

1 Involvement extends proximally from rectum and is mainly of left colon.
2 The disease usually begins in the rectum and sigmoid and spreads upwards, eventually involving the entire colon.
3 There is a tendency for patient to experience remissions and exacerbations.
4 Very high frequency of secondary and often multiple colon cancer.
5 It is a serious disease accompanied by systemic complications (see below) and high mortality rate.

Diagnosis

1 Stool examination to rule out bacillary or ameobic dysentery.
2 Sigmoidoscopy; proctoscopy.
3 Barium enema x-ray.

NOTE: If disease is in acute stage, laxatives may be contraindicated because it may cause exacerbation and lead to toxic megacolon.

4 Review of nursing history for patterns of fatigue and overwork.
5 Assessment of behavioural manifestations indicative of emotional concerns.
6 Assessment of food habits that may have a bearing on triggering symptoms (milk intake may be a problem).
7 Careful clinical assessment to rule out diverticulitis, cancer, etc.

Complications

1 Skin ulcers.
2 Arthritis.
3 Malnutrition.
4 Anaemia.
5 Abscess formation.

6   Stricture, anal fistula.
7   Erythema nodosum.
8   Amyloidosis.
9   Electrolyte imbalance.
10 Malignancy (colonic cancer).

Objectives of Treatment and Nursing Management

NOTE: There is no cure for ulcerative colitis because the cause is unknown; the *chief objective* of treatment is to control the disease to achieve patient comfort and improve the quality of life.

This can be done by:

1   Initiating early, effective management of exacerbations.
2   Prolonging remissions with appropriate therapy.
3   Subjecting the patient to surgery only when judiciously necessary.

To Promote Rest and Relaxation of the Intestinal Tract

1   It may be necessary to reduce or eliminate food and fluid and then to resort to parenteral feeding or to low-residue diets.
2   Give sedatives and tranquillizers not only to provide general rest but also to allow peristalsis to slow down and afford rest to the inflamed bowel.
3   Be aware of the possibility of pressure sores in this patient because of malnourishment and enforced inactivity, especially if he is thin.
4   Administer tincture of belladonna, atropine or Lomotil, as prescribed to lessen intestinal motility. Antispasmodics, if prescribed, must be given with caution, since they may be instrumental in producing toxic megacolon.
5   Relieve painful rectal spasms (produced by frequent diarrhoeal stools) with anodyne suppositories.
6   Report any evidence of sudden abdominal distension, since it may indicate toxic megacolon.
7   Reduce physical activity to a minimum or provide frequent rest periods.
8   Provide commode or bathroom next to bed, since urgency of movements may be a problem.

To Combat Infection and Toxic State

1   Give sulpha drugs as prescribed: nonabsorbable sulphasalazine (Salazopyrin) may be prescribed as an oral medication.
2   Administer corticosteroids as prescribed: the type depends upon the condition of patient—mode of administration may be oral, intravenous or rectal. Rectal administration may be in the form of hydrocortisone-retention enemas (Predsol enemas)
3   For severe proctitis, nightly rectal instillations of steroids as prescribed (dissolved in tap water, or as suppositories) may produce a remission of symptoms.

To Meet Nutritional and Fluid Needs of the Body

1   If patient is acutely ill, maintain him on parenteral replacement of vitamins, fluids and electrolytes (potassium is very important).

Table 4.1. Diets Varying in Residue*

Foods	Residue-Restricted Diet	Moderate Residue Diet	Minimal Residue Diet
Milk†	Milk, buttermilk, yogurt, cream	Same	Same
Cheese	Cottage, cream,† Cheddar	Same	Cottage, cream only†
Fat	Butter, margarine	Same	Same
Eggs	Cooked, poached, scrambled in double boiler	Same	Same
Meat, fish, fowl	Tender chicken, fish, sweetbreads, ground beef and lamb	Same	Ground, tender meat; minced chicken and fish
Soups and broths	Broth, strained meat-base soups	Same	Broth only
Vegetables	Cooked vegetables: asparagus, peas, string beans, spinach, carrots, beets, potatoes—boiled, mashed, baked	Vegetable juice; vegetable purée, cooked asparagus tips, carrots, potatoes—boiled, mashed baked	Unseasoned vegetable juices in limited amounts†
Fruits	Fruit juices, cooked and canned fruits (without skins, seeds or fibre), bananas	Fruit juice, fruit purée, ripe bananas, cooked, peeled apples, apricots, peaches, pears, plums	Fruit juices preferably citrus in limited amounts†
Bread, cereals	Refined, enriched bread and cereals; macaroni, spaghetti, noodles, rice, crackers	Refined, enriched bread and cereals only, macaroni, spaghetti, noodles, rice, white crackers	As in moderately low residue
Desserts	Ices, ice creams,† junket,† cereal puddings,† custard,† gelatin, plain cake and biscuits; all without fruit and nuts	Same	Same
Beverages	Tea, coffee, carbonated beverages	Same	Tea, coffee as permitted
Condiments	Salt, moderate amounts of pepper, other mild spices, sugar	Salt and sugar	Salt and sugar

* From Mitchell, et al. (1976) Nutrition in Health and Disease, 16th edition, Philadelphia, J B Lippincott
† If tolerated.

2 Consider a milk-free diet, since studies have shown that fewer relapses occur on a milk-free diet; the incidence of lactase deficiency is more frequent in patients having attacks than in those in remission.
3 Provide a well-balanced, low-residue, high-protein diet to correct malnutrition (Table 4.1).
4 Determine which foods agree with this patient and which do not. Modify diet plan accordingly.
5 Bolster with supplemental vitamin therapy, including vitamin K.
6 Avoid cold fluids because they increase intestinal motility.
7 Administer proper electrolytes which have been lost in diarrhoeal bouts, especially potassium.
8 Administer dephenoxylate (Lomotil) as prescribed for symptomatic relief of diarrhoea.
9 Prohibit smoking because it also increases intestinal motility.

Nursing Alert: Since opiates may precipitate toxic megacolon, use only for brief periods, if at all, in acutely ill patients.

10 Administer blood transfusions and iron to correct existing anaemia.
11 Carefully note fluid intake and output and character of bowel movements.

To Cope With and Correct Psychological Disturbances

1 Offer psychological support
2 Educate the patient to accept and learn to live with this chronic disease. This is done on a long-range basis.
3 Recognize that psychotherapy during the acute phases of this illness may do more harm than good.
4 Indicate by actions and expressions that you, the nurse, are responsible for and care for him. Good nurse–patient relationship enables him to satisfy his dependency needs.
5 Solicit the assistance of the family in helping to understand the patient: assist the family in understanding the patient.
6 If patient is to have an ileostomy, before surgery it is helpful to have patient visited by someone who has had a similar operation and has made a good adjustment. After surgery, these persons can also help with management problems (Apply to the Ileostomy Association).

NOTE: It is not infrequent that impotence occurs in males after a colectomy because of damage to pudendal nerves.

To Prevent Complications

1 Observe for signs of colonic perforation and haemorrhage.
2 Assess carefully the behaviour of the patient and all his complaints.

Surgical Treatment and Nursing Management

Indications and Contemplated Surgery

1 Recommended when no improvement occurs through conservative means: evidenced by impending perforation, actual perforation, deteriorating clinical

course after 24–48 hours on maximum medical regime, severe haemorrhage or persistent colonic dilation for longer than 1 week.

2   Total proctocolectomy and permanent ileostomy recommended.

Preoperative Physical and Psychological Preparation

1   Institute an intensive programme of fluid, blood and protein replacement.
2   Administer chemotherapy and antibiotics to reduce intestinal organisms.
3   Recognize psychological needs of this patient:
   a. Fear, anxiety and discouragement accompany diarrhoea.
   b. Hypersensitivity may be evident.
   c. Let him know his complaints are understood.
4   Encourage patient to talk; listen to what he says is bothering him.
5   Answer his questions relative to the permanent ileostomy he is about to have.

Postoperative Care Including Ileostomy Management

See Management of Patient Undergoing Major Intestinal Surgery, p. 441.
See Conditions: Caring for a Patient with an Ileostomy, p. 456.

Health Teaching

1   It is important to involve the patient in understanding chronic ulcerative colitis and each component of care prescribed; he should be made to feel that he is sharing responsibility for maintaining his health.
2   This patient needs encouragement and support postoperatively even though surgery is considered curative; there may be problems with skin care; there may also be aesthetic difficulties, surgical revisions.
3   When early indications of relapse are noted, such as bleeding or increased diarrhoea, the patient should report these findings early so that steroid treatment may be initiated.
4   Monitoring of the patient's condition should continue when new symptoms suggest it or on a regular annual basis.
5   Let the patient know that he has a valuable resource person in the stoma therapy nurse and that he should not hesitate to call her about his ileostomy problems.

Crohn's Disease (Regional ileitus, Granulomatous colitis, Transmural colitis)

Crohn's disease is a chronic inflammatory disease of the small intestine usually affecting the terminal ileum at the region just before the ileum joins the colon. The aetiology is unknown.

Incidence

1   Affects both sexes equally.
2   Appears more often in Jewish persons of Eastern European origin.
3   A familial tendency exists.
4   May occur at any age, but occurs mostly between 15 and 35 years of age.

Clinical Features

1 Intestinal tissue thickens first by oedema and later by formation of scar tissue and granulomas.
2 At times, 'skip lesions' occur with normal intestine in-between.
3 This condition interferes with the ability of the intestine to transport the contents of upper intestine through the constricted lumen; this causes crampy pains after meals.
4 Inflammation and ulcers form in the lining membrane, producing a constant irritating discharge.
5 In some patients, the inflamed intestine may perforate and form intra-abdominal and anal abscesses.

Clinical Manifestations

These are characterized by exacerbations and remissions—may be abrupt or insidious:

1 Crampy pain after meals; this causes patient to eat in small amounts or to even avoid eating, which then results in malnutrition, weight loss and possibly anaemia (hypochromic or macrocytic).
2 Chronic diarrhoea due to irritating discharge may occur.
3 Milk products and chemically or mechanically irritating food may aggravate the problem.
4 Melaena and malabsorption syndrome may occur; occult blood may appear in stool.
5 Low-grade fever occurs if abscesses are present.
6 Lymphadenitis occurs in mesenteric nodes.
7 Abdominal tenderness, especially in right lower quadrant.

Clinical Complications

1 Stricture and fistulae formation (ischiorectal, perianal—even to bladder or vagina).
2 Mechanical intestinal obstruction.
3 Incidence of colorectal cancer is higher in these patients.

Clinical Evaluation

1 Regional ileitis may simulate acute appendicitis.
2 Upper gastrointestinal barium studies—classic 'string sign' is noted at terminal ileum that suggests a constriction of a segment of intestine.

Medical and Nursing Therapeutic Regime

Objectives

To promote patient comfort and maintain adequate hydration and nutrition.
To employ safeguards to prevent transmission of pathogenic organisms from one patient to another—conscientious hand washing as well as proper linen and equipment care.

To transmit feelings of understanding, concern and helpfulness to this patient who is often dejected, debilitated, embarrassed about frequent and offensive stools and even fearful of eating.

1 Administer a low-residue, bland, high-caloric diet with vitamin supplements to improve nutritional status.
2 Provide iron medications if anaemia is present.
3 Treat diarrhoea symptomatically.
4 Consider antibiotics and sulphonamides such as Sulphasalazine. Steroids for control of inflammatory process.
5 If patient does not respond to conservative medical and pharmacotherapy (sulpha drugs, steroids, azothioprine), surgery may be necessary.
6 Surgery is determined specifically for each patient. The involved segment may be resected with anastomosis. Bypass procedures may be done. Unfortunately, recurrence of the disease is possible following surgery.

Differences Between Crohn's Disease and Ulcerative Colitis

Table 4.2. Differences Between Crohn's Disease and Ulcerative Colitis

	Crohn's Disease	Ulcerative Colitis
Pathology		
Early	Transmural thickening	Mucosal ulceration
Later	Deep penetrating granulomas	Mucosal minute ulcerations
Clinical Manifestations		
Bleeding	Generally no, but may occur	Common
Perianal disease	Common	Rare
Fistula	Common	Rare
Perforation	Common	Rare
X-ray: Barium studies		
Stricture	Common	Rare
Distribution	Segmental	Continuous
Associated with malignancy	Not common	Common

Ileostomy

An *ileostomy* is an opening in the ileum for the purpose of treating intractable granulomatous or ulcerative colitis, of diverting intestinal contents in colon cancer, or acting as a conduit for ureteral drainage in patient with a nonfunctioning urinary bladder (ileal conduit). The opening (*stoma*) is brought out through the abdominal wall, usually the lower right section of the abdomen. This stoma becomes the outlet for discharge of intestinal contents.

Implications for the Patient

See also Colostomy for Pre- and Postoperative Nursing Management, pp. 468, 470

1   Some patients welcome the ileostomy, since it means the removal of a long-standing incapacitating disease process; in general, however, many patients experience psychological problems that are often overwhelming. Preoperative counselling by the medical and nursing team as well as by Ileostomy Association members is most helpful.

2   The patient appreciates that now he has the prospect of enjoying a normal diet, as against the low-residue diet to which he was restricted.

3   Patient wears a two-piece rubber or disposable soft vinyl pouch with an open-end bottom; a clamp fitted on the bottom of the bag permits emptying. He empties the bag 4–5 times a day, usually when he goes to the bathroom to urinate.

4   The patient with an ileostomy requires instruction—first from the nurse in the hospital, then from a stoma therapist, and finally from the health visitor or Ileostomy Association member.

5   Appliances are held in place in several ways—cement, double-faced adhesive discs, karaya rings.

6   Waterproof paper tape is effective in anchoring the appliance when the patient showers or swims.

7   At first the discharge will be liquid, but later the small intestine will begin to take on its water-absorbing function to permit a more semisolid, pasty discharge.

8   Because the discharge is rich in enzymes, it may cause skin irritation; therefore optimum skin care becomes a top priority consideration for the patient.

Discharge Planning and Health Teaching

1   Because an ileostomy can bleed easily, it should be cleansed gently.

2   Early in his experience, the patient may notice his new ileostomy may be noisy because of gas accumulations; as time goes on it becomes quieter.

3   Fluids are to be increased in warm weather months inasmuch as the colon is no longer functioning to conserve water and electrolytes.

4   The intake of too much salt is to be avoided, because salt increases ileal output.

5   Cellulose products such as peanuts are to be avoided, since their digestion depends upon colon bacteria. (Dietary considerations are similar to those suggested for patients with colostomy, p. 471.

6   Foods which seem to increase ileal output are prunes, dates, stewed apricots, strawberries, grapes, bananas, cabbage, beans and nuts. Avoid these foods.

7   For *food blockage*, an ileostomy lavage can be taken using a 120 ml (4 oz) syringe or funnel and tubing and injecting approximately 400 ml of saline every 10 min until relief is obtained. *This procedure is usually prescribed by a doctor and supervised.*

8   After 3 weeks—and later after 6 weeks—this person may have to be refitted for an appliance; the permanent appliance is fitted after 3 months. At all times, the faceplate opening should be approximately 0.15–0.3 cm (0.0625–0.125 in) larger than the stoma itself.

9   The problem of odour appears to be a personal problem; some patients have it, others do not. Utilize conscientious care in keeping body, clothing, and pouch clean. Observe that ingestion of certain foods is more likely to cause odours than other foods (beer and beans are chief offenders).

10   Swallowing air may produce gas, so the patient should be instructed to chew

food with a closed mouth, to eat leisurely and to avoid talking while eating; smoking and chewing gum often permit swallowing of air.

11 For men, a broad athletic support is an effective device worn under the trunks to keep ileostomy bag supported.

12 For women, a light pantygirdle over pantihose provides comfort and support; however, rigid stays in a girdle are to be avoided.

13 Whether the patient tells his friends that he has an ileostomy is a purely personal decision.

14 Karaya gum powder as well as skin shields, Stomahesive (Squibb) are effective agents in keeping the skin healthy (see p. 470).

GUIDELINES: Changing an Ileostomy Appliance

Purposes

1 To prevent leakage (bag is usually changed every 2–4 days).
2 To permit examination of skin around stoma.
3 To assist in controlling odour if this presents a problem.

Time

1 Early in morning before breakfast or 2–4 hours after a meal when the bowel is least active.
2 Immediately if patient is complaining of burning or itching underneath the disc or has pain around the stoma.

Equipment

Duplicate ileostomy appliance with belt.
Soap, water and washcloth
Karaya powder, karaya ring (self-adhering appliance); double-faced adhesive discs are best.
Gauze dressings
Paper bag for soiled dressings.

Procedure

Nursing Action	Reason
Preparatory Phase	
1 Have patient assume a relaxed position.	1 Encourage patient participation and understanding so that eventually he will be able to change appliance himself.
2 Explain details of this activity to patient.	
3 Expose ileostomy area; remove ileostomy belt.	
4 Position lamp; wash hands.	

Nursing Action	**Reason**

Performance Phase

1	Remove disc slowly from skin.	1	Solvent is not used, because it is damaging to skin.
2	Wash skin with warm water and soap using a soft washcloth. Observe stoma for its colour and condition.	2	Patient could take a shower or bath at this time. If stoma is discharging, cover with a dressing and plastic such as clingfoil; seal with Micropore tape.
3	Moisten a karaya gum washer; wait until it is tacky and then apply over the stoma.	3	Gum karaya protects the skin while permitting healing underneath.
4	If Stomahesive or Karaya gel are used, follow specific instructions in package insert. Be sure skin is thoroughly dry.	4	These are effective hypoallergenic skin barriers.
5	Apply adhesive disc on the faceplate of the pouch against washer; press firmly for a few minutes until adherence is assured.	5	Seal-tight adherence results only when both parts are tacky before being pressed together.
6	Check the pouch bottom for closure; use rubber band or clip provided.	6	Proper closure controls leakage.

Follow-up Phase

1	Dispose of waste materials.		
2	Clean ileostomy bag by washing in soap and water.	2	Preserve life of appliance and control odour.
3	Soak in deodorant solution; or rinse in solution of 60 ml (2 oz) distilled vinegar to 1 litre water.	3	Deodorizing agents should be effective but not destructive to rubber.

Diverticulosis and Diverticulitis

A *diverticulum* is a pouch or saccular dilatation leading out from a tube or main cavity (Fig. 4.13).

Diverticulitis is an inflammation of diverticula.

Diverticulosis is the condition in which an individual has multiple diverticula.

Predisposing Factors

1   Probable congenital predisposition.
2   Weakening and degeneration of muscular wall of the intestine causing herniation of the lining mucous membrane through a muscle at site of artery penetration.
3   Increased mechanical pressure due to abnormal high-pressure contractions of sigmoid colon in response to neurohumoral stimuli.
4   Chronic overdistension of the large bowel.

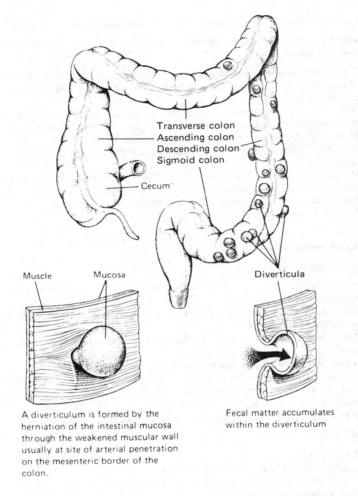

Transverse colon
Ascending colon
Descending colon
Sigmoid colon

Cecum

Muscle   Mucosa

Diverticula

A diverticulum is formed by the
herniation of the intestinal mucosa
through the weakened muscular wall
usually at site of arterial penetration
on the mesenteric border of the
colon.

Fecal matter accumulates
within the diverticulum

Figure 4.13.   Diverticula are most common in the sigmoid colon; they diminish in number and size as the colon approaches the caecum. Diverticula are rarely found in the rectum.

Incidence

1   Usually occurs in individuals over 40 years of age.
2   Diverticula of the large bowel occurs in 5–10% of adults; of these, one-third may experience diverticulitis. The condition is most common in sigmoid colon.
3   Small bowel diverticula are unusual but when they occur they are often multiple. They may act as areas of stasis and bacterial overgrowth, leading to malabsorption of fat and vitamin B_{12}.

Altered Physiology (colon diverticulosis and diverticulitis)

Constipation from spastic colon syndrome often precedes development of diverticulosis by many years.

1   Following local inflammation of the diverticula, there may be narrowing of the colon with fibrotic stricture, which then leads to cramps and increasing constipation.
2   With the development of granulation tissue, occult bleeding may occur, producing iron-deficiency anaemia; fatigue and weakness are then evident. However, massive bleeding is more common.
3   Abscess development causes a tender palpable mass; fever and leucocytosis also occur.
4   If the diverticulum perforates, local abscess or peritonitis results; peritonitis causes rigidity, abdominal pain, loss of bowel sounds and eventually shock.
5   Uninflamed or minimally inflamed diverticula may erode adjacent arterial branches, causing acute massive rectal bleeding.

Clinical Manifestations

General Clinical Signs

1   May occur in acute attacks or may persist as a long, drawn-out smouldering infection.
2   Tends to spread into surrounding bowel wall, increasing the irritability and spasticity of the colon.
3   When infections are severe, perforation of the colon can occur, leading to peritonitis.
4   When infection is less acute but slowly progressive, extensive scarring and abscess formation involving the bowel wall may occur, with the possibility of lower bowel obstruction. Sometimes, fistulae form with the bladder, the adjacent small bowel, the vagina or even the skin.
5   Sepsis may spread via portal vein to liver, causing liver abscesses.

Specific Clinical Signs

1   Diverticulosis:
    a. Bowel irregularity, constipation, and diarrhoea.
    b. Sudden massive haemorrhage (occurs in 10–20% of patients).
2   Milder forms of diverticulitis:
    a. Bouts of soreness, mild lower abdominal cramps.
    b. Bowel irregularity, constipation and diarrhoea.
3   Moderately severe acute diverticulitis:
    a. Crampy pain in lower left quadrant of abdomen.
    b. Low-grade fever, chills, leucocytosis.

Diagnosis

1   Sigmoidoscopy; possible colonoscopy.
2   Fluoroscopy and x-ray with barium enema.

Treatment and Nursing Management

Objective

To provide rest for the intestinal tract and to alleviate constipation.

1   During acute episode, maintain fluid and nutritional requirements with intra-venous therapy; give nothing by mouth.
2   Maintain antibiotic therapy as prescribed to reduce infection.
3   When indicated, employ stool softeners such as diocytl sodium sulphosuccinate (Normax).
4   Administer bulk additives to counteract tendency toward constipation; a frequently prescribed hydrophilic mucilloid smooth bulk laxative is psyllium (Metamucil).
5   Warm oil-retention enemas may be used to treat inflammation locally.

NOTE: In some patients, an increase in bulk results in an increase in symptoms.

6   Check with doctor as to type of diet to be followed. Some authorities prefer fibre-content in the diet rather than a low-residue diet. With increased fibre, more bulk is added to give the stool proper consistency. With a low-residue diet, the colon may work harder to propel contents, thereby producing high pressure on the intestinal wall, which in turn promotes diverticula formation.
7   *Surgical:*
   a. If there is little response to medical treatment, or if complications such as haemorrhage, obstruction or perforation occur, surgery is necessary.
   b. Preparation for surgery:
      (1) Low-residue diet or nothing by mouth.
      (2) Antibiotics, systemic and intestinal surface-acting, to reduce bowel bacterial flora, diminish bulk of stool and soften faecal mass for easier movement.
      (3) Cleansing enemas may be ordered.
   c. Resection of segment of intestine involved with diverticula, reuniting (anastomising) two ends to maintain continuity.
   d. Temporary colostomy is sometimes performed to divert faecal stream (see p. 468), with continuity restored in later second-stage procedure.

Health Teaching

Objective

To prevent recurrence of diverticular disease.

1   Maintain a diet that is high in soft residue and low in sugar; obtain lists of these foods in order to be familiar with proper dietary control; how well the intestinal tract functions in great measure depends upon proper food intake.
2   Bran products will add bulk to the stool and can be taken with milk or sprinkled over cereal.
3   Establish regular bowel habits to promote regular and complete evacuation; mineral oil can be used nightly if necessary, but dependence on it should be discouraged.

4   Have patient continue periodic medical supervision and follow-up; report problems and untoward symptoms.

Intestinal Obstruction

Intestinal obstruction is an interruption in the normal flow of intestinal contents along the intestinal tract.

The block may occur in the small or large intestine, may be complete or incomplete, may be mechanical or paralytic, and may or may not compromise the vascular supply. Obstruction most frequently occurs in the very young and the very old.

Treatment of Obstruction

1   Mechanical—a physical block to passage of intestinal contents without disturbing blood supply of bowel.
   a. Location:
      (1) Extrinsic, e.g., adhesions, hernia, intussusception.
      (2) Intrinsic, e.g., haematoma, tumour.
      (3) Intraluminal, e.g., foreign body, faecal or barium impaction, polyp.
      b. Clinical pattern:
         (1) High small-bowel (jejunal); 80% incidence.
         (2) Low small-bowel (ileal); 80% incidence.
         (3) Colonic: 20% incidence.
2   Paralytic (adynamic, neurogenic) ileus:
      Peristalsis is ineffective (diminished motor activity perhaps because of toxic or traumatic disturbance of the autonomic nervous system); there is no physical obstruction and no interrupted blood supply.
3   Strangulation:
      Obstruction also compromises blood supply, leading to gangrene of the intestine.

Causes

1   Mechanical (extramural):
   a. Adhesions—postoperative.
   b. Hernia.
   c. Malignancy.
   d. Volvulus (loop of intestine that has twisted).
2   Mechanical (intramural):
   a. Carcinoma.
   b. Haematoma.
   c. Intussusception (telescoping of intestine).
   d. Stricture or stenosis (scarring).
3   Paralytic:
   a. Spinal cord injuries, vertebral fractures.
   b. Postoperatively after any abdominal surgery.
   c. Peritonitis, pneumonia.
   d. Wound breakdown.
   e. Gastrointestinal tract surgery.

NOTE:
1 In postoperative patients, approximately 90% of mechanical obstructions are due to adhesions.
2 In nonsurgical patients, hernia (most often inguinal) is the most common cause of mechanical obstruction.

Altered Physiology

1 Disturbed physiological responses as a result of mechanical small-intestine obstruction results in increased peristalsis, distension by fluid and gas and increased bacterial growth proximal to obstruction. The intestine empties distally.
2 Increased secretions into the intestine are associated with diminution in the bowel's absorptive capacity.
3 The accumulation of gases, secretions, and oral intake above the obstruction causes increasing intraluminal pressure.
4 Venous pressure in the affected area increases, and circulatory stasis and oedema results.
5 Bowel necrosis may occur because of anoxia and compression of the terminal branches of the mesenteric artery.
6 Bacteria and toxins pass across the intestinal membranes into the abdominal cavity, thereby leading to peritonitis.
7 'Closed-loop' obstruction is a condition in which the intestinal segment is occluded at both ends, preventing either the downward passage or the regurgitation of intestinal contents.

Clinical Manifestations

Fever, peritoneal irritation, increased white blood cell count, toxicity and shock may develop with all types of intestinal obstruction.

1 Simple mechanical—high small bowel:
     Colic (cramps) mid to upper abdomen, some distension, early bilious vomiting, increased bowel sounds (high-pitched tinkling heard at brief intervals), minimal diffuse tenderness.
2 Simple mechanical—low small bowel:
     Significant colic (cramps) midabdominal, considerable distension, vomiting—slight or absent—later faecal, increased bowel sounds and 'rush' sounds, minimal diffuse tenderness.
3 Simple mechanical—colon:
     Cramps (mid-to-lower abdomen), later-appearing distension, then vomiting may develop (faecal), increase in bowel sounds, minimal diffuse tenderness.
4 Partial chronic mechanical obstruction—may occur with granulomatous bowel (Crohn's) disease:
     Symptoms are cramping abdominal pain, mild distension, and diarrhoea.
5 Strangulation:
     Symptoms are initially those of mechanical obstruction but later progress rapidly: Pain is severe, continuous and localized. There is moderate distension, persistent vomiting, usually decreased bowel sounds and marked localized tenderness. Stools or vomitus contain fresh or occult blood.

6   Paralytic ileus:
    Gaseous distension is prominent; abdomen is tense; pain is dull, continuous and diffuse; constipation is rarely complete, since small amounts of flatus may be passed; peristalsis is usually depressed, and bowel sounds are infrequent or absent; vomiting occurs only after eating (vomiting may later become faecal).

Nursing Alert: Because of loss of water, sodium and chlorides, signs of dehydration become evident: intense thirst, drowsiness, general malaise, aching; tongue becomes parched, face appears pinched, abdomen becomes distended. Shock may result (pulse increasingly rapid and weak, temperature and blood pressure lowered, skin pale, cold, clammy) ending in death.

Treatment and Nursing Management

Objective

To remove the obstruction, treat the fluid and electrolyte imbalance, relieve the distension, and prevent or detect early the complications of shock and peritonitis.

Initial Nursing Assessment and Care

1   Describe accurately the nature and location of the patient's pain, the presence of distension, the absence of flatus or defaecation. The overview of symptoms is important in differentiating intestinal obstruction from other more benign conditions.
2   Elderly patients with poor bowel tonus who often remain in the recumbent position for extended periods are likely to experience air-fluid lock syndrome, which is described below.
    a. Fluid collects in dependent bowel loops.
    b. Peristalsis is too weak to push fluid 'uphill'.
    c. Obstruction occurs primarily in the large bowel.
    d. Management consists simply of alternately turning the patient from supine to prone position every 10 min until enough flatus is passed to decompress the abdomen. A rectal tube may help.
3   Monitor and record vital signs (including blood pressure) every 4 hours.
4   Measure and record accurately all intake and output.
5   Save any stool that may be passed; this is to be tested for occult blood.
6   Anticipate doctor's request for urinalysis, haemoglobin determination and blood cell counts.
7   Frequently determine the patient's level of consciousness; decreasing responsiveness may offer a clue to an increasing electrolyte imbalance.
8   Institute long-tube decompression of intestine proximal to block.
9   Recognize the patient's concern and initiate measures to secure his cooperation and confidence in the staff; these measures include ascertaining his specific anxieties and providing him with therapeutic responses.
10 Compare the patient's state of orientation with his admission status; a lessening awareness of his environment may suggest his going into shock.
11 Minimize those factors that would enhance gastric secretions in order to prevent fluid loss (via nasogastric suction); avoid conversation about enticing meals and eliminate meals being served within his range of seeing or smelling.

12   Observe for evidence of postural hypotension as patient is moved from a semirecumbent position to an upright position; this may be suggestive of circulatory insufficiency.
13   Undertake measures to prepare the patient for surgery, since most problems of mechanical obstruction require surgical correction.

Medical, Surgical and Nursing Management

1   Relieve distension by introducing a long gastrointestinal tube by the Medical Officer (see p. 432); this can be passed more effectively with the patient lying on his right side; begin decompression to remove gas and fluid.
2   Correct fluid imbalance by initiating as directed by the Medical Officer.
     a. Na^+, K^+, plasma substitutes.
     b. Ringer's lactate to correct interstitial fluid deficit.
     c. Dextrose–water to correct intracellular fluid deficit.
3   Administer antibiotics (neomycin and kanamycin) and possibly a broad spectrum agent to lessen the possibility of infection, particularly peritonitis.
4   Recognize that giving an enema may distort an x-ray picture by introducing gas into the tract distal to the obstruction. An enema may make a partial obstruction worse, hence it is contraindicated.
5   Prevent infarction by carefully assessing status of patient; if pain increases in intensity, localizes or becomes continuous, it may herald strangulation.
6   Detect early signs of peritonitis, such as rigidity and tenderness, in an effort to minimize this complication.
7   Relieve obstruction by releasing, removing or repairing the cause of the obstruction; this is done surgically in most instances. Complete small bowel obstruction and colon obstruction requires an operation for relief. When tube suction therapy does not help after 12 hours, surgery is indicated.
     a. *Resection* of obstructing lesion and end-to-end anastomosis is done when no evidence of peritonitis and only minimal oedema exist; this requires a proximal colostomy to decompress new anastomosis.
     b. Resection of all necrotic intestine is necessary.
     c. A tube *enterostomy* may be done by introducing a catheter into distended bowel; the other end of catheter is brought out through the abdominal wall via a separate incision. This is a palliative measure.
     d. A *loop colostomy* is done when relief is sought by drawing a proximal loop or segment of colon up to the skin surface and opening it as a colostomy; the distal portion of colon is treated later.

Postoperative Nursing Care

1   To meet fluid, electrolyte and nutritional needs, administer prescribed amounts of fluids; keep accurate intake and output records.
2   For an enterostomy, connect tube to drainage bottle at side of bed; expect considerable amout of faecal drainage during the first 12–15 hours (500–1000 ml).
     a. Observe frequently the patency of drainage equipment.
     b. If there is difficulty with drainage, it may be necessary to inject 15 ml of warm saline into the enterostomy tube every 2–4 hours with approval of doctor.
     c. Protect skin around enterostomy tube with Stomahesive or karaya gel.

3   Follow additional postoperative care described on p. 441, Major Intestinal
Surgery.

Cancer of the Colon

Incidence

1   Males are affected slightly more often than females.
2   The highest incidence occurs in patients about 50 years old.
3   Five-year-survival is 40–50% (best of visceral cancers).

Aetiology

1   Familial polyposis (numerous pedunculated growths arising from mucosa and
extending into lumen of intestine).
2   Chronic ulcerative colitis—definite risk of colon cancer (up to 20% after 20 years
of age with active disease).
3   Diverticulosis and cancer may be found together and simulate each other—no
definite evidence that the presence of diverticula is significant in the development
of cancer.
4   Cancer of the colon occurs much more frequently in developed countries and
rarely in underdeveloped countries. The increased incidence of colon cancer in
developed countries is probably related to the relatively lower fibre content of
diet in these areas.
5   Unabsorbable fibre deficit appears to be related to intestinal transit time, stool
bulk and consistency.
6   The effect of diet on the colon bacterial flora is a factor possibly contributing to
cancer.

Clinical Manifestations

1   Distribution of cancer in the colon is shown in Fig. 4.14.
2   Most common symptoms:
   a. Blood in stools (usually occult)—causing anaemia.
   b. Partial obstruction—causing constipation alternating with diarrhoea, lower
abdominal pains (crampy), distension.
   c. Additional signs—progressive weakness, anorexia, weight loss, shortness of
breath, anginal pain, anaemia.

Diagnosis

1   Digital rectal examination—half of all colon and rectal cancers are found this
way.
2   Endoscopy (proctosigmoidoscopy/colonoscopy)—two thirds of all colon and
rectal cancer can be seen and biopsied via proctoscope alone.
3   Stool examination for blood—often reveals evidence of carcinoma when the
patient is otherwise asymptomatic.
4   Blood-haemoglobin determination for anaemia.
5   Barium enema—especially significant in unexplained abdominal mass.
   Napkin-ring-type outline clearly indicates obstruction and possible tumour.

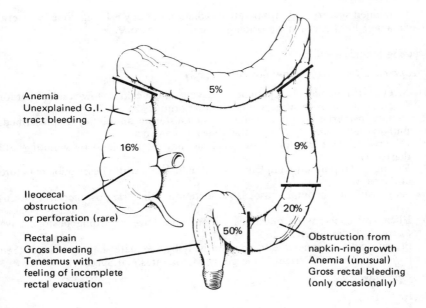

Anemia
Unexplained G.I.
tract bleeding

5%

16%

9%

Ileocecal
obstruction
or perforation (rare)

Rectal pain
Gross bleeding
Tenesmus with
feeling of incomplete
rectal evacuation

50%

20%

Obstruction from
napkin-ring growth
Anemia (unusual)
Gross rectal bleeding
(only occasionally)

Figure 4.14.   Distribution of cancer in the colon.

6   Silicone foam enema—expelled silicone cast may show indentations suggestive of cancer of polyps.
7   Intravenous pyelography (urography) and possible cystoscopy may be indicated to assess whether malignancy has spread locally to involve ureter or bladder.

Treatment

Diagnosis Confirmed By

1   Removing rectosigmoid polyps through sigmoidoscope for histologic study.
2   Removing polyps above rectosigmoid by colonoscopy or laparotomy (if other symptoms are present) to verify diagnosis.

Surgical Therapeutic Plan

1   Recommend total colectomy for patient with familial history of polyposis or prolonged, universal, chronically active colitis, even before cancer is confirmed.
2   Most common operative procedures:
    a. Wide segmental resection of colon and mesentery with anastomosis, or
    b. Abdominoperineal resection with colostomy (if lesion is in rectum).
    c. Even more extensive surgery involving removal of other organs if cancer has spread—such as to the bladder, uterus, small intestine, groin, etc.
    d. If cancer is extensive and it may not be in the patient's best interest to do radical surgery, palliative treatment may be done using radon seed implantation

(combined surgery and preoperative radiation therapy is being done in several areas) or local excision via colonoscope or proctoscope.

Nursing Management

Preoperative Care (colostomy not anticipated)

1   Meet nutritional needs of patient by serving a high caloric, low-residue diet for several days prior to surgery if condition permits.
2   Reduce bacterial count of colon by administering antibiotics as prescribed: phthalylsulphathiazole (Sulphathalidine), kanamycin.
3   Observe and record fluid losses such as may be sustained by vomiting and diarrhoea.
4   Record and report any complaints of abdominal pain with a description of nature and location.
5   Assist with and maintain nasogastric suction to minimize postoperative distension.
6   Elicit any concerns or questions patient may have regarding postoperative discomfort, dependency, etc.
7   Prepare patient immediately preoperatively by adequate shaving of area. (See p. 441 for Care of Patient Undergoing Major Intestinal Surgery).

Postoperative Care

See p. 441.

Colostomy

A *colostomy* is a temporary or permanent opening of the colon through the abdominal wall (an abdominal anus). Placement of colostomy will influence the nature of the discharge (Fig. 4.15). The *stoma* is that part of the colon that is brought above the abdominal wall in a colostomy.

Purposes

1   It may be part of an abdominoperineal resection for cure or palliation of cancer.
2   It may be palliative when unresectable malignancy is present.
3   It can be a temporary measure to protect an anastomosis.
4   It may be temporary to divert faecal stream during radiation or other therapy.

Nursing Management

Preoperative Care

1   Determine the nature of anticipated surgery; the colostomy must be positioned where the patient can see and care for it (this is determined by the surgeon).
    a. The colostomy should not be placed in the laparotomy incision.
    b. It should be placed where it will not interfere with proper fitting and comfortable wearing of an appliance—away from iliac crest, costal margin, umbilicus, scars, deep folds.
    c. It is preferable to leave the anal sphincter intact, if possible.

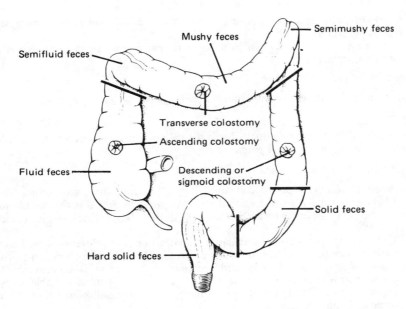

Semimushy feces

Mushy feces

Semifluid feces

Transverse colostomy

Ascending colostomy

Fluid feces

Descending or sigmoid colostomy

Solid feces

Hard solid feces

Figure 4.15.   A diagrammatic representation of the placement of permanent colostomies and the nature of the discharge at these sites.

    d. Apply several types of skin adhesives or cement to the abdomen to determine possible contact allergy.
    e. If possible, show patient the intended appliance and have him try it on.
2 Make specific plans for the patient's understanding and acceptance of a colostomy.
    a. Collaborate with the surgeon in ascertaining the nature of communication and information exchanged between surgeon and patient, including initial patient contact, in-hospital experience, plans for rehabilitation.
    b. Reinforce the patient's hope for a future that will be manageable and will lead to independent functioning.
    c. Develop with the stoma therapist a plan to include short- and long-term goals for the patient.
    Provide the patient with literature and information according to his level of understanding.
3 Preparation for surgery—follow usual preoperative procedures and modify to meet individual needs.
    a. Follow low-residue diet to limited liquids to nothing by mouth in the prescribed time frame.
    b. Administer antibiotic agents (neomycin, kanamycin) for bowel disinfection to reduce pathogenic bacterial flora.
    c. Give enemas for mechanical cleansing of intestinal tract.

d. Maintain hydration by assisting with intravenous infusion and observing and recording urinary output.

e. Prepare patient and assist in nasogastric intubation for decompression of intestinal tract.

Postoperative Care

Also see p. 441 and below, and Health Teaching (below).

Objective

To educate the patient to gradually learn the care of his colostomy and to carry on with diminishing professional guidance.

Initial Care of the Colostomy

1   Apply a temporary plastic colostomy bag to control odours and soiling.
2   Begin to irrigate when the immediate postoperative period is past and bowel function has resumed (usually fifth or sixth day) (see Guidelines, p. 472), if required.
3   Utilize the treatment time of irrigating the colostomy as the learning time for the patient to begin to master the art of controlling his colostomy independently.
4   Although irrigation is widely used, recognize that there are some persons who cannot control the colostomy this way, i.e., the patient with an 'irritable' colon, excess gas or unpredictable bowel movements. He will use a dressing or disposable bag.
5   Often the recognition of a bowel movement is when the patient's bag or dressing is checked; for others, it may be the awareness of the escape of flatus or the contact of stool on the skin.
6   For some there is an awareness of motility which enables them to get to the bathroom in time for discharging stool into the toilet.
7   Frequency and number of movements vary from person to person.
8   Irrigations for most persons are done every other day.
9   The cone-tip (Hollister) is excellent to prevent insertion of a catheter into insensitive mucosa with risk of perforating the bowel wall. The cone-tip is plugged into the stoma for about 2.5 cm and permits irrigation without perforation or leakage.
10   Regulation is enhanced when there is systematic planning: balanced meals eaten at regular intervals; a regular time for irrigation and evacuation.

Discharge Planning/Health Teaching

Irrigation of Colostomy (see p. 472).

Skin Care

1   Effective skin barriers are karaya gum or tincture of benzoin. Karaya is available in powder form or discs that can be shaped into rings for individual stomas; this can be placed on excoriated peristomal skin (i.e., new skin can grow under it).
2   Hypoallergenic skin shield is Stomahesive (Squibb), which tends to deteriorate less quickly than the karaya washers and often can be worn in areas where there are creases and wrinkles.

Stomahesive can be used as a 3″ × 4″ sheet or can be cut into washer size. The side of the Stomahesive shield that is attached to the waste-collecting bag is not sticky and therefore must be attached to the faceplate with an adhesive.

NOTE: Stomahesive is unsuitable for draining wet skin.

3   Coverings over the stoma may be disposable pouch, gauze, clingfoil or wax paper over a dressing. Adhesive tape may be used.
4   For peristomal excoriation, corticosteroid aerosol sprays or creams are useful when used sparingly.
5   For allergic reactions, try other products until a compatible one is found; antacid suspensions are found practical for some patients.

Odour Control

1   Avoid foods known to cause odours—for example, onions, members of the cabbage family, eggs, fish and beans.
2   Note that faecal odours are lessened with yogurt and buttermilk.
3   Odours can be controlled by taking one or two tablets of bismuth bicarbonate or Celevac or charcoal biscuits at mealtimes and bedtime.

Control of Gas

1   Most gas is due to swallowed air (often taken in while chewing gum) or beer, highly spiced foods and carbonated beverages.
2   Avoid gas-forming foods: beans, cabbage family, onions, radishes, cucumbers, fish and highly seasoned foods.

Diet

1   Avoid overeating and eating irregularly; chew food well.
2   Individualize the diet so that it is balanced and will not cause diarrhoea and constipation. A daily diary is effective in determining what foods cause difficulty and can then be eliminated from the diet.
3   Note that fruits, fruit juices and tomatoes may cause frequent bowel movements. Beer may be a laxative as well as a gas-producer.

Enhanced Daily Living

1   Approximately 10–12% of male ostomates suffer impairment of sexual function and potency; fortunately, this impairment is temporary in most cases. Male colostomates vary in degree of potency from full potency to complete impotence. Some patients take up to 2 years to regain potency.
2   An ostomy in a woman does not preclude a successful pregnancy; close medical care is required.
3   There is no contraindication to any form of travel, including horseback riding.
4   Participation in any type of sport is possible.
5   Showering is possible; remove appliance, cleanse with soap and water, and apply dressings after bathing. Sterile technique is unnecessary.
6   Girdles, swim trunks and pantihose may all be worn, provided there is no discomfort or too much constriction.
7   Promote patient's acceptance of the colostomy by building up self-esteem; encourage the family to assist the patient during the period of adjustment.

8   Contact the health visitor who will serve as a liaison between hospital, doctor and home as a follow-up while the patient continues to adjust to the colostomy at home.
9   Inform the patient of ostomy clubs and enroll him in the local group so that he may obtain information and exchange ideas with other ostomates.
10 Provide the patient with literature, addresses, and phone numbers of local organizations.

Pertinent References

1   For the patient:
    a. Colostomy Welfare Group, 38 Ecclestone Square, London SW1 1PB.
    b. Ileostomy Association of Great Britain, 1st Floor, 23 Winchester Road, Basingstoke, Hants RG21 1VE.

GUIDELINES: Irrigating a Colostomy

Purposes

1   To empty the colon of its contents: faecal, gas, mucus.
2   To cleanse the lower intestinal tract.
3   To establish a regular pattern of evacuation so that normal life activities may be pursued.
4   To prevent intestinal obstruction.
5   To prevent skin excoriation due to irritating faecal contents.

Equipment

1   Reservoir for irrigating fluids: enema bag, irrigating can, large bulb syringe.
2   Irrigating fluid: tap water or warm saline—4 ml of salt to 500 ml of water (1 tablet salt to 1 pint water); total solution—1000–2000 ml at 40.5°C (105°F).
3   Tubing, connecting tubes and clamp: rubber or plastic tubing; preferable clamp—one that can be opened with one hand.
4   Irrigating tip: soft rubber catheter—No. 22 or No. 24 with or without wide-cone irrigating tip.
5   Irrigating bag or kidney dish: self-adhesive (adhering) or held in place with a belt. (A plastic or rubber sheet can be used as a trough in place of bag or kidney dish.
6   Newspaper or plastic bag: to collect soiled dressings and disposable bag.
7   Petroleum jelly and toilet tissues.
8   Elastic belt to hold bag or dressings in place.

Procedure

Preparatory Phase

1   Select a suitable time, preferably after a meal, so that this hour fits into patient's posthospital pattern of activity.
2   Hang irrigating reservoir with solution 45–50 cm (18–20 in) above stoma.
3   Have patient sit in front of toilet commode or side of bed.
4   Remove soiled dressings and place in bag.

Nursing Action	Reason

Irrigation

1 Apply irrigating vessel to stoma.

2 Attach tubing to bag and irrigating tip; allow some of solution to flow through catheter.

3 Insert catheter gently about 10–15 cm (4–6 in); move it in and out a number of times while solution slowly flows.

1 Unnecessary; however, if available, it helps to control odour and splashing.

2 By releasing air bubbles in the set-up, air is not introduced into the colon to cause crampy pain.

3 This cleanses and clears terminal end of colon up to 15 cm (4 in). Solution flowing slowly helps to relax bowel and facilitates passage of tube.

Nursing Alert: Finger dilatation of any stoma is not advised (it may be done by the doctor on rare occasion). Dilatation may cause tearing of mucosa and skin leading to infection, fibrosis and stricture formation.

4 Allow fluid to enter colon; if cramping occurs, clamp off tubing and allow patient to rest before progressing.

5 Remove catheter when the patient has taken as much solution as possible—about 5–10 min.

6 Allow faecal material to flow into toilet; most of faecal material will be expelled in 15–20 min.

7 If available, apply sealable type bag to permit his moving about.

8 If fluid is not evacuated, siphon off.

4 Painful cramps are usually caused by too rapid flow or two much solution.

6 Gravity and peristaltic action will promote expulsion in about 20 min; however, it may require longer time.

Follow-up Phase

1 Cleanse area with mild soap and water; pat dry.

2 Replace colostomy dressing or pouch; karaya powder or karaya ring may be used.

3 Clean equipment with soap and water; dry before being stored in well-ventilated area.

1 Cleanliness and dryness will provide patient with hours of comfort.

2 This will protect skin from irritation.

3 This will control odour and prolong life of equipment.

ANORECTAL CONDITIONS AND TREATMENTS

Perianal Abscess; Fistula in Ano; Fissure in Ano

Condition	Description	Treatment
Perianal abscess	Localized infection in fatty tissue near rectum.	Incision and drainage (see Nursing Management, p. 476).

Condition	Description	Treatment
	Condition should raise suspicion of granulomatous bowel disease.	
Fistula in Ano	Abnormal opening from the skin near the anus that winds tortuously into the anal canal. Because it is an infectious area, pus leaks outward. Condition should raise suspicion of granulomatous bowel disease.	1. Surgical identification of the path of a fistula. 2. Cutting fistula open followed by insertion of packing (see Nursing Management, p. 476).
Fissure in Ano	Longitudinal ulcer (a crack that does not heal in the anal canal) frequently associated with constipation, as well as excruciating pain and blood streaking on defaecation.	1. Dilation of anal sphincter. 2. Excision of fissure (see Nursing Management, p. 476).

Haemorrhoids

Haemorrhoids are varicose veins of the anal canal; *external* haemorrhoids appear outside the external sphincter, whereas *internal* haemorrhoids appear above the internal sphincter. When blood within the haemorrhoids becomes clotted and infected, the haemorrhoids are referred to as *thrombosed*.

Predisposing Factors

1 Pregnancy
2 Straining at stool
3 Chronic constipation
4 Prolonged sitting
5 Anal infection
6 Hereditary factor
7 Portal hypertension (cirrhosis)

Clinical Manifestations

1 Pruritus (itching)
2 Protrusion
3 Constipation
4 Bleeding during defaecation
5 Infection or ulceration
6 Pain noted more in external haemorrhoids.

Diagnostic Evaluation

1   History and visualization by external examination and the use of an anoscope or proctoscope.
2   Barium enema also should be performed, since haemorrhoids are often warning signs of more serious colonic lesions, which may be the actual source of observed rectal bleeding

Treatment

Medical

1   Patient should adhere to a low-roughage, high fibre diet to keep stool soft. Some authorities suggest a diet that includes 30 g miller's bran per day or replacing white bread with whole wheat.
2   Bowel habits should be regulated with nonirritating laxatives (e.g., mineral oil or milk of magnesia) to keep stools soft.
3   Frequent hot salt baths.
4   Insertion of soothing anal suppository 2–3 times daily.
5   Application of witch hazel compresses for comfort.
6   Control of itching by placement of a cotton pledget on folded soft tissue between the buttocks against the anus to absorb moisture.
7   Do not use topical anaesthetics chronically on haemorrhoids or fissures as they often produce hypersensitivity (allergic) perianal skin rashes with severe itching.
8   If haemorrhoids are prolapsed and the patient is unable to reduce them himself, the nurse may have to reduce them manually:
    a. Apply cold compresses to anal area.
    b. Gently apply anaesthetic ointment with a gloved finger.
    c. Very gently manipulate haemorrhoids back through rectal sphincter.
    d. Apply an anaesthetic ointment on a dressing to rectal area.
9   Surgery may be indicated when the following conditions exist:
    a. Prolonged bleeding
    b. Disabling pain
    c. Intolerable itching
    d. General unrelieved discomfort.

Surgical

1   Incision and removal of clot from acutely thrombosed haemorrhoid.
2   Excision of haemorrhoids includes the following procedures:
    a. Dilatation of rectal sphincter.
    b. Ligation and excision of haemorrhoid under local or spinal anaesthesia.
    c. Insertion of drainage tube to permit escape of flatus and blood.
3   Alternate technique—injection of haemorrhoids with a sclerosing agent.
    a. This technique is especially indicated for a nonprolapsed internal haemorrhoid that bleeds following each bowel movement.
    b. The patient should report any evidence of bleeding following injection therapy; electrocoagulation may be necessary.
4   Dilatation—forced dilatation of the anal canal and lower rectum under general anaesthesia is another advocated treatment.

This procedure is not advocated for patients whose main complaints are prolapse or incontinence. It also is not recommended for ageing patients with weak sphincters.

5   Cryodestruction—freezing of haemorrhoids.

It is claimed to be painless; some patients have a foul-smelling discharge for about a week following cryosurgery.

Pilonidal Sinus

A *pilonidal sinus* is a congenital sinus located in the intergluteal cleft on the posterior surface of the lower sacrum; hair frequently protrudes from the sinus openings giving its name—pilonidal (a nest of hair).

Clinical Manifestations

1   Rarely produces symptoms until early adult life when infection produces drainage followed by the development of an abscess.
2   Trauma may be a factor in sinus development.

Treatment

1   Antibiotics are administered.
2   When abscess develops, incision and drainage is indicated.
3   Radical dissection indicated when abscesses recur or secondary sinus infection develops.
4   Healing takes place by granulation, since defect may be too large to heal with suturing.

Nursing Objectives and Management in Caring for Patients with Rectal Problems

Preoperative Care

To Recognize the Psychosocial Concerns of the Patient with a Rectal Problem

1   Be an understanding and concerned listener when this patient relates problems of a personal nature.
2   Ensure and respect his privacy when attending to personal hygiene, examinations and treatments.
3   Do not minimize complaints of discomfort.

To Assess Nature of the Rectal Problems in Order to Assist Doctor in Approaching an Accurate Diagnosis

1   Observe the stool for evidence of bleeding. Is stool mixed or coated with blood?
2   Determine presence of pain during and after evacuation. Is there associated abdominal pain? How long does it last?
3   Describe the problem in the patient's words when recording.
4   Note presence of a discharge. Is it purulent, bloody?

Postoperative Care

To Promote Comfort of Patient and Healing of Wound

1   Be gentle in changing dressings, shaving, irrigating or administering perineal care.
2   Use tullegras in protecting edges of wounds (e.g. following incision and drainage of ischiorectal abscess, excision of pilonidal sinus) to prevent crusting and the dressings from sticking to wound.
3   Provide salt baths when recommended; adjust temperature and provide a comfortable position for the patient.
4   Use caution in applying analgesic or anaesthetic ointments since this often leads to secondary skin rashes from allergy.
5   Keep the perineal area clean to minimize or eliminate infection; presence of *E. coli* demands meticulous cleanliness to prevent infection and promote healing.
6   Change patient's position from side to side to prevent added discomfort of pressure area; use a sorboring.
7   Prevent constipation by proper attention to diet needs of patient, give mild laxative only as prescribed.
8   Encourage voluntary micturition to avoid catheterization; this may be facilitated by getting patient out of bed.
9   Observe vital signs and dressings for evidence of haemorrhage, particularly following haemorrhoidectomy.
10 Daily rectal sphincter dilatation may be needed to relieve pain from spasm, to assure granulation of incisional wounds from bottom out and to prevent postoperative stricture.

Health Teaching

To prepare patient for convalescence.

1   Instruct patient on perianal hygiene to minimize the possibility of infection; avoid rubbing area with toilet tissue; instead, pat the area dry.
2   Apply wet dressings (equal parts of witch hazel and water) to relieve oedema.
3   Advise patient regarding the effect of diet on stool formation; plant fibres of leafy vegetables and the roughage of bran flakes, whole grains and whole wheat bread add roughage to the diet to form cellulose. Cellulose absorbs water, swells and softens stool, thereby stimulating peristalsis and aiding in intestinal elimination. Encourage patient to eat fresh fruits, fruit juice and fresh vegetables except for seeds, skins, corn and nuts.
4   Avoid laxatives so that stool is formed rather than being soft or liquid.
5   Recommend hot salt baths or hot compresses to relieve painful sphincter spasm.
6   Suggest adequate fluid intake and daily exercise to prevent constipation; encourage patient to have a regular time each day for having a bowel movement.
7   Stool softeners are often given until good bowel habits are established.
    a. 'Wetting agents' contain dioctyl sodium sulphosuccinate (Normax), a substance that penetrates, moistens and softens hard dry stool.
    b. 'Bulk producers' such as psyllium (Metamucil) and agar preparation absorb water, add bulk and add moisture to stool.
    c. Mineral oil tends to destroy oil-soluble vitamins A, D, E and K and intereferes

with absorption of calcium and phosphorus. It should be given at least 3 hours after the evening meal. (Do not give mineral oil to elderly patients because of aspiration pneumonia.)

8   Administer enemas only when absolutely necessary; rectal suppositories may be helpful.

GUIDELINES: Removal of Faecal Impaction

A *faecal impaction* is the retention of hardened faeces in the rectum or lower sigmoid.

Manifestations and Occurrence

1   The patient may say he is constipated; often he has a desire to defaecate but is unable to do so.
2   Diarrhoea or liquid faecal seepage may occur around the obstructing impaction.
3   The patient may complain of rectal pain.
4   This condition may occur in elderly persons following chronic constipation, insufficient hydration or ingestion of fibrous foods.
5   Orthopaedic patients who have been in traction or in body casts may develop an impaction.
6   Occasionally, impaction occurs in patients following rectal surgery or when barium has not been adequately removed following radiologic examination.
7   Impaction is also common in patients with neurologic or psychotic disorders.

Purpose of Faecal Disempaction

To remove hardened faeces in the rectum or lower sigmoid.

Equipment

Clean (not necessarily sterile) rubber or plastic glove
Water-soluble lubricant
Bedpan
Plastic or rubber sheet with cloth protection
Soap, water, washcloth

Procedure

Nursing Action	Reason
Preparatory Phase	
1 Explain procedure to patient.	
2 Position patient on left side with upper knee flexed.	2 To permit access to rectum and lower sigmoid.
3 Drape patient and place protecting pad under buttocks.	3 To prevent chilling and undue exposure.
4 Place bedpan in a convenient place.	4 To serve as receptacle.
5 Put on glove and lubricate index finger generously (some prefer the middle finger because it is longer).	

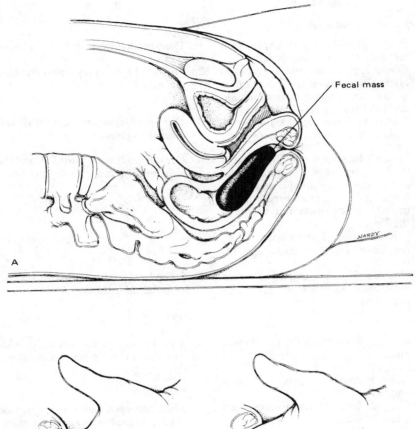

Fecal mass

A

B

C

Figure 4.16. Faecal impaction. a. Note shaded areas inside rectal sphincter—this indicates faecal impaction. b. By gently stimulating the rectal wall with a gloved index finger and using a circular motion, it is possible to loosen faecal material. c. It may be necessary to gently insert two fingers in an attempt to crush the faecal mass. A scissor-like motion is used.

Nursing Action	**Reason**

Performance Phase (Fig. 4.16)

1   Insert gloved finger *gently* into rectum until impaction is felt.

1   This stimulation may increase peristalsis.

2   *Gently* remove or break faecal material within reach and deposit in bedpan; work finger around and into mass to break it up if possible.

2   The emphasis is on *gentleness*, since this may be painful.

3   Gently stimulate rectal sphincter by making a circular motion once or twice.

3   This may stimulate peristalsis and relax the sphincter.

4   If step 3 does not result in removal of the impaction, it may be necessary to *gently* insert the middle and index finger and attempt to break up the mass by a scissorlike movement of the fingers.

Repeat steps 2 or 4 until all easily reachable faecal masses are removed.

4   Greater leverage is afforded, and the mass may be more easily broken.

5   Note any bleeding or pain; observe patient for shortness of breath or perspiration.

5   Should any of these responses occur, stop the procedure.

Follow-up Phase

1   Gently wash and dry the rectal area; make the patient comfortable and have him rest.

1   Drying the area prevents skin excoriation and promotes comfort.

2   Note bedpan contents and then empty.

3   Record colour, consistency and odour of stool.

3   These characteristics may provide clues as to the nature of the problem.

4   Plan health instruction measures in an effort to prevent a recurrence.

Explore nutritional and fluid needs of the patient; determine activity level and encourage suitable exercises to promote adequate elimination.

4   Investigate the possibility of using stool softeners; suggest periodic use of an enema.

3. Conditions of the Hepatic and Biliary System

MANIFESTATIONS OF DISORDERS OF THE LIVER

Jaundice (Icterus)

The condition of the body when all tissues including the sclerae and skin assume a yellow or greenish-yellow tinge due to an increased concentration of bilirubin. (See p. 483 for types of jaundice.)

1 Normal bilirubin concentration in blood 3–17 μmol/l (0.2–1.0 mg/100 ml) of blood.
2 Over 50 μmol/l (3.0 mg/100 ml) of blood, jaundice can be detected.

Abnormal Bleeding Tendencies

1 Because of blood coagulation defects, gastrointestinal haemorrhage may occur as well as bleeding gums, blood in urine, rectal bleeding, tarry stool.
2 Minor skin trauma may produce ecchymosis (black and blue marks).
3 Following all types of intramuscular and intravenous injections, it is necessary to apply pressure for longer than usual and to observe for haematoma.

Excessive Water Retention, Oedema and Ascites

1 Tissue oedema and intra-abdominal fluid are manifestations of intense sodium and water retention combined with potassium excretion.
2 Hypoalbuminaemia, iron-decreased hepatic synthesis and disturbed kidney function are also instrumental in causing fluid retention.

Impairment of Central and Peripheral Nervous System

1 Pyridoxine deficiency can result in nervous irritability and in convulsive seizures in children.
2 Thiamine deficiency may lead to polyneuritis and Wernicke–Korsakoff psychosis.
3 Stupor, somnolence and confusion from failure to metabolize ammonia arriving from intestine in portal venous system, and from impaired metabolism of sedative drugs.

DIAGNOSIS OF LIVER DISEASE

GUIDELINES: Assisting with Liver Biopsy

Liver biopsy is the sampling of liver tissue by needle aspiration.

Purpose

To establish a diagnosis of liver disease by histological study of liver tissue.

Equipment

Sterile aspiration syringe and biopsy needle (Silverman)
Local anaesthetic
Skin antiseptics, sterile towel, gloves
Glass slides, specimen bottles containing fixative and/or test tubes

Procedure

Preparatory Phase

1 Verify that the patient has had prothrombin tests and blood typing by checking the chart.
2 Determine availability of compatible blood inasmuch as these patients often have clotting defects (i.e. blood grouping and cross matching).
3 Determine and record patient's pulse, respiration, arterial pressure and prothrombin time immediately before the biopsy in order to have a base line of comparison with the postbiopsy condition of the patient.
4 Explain the steps of this procedure to the patient to reduce his concerns and gain his co-operation.

Nursing Action	**Reason**
Performance Phase	
1 Place patient flat in bed with arm under head and face turned left.	
2 Expose the upper abdomen in readiness for skin disinfection and local anaesthetic injection.	2 For optimum exposure and comfort of patient the right hypochondriac region is treated as a surgical area to minimize danger of infection.
3 Determine biopsy site—one interspace below upper border of liver dullness 2 cm behind anterior axillary line.	
4 Doctor anaesthetizes the skin, intercostal tissues and liver capsule with local anaesthetic.	4 To promote local comfort.
5 Doctor introduces biopsy needle into intercostal tissues but not into liver.	5 To prevent tearing of diaphragm or liver.
6 Instruct patient to inhale and exhale deeply three or four times, then to exhale and hold his breath.	6 Holding one's breath immobolizes the chest wall and diaphragm; this helps to prevent the needle from tearing the diaphragm or the liver.
7 The doctor rapidly introduces biopsy needle into the liver, aspirates tissue and withdraws.	
8 As soon as needle is withdrawn, inform patient to resume normal breathing.	8 Actual insertion and withdrawal of needle takes about 10 s.
Follow-up Phase	
1 Following a biopsy, assist the patient to turn on his right side, place a pillow under his lower rib cage and advise him to remain quiet for several hours. Cover needle site with dry dressing.	1 Compressing the liver against the chest wall near the biopsy site, reduces the possibility of bleeding.

Nursing Action	Reason
2 Determine and record the patient's pulse and respiratory rates and his blood pressure at frequent intervals until they stabilize.	2 The nurse needs to be aware of the possible complications of liver biopsy; haemorrhage and bile peritonitis. Anticipatory nursing includes early recognition of symptoms.
3 Recognize that an increasing pulse and falling blood pressure may be indicative of haemorrhage; note any indication of pain.	

Liver Diagnostic Studies (Liver Function Tests)

See Table 4.3.

JAUNDICE

Haemolytic Jaundice

Haemolytic jaundice is attributable to abnormally high concentration of bilirubin in blood exceeding the capacity of normal liver cells to excrete it.

1 Encountered in patients with haemolytic transfusion reactions, hereditary spherocytosis, autoimmune haemolytic anaemia, erythroblastosis foetalis, and other haemolytic disorders.
2 Bilirubin in the blood is unconjugated (indirect-reacting).
3 In faeces and urine, urobilinogen is increased; urine is free of bilirubin.
4 Prolonged jaundice leads to formation of 'pigment stones' in gallbladder. Extremely severe jaundice causes brain-stem damage in neonates. A serum bilirubin for over 360 μmol/l in a full term baby may indicate the need for an exchange transfusion, but each case is assessed individually.

Hepatocellular Jaundice

Hepatocellular jaundice is due to an inability of diseased liver cells to clear the normal amount of bilirubin from the blood.

Causes

1 Infection—infectious hepatitis, homologous serum hepatitis, yellow fever virus.
2 Drug or chemical toxicity—carbon tetrachloride, chloroform, phosphorus, arsenicals, ethanol, halothane, isoniazid, mushroom poisoning.

Clinical Manifestations

1 Mildly or severely ill patient.
2 Lack of appetite, nausea, loss of vigour and strength, weight loss.
3 Elevated SGOT (serum glutamic oxaloacetic transaminase) and SGPT (serum glutamic pyruvic transaminase)—two enzymes that are liberated with cellular necrosis and rise in bloodsteam.

Table 4.3. Liver Diagnostic Studies

Test and Purpose	Normal	Clinical and Nursing Significance
Bile Formation and Secretion		
1 *Serum bilirubin (van den Bergh reaction)* Measures bilirubin in the blood; this determines the ability of the liver to take up conjugate and excrete bilirubin. Bilrubin is a product of the breakdown of haemoglobin		
Total serum bilirubin	3–17 μmol/l	
2 *Urine bilirubin* Not normally found in urine, but if direct serum bilirubin is elevated, some spills into urine	None	Mahogany-coloured urine; when specimen is shaken, yellow tint to foam can be observed. Confirm with Ictotest tablet or dipstick If pyridium (Phenazopyridine) is being taken, there may be a false positive bilirubin. (Mark lab slip if this medication is being taken)
3 *Urobilinogen* Formed in small intestine by action of bacteria on bilirubin. Related to amount of bilirubin excreted into bile	Urine urobilinogen up to 0–6.7 μmol/l Faecal urobilinogen 50–504 μmol/24 hours	Urine specimen is collected over 2-hour period after lunch. Place specimen in dark brown container and send it to lab immediately to prevent decomposition If patient is receiving antibotics, mark lab slip to this effect since production of urobilinogen can be falsely reduced
Protein Studies		
1 *Albumin and globulin measurement* Is of greater significance than total protein measurement		As one increases, the other decreases; hence,
Albumin—produced by liver cells	35–50 g/l	Albumin cirrhosis chronic hepatitis
Globulin—produced in lymph nodes, spleen and bone marrow and Kupffer cells of liver	23–35 g/l	Globulin cirrhosis chronic obstructive jaundice viral hepatitis
Total serum protein	60–80 g/l	

(continued)

Table 4.3. (*cont.*)

Test and Purpose	Normal	Clinical and Nursing Significance
2 *Prothrombin test* Prothrombin and other clotting factors are manufactured in the liver; its rate is influenced by the supply of vitamin K	Less than 2 prolonged versus control samples	Prothrombin time may be prolonged in liver disease, in which case it will not return to normal with vitamin K. It may also be prolonged in malabsorption of fat and fat-soluble vitamins, in which case it will not return to normal with vitamin K
Fat Metabolism		
1 *Cholesterol* It is possible to measure lipid metabolism by determining serum cholesterol levels	3.6–5.7 mmol/l	Serum cholesterol level is lower in parenchymal liver disease Serum lipid level is increased in biliary obstruction
Liver Detoxification		
1 *Bromsulphalein excretion (BSP test)* Liver serves to excrete this dye from the body via bile. The dye may rarely cause an anaphylactic reaction. Given intravenously, it is removed from the blood, stored, conjugated and excreted by the liver cells		Administer dye according to body weight: 5 mg/kg body weight Observe patient closely for: urticaria, nausea, vomiting, dizziness, allergic reaction Have available adrenalin in case of anaphylactic reaction
Draw blood from opposite arm just before and 45 min after injection	After 45 min less than 5% of dye should be retained	Recognize that local reaction at injection site may occur; instruct patient not to bend arm after injection, and apply gentle pressure to prevent extension of irritation If local reaction: Apply hot pack for comfort and to hasten absorption Note: Since Telepaque interferes with liver uptake of this substance, notify laboratory if patient has taken Telepaque within past 36 hours *Abnormalities*: Increased retention occurs in all forms of hepatobiliary disease including impaired liver circulation in portal hypertension or right-sided congestive heart failure

(*continued*)

Table 4.3. (*cont.*)

Test and Purpose	Normal	Clinical and Nursing Significance
2 *Serum alkaline phosphatase* Since bile disposes this enzyme, any impairment of liver cell excretory function will cause an elevation. In cholestasis or obstruction, increased synthesis of enzyme causes very high levels in blood	Varies with method: 20–105 IU/l 3–13 King Armstrong units 1–4 Bassey–Lowry units	*Abnormalities*: The level is elevated to more than three times normal in obstructive jaundice, intrahepatic cholestasis, liver metastasis or granulomas. Also elevated in osteoblastic diseases, Paget's disease and hyperparathyroidsm
Enzyme Production		
1 SGOT—serum glutamic oxaloacetic transaminase	10–45 IU/l	An elevation in these enzymes indicates live cell damage
2 SGPT—serum glutamic pyruvic transaminase	10–45 IU/l	Note: Opiates may also cause a rise in SGOT and SGPT
3 LDH—lactic dehydrogenase. All three are useful in measuring extent of liver damage	50–300 IU/l	

Normal values vary considerably from one laboratory to another according to conditions under which enzyme estimates are performed. All figures are approximate and vary from centre to centre.

4   Rise in BSP (bromsulphalein) and bilirubin. Alkaline phosphatase mildly elevated.
5   Abnormal serum proteins in prolonged illness; prothrombin time increased.
6   Headache and chills possible in infectious condition.
7   Cholesterol decreased in serum.

Cholestatic Jaundice

Causes

1   Extrahepatic obstruction—blockage of bile ducts by gallstone(s), tumour(s), an inflammatory process or an enlarged pancreas pressing on the duct.
2   Intrahepatic cholestasis—caused by injury to bile canaliculi or blockage of intrahepatic ducts due to tumours or granulomas.
     Certain drugs may cause this, e.g., 'cholestatic' agents: phenothiazine derivatives, perphenazine (Fentazin), sulphonamides, tolbutamide (Orinase) and other antidiabetic drugs, thiouracil and para-aminobenzoic acid (PABA).

Clinical Manifestations

Due to damming back of bile, it is reabsorbed by blood. The following responses may be noted:

1   Skin jaundice, sclera yellow.
2   Deep orange-coloured urine.
3   White or clay-coloured stools.
4   Itchy skin and dyspepsia due to impaired bile acid excretion.

Laboratory Evidence

1   SGOT and SGPT rise relatively little.
2   Bilirubin and BSP are increased.
3   Alkaline phosphatase is strikingly elevated.
4   Cholesterol is elevated.

Objectives of Nursing Management

To Control Pruritus and Make the Patient More Comfortable

1   Use starch or baking soda baths, soothing lotions such as calamine.
2   Administer antihistamines, tranquillizers and sedatives if ordered.
3   Administer cholestyramine (Cuemid or Questran) to deplete retained acids which cause itching.
4   Assist patient in reducing the strong tendency to scratch his skin:
    a. Resort to activities which can divert his attention.
    b. Keep nails trimmed and clean.
    c. Avoid excessive top bedding.
    d. Give soothing massages particularly at night in preparing patient for sleep since this is an especially likely time to scratch.
    e. Provide clean white gloves to use at night if he scratches subconsciously.

To Support the Patient Psychologically

1   Instruct staff to avoid remarks or facial expressions which the patient can interpret as referring to his unusual appearance.
2   Notify visitors in a like manner to avoid embarrassing the patient.
3   Encourage patient to talk about his problems and listen to his expressions of concern.
4   Use discretion by not placing patient's bed in a position where he can look at himself in the dresser mirror.

HEPATITIS

Hepatitis is an inflammation of the liver caused by viruses.

Significance

1   From a community health point of view one is concerned with ease of disease transmission and morbidity.
2   From a socioeconomic point of view one is concerned with prolonged loss of time from school and employment.

Preventive Measures

1   Stress importance of proper public and home sanitation.

2 Recognize merits of conscientious surveillance in the proper and safe preparation and dispensation of food.
3 Promote effective health supervision in schools, dormitories and camps.
4 Initiate and support health education programmes.

Types of Hepatitis

1 Type A hepatitis (infectious hepatitis, IH virus).
   Also called epidemic hepatitis, catarrhal jaundice, short-incubation hepatitis.
2 Type B hepatitis (serum hepatitis, SH virus).
   Also called homologous serum jaundice.

Diagnosis

1 By radioimmunoassay test, the presence of hepatitis B antigen, (HBsAg, Australia antigen) is detected in individuals who have infectious or serum hepatitis.
2 By the (HB_SAg) test, detection of hepatitis is possible before the patient becomes clinically ill.
3 SGPT levels also rise 1–2 weeks before clinical jaundice occurs.

Type A Hepatitis

Epidemiology

1 Causative agent—filtrable virus.
2 Mode of transmission:
   a. Faecal–oral route; respiratory possible.
   b. Blood transfusion, blood serum or blood plasma from a carrier or infected person.
   c. Contaminated equipment: syringe and needles.
   d. Contaminated food, milk or shellfish, polluted water.
3 Incubation—3–7 weeks; average 4 weeks.
4 Occurrence:
   a. Worldwide—sporadic or epidemic.
   b. Autumn and winter months.
   c. Usually in children and young adults.

Clinical Manifestations

1 Pre-icteric (prior to period of jaundice) phase:
   a. Headache, fever, anorexia, nausea, vomiting, abdominal tenderness, pain over liver, backache, muscle cramp.
   b. Respiratory manifestations.
2 Icteric phase:
   a. Urine—dark; stool often light for several days.
   b. Liver—enlarged, often tender.
   c. Nausea, vague epigastric distress, heartburn, flatulence, anorexia.

Type B Hepatitis

Epidemiology

1 Causative agent:
   a. Filtrable virus.
   b. Hepatitis B antigen (HB_SAg).
2 Mode of transmission:
   a. Parenteral route:
      (1) Blood—blood components transfusion from an infected person.
      (2) Contaminated needles, syringes, e.g; drug addicts.
   b. Skin puncture—medical instruments (tattooists).
   c. Mucosal transmission; dental instruments, venereal contact.
3 Incubation—6 weeks to 6 months (average 2.5–3 months).
4 Occurrence:
   a. Worldwide.
   b. Recipients of blood and blood products (especially in haemodialysis units).

Diagnosis

1 Counterelectrophoresis (CEP).
2 'Sandwich' counterelectrophoresis (SCEP).
3 Radioimmunoassay.

Clinical Manifestations

1 Symptoms and signs similar to infectious hepatitis, but usually more insidious in onset.
2 Respiratory manifestations minimal or absent; rarely fever.

Treatment and Nursing Management

1 Isolate patient to minimize contacts; allow activity as tolerated.
2 Wear gloves; wash hands thoroughly.
3 Assist with laboratory diagnostic studies such as of transaminase and serum bilirubin levels.
4 Provide tissues and paper bags for nasal and throat secretions; incinerate.
5 Handle bedpan carefully; clean thoroughly and restrict its use to the same patient. Continue this pattern for at least 3 weeks.
6 Ascertain nature of sewage disposal; if questionable, after diagnosis is verified, utilize chemical disinfection before disposal.
7 Instruct and supervise patient to ensure meticulous personal hygiene habits.
8 Use disposable syringes and needles; label clearly all laboratory specimens as coming from a patient with hepatitis.
9 Provide diet that is nutritious and appealing to the patient; small, frequent feedings may be in order.
   a. Offer a large breakfast inasmuch as anorexia worsens later in the day.
   b. Prohibit use of alcohol.
10 Administer alkalies to counteract gastric acidity.
11 Avoid sedatives; they are poorly handled by an inflamed liver.

12 Admonish patient not to give blood as a donor until blood tests reveal no evidence of the virus.
13 Impress on the patient the importance of careful follow-up visits including laboratory and physical examinations until laboratory results have returned to normal levels.
14 Correct any unsanitary condition in patient's area of contact.
15 Recognize that recovery is slow and prolonged; increase activities as tolerated.
16 Type A only: Give gamma globulin to close contacts of the patient, particularly members of the family.

Health and Teaching and Preventive Measures

Type A Hepatitis	Type B Hepatitis
Encourage optimum sanitation practices.	Reject blood donors who have had serum hepatitis.
Instruct patient to practise good personal hygiene.	Instruct patient to maintain a 6-month interval of time since last serving as a donor.
Employ proper safeguards to prevent use of blood and its components from infected donors.	Transfuse a patient only when justified. Use blood substitutes when feasible.
Screen food handlers carefully.	Use disposable needles and syringes; dispose of these carefully.
Practise safe preparation and serving of food.	Use hyperimmune globulin.
Administer Immune Serum Globulin (ISG) intramuscularly within a few of exposure	Routine screening for Australia antigen of all members working in or entering haemodialysis units.
Use disposable needles and syringes; dispose of these carefully.	

Nursing Alert: Although type A hepatitis is usually spread by faecal and oral routes and type B hepatitis is usually spread by the parenteral route, BOTH TYPES MAY BE SPREAD BY ALL ROUTES!

HEPATIC COMA

Two Major Types

1 Fulminant—Due to acute massive liver cell necrosis, usually in previously healthy liver. Mortality in adults is 50–60%, but it is lower in younger age groups.
2 Subacute—Due to acute metabolic insult in a cirrhotic patient with borderline compensation of hepatic function. Mortality is only 10–20% and usually reversible if the precipitating cause is withdrawn (see below).

Causes

1 Incomplete metabolism of nitrogenous compounds by the diseased liver—manifestation of profound liver failure.
2 Biochemical abnormalities responsible are not known; however, the accumula-

tion of significant amounts of nitrogenous substances, particularly ammonia, in the blood are believed to be highly suspect.
3   Shunting of portal blood that contains ammonia and other bacterial metabolites of protein, around the liver.

Precipitating Factors

1   Progressive hepatocellular diseases are not associated with any acute irritation of the liver.
2   Increased sources of ammonia in the blood; high protein diet, gastrointestinal bleeding, following administration of ammonium chloride, thiazides.
3   Infections, paracentesis, acute alcoholism, hypotension, shock, general anaesthesia, minor surgery, hypokalaemia, alkalosis, administration of sedatives or narcotics.
4   Portacaval shunts, especially if protein is not restricted postoperatively in the diet.

Clinical Manifestations

Five Stages

1   Minor mental aberrations—patient slightly confused, untidy and displaying inappropriate behaviour and defective abstract thinking.
2   Motor disturbances—coarse or 'flapping' tremor (especially of hands), hyperreflexia.
3   Progression to gross disturbances of consciousness—somnolence or stupor, hepatic encephalopathy (HE).
4   Complete disorientation to time and place; eventual coma.
5   Decerebrate rigidity, hypoventilation→apnoea.

Altered Physiology

Problems

1   Disruption of enzymatic function in liver cells, muscle and brain.
2   Failure of liver cells to detoxify the ammonia (by converting it to urea).
3   Accumulation of sympathomimetic amines (false neurotransmitters) from abnormal metabolism of aromatic amino acids.

Sources of Ammonia

It comes from bloodstream as a result of the following:

1   Its absorption from the *gastrointestinal tract* (largest source).
      Enzymatic and bacterial digestion of ingested protein and of urea passing from blood into the gastrointestinal tract; increases blood ammonia
   a. Increases result from:
      (1) Gastrointestinal bleeding.
      (2) High protein diet.
      (3) Ingestion of ammonium salts (diuretic: ammonium chloride).
      (4) Bacterial overgrowth in small bowel (infection).
      (5) Uraemia.

b. Decreases result from:
   (1) Elimination of protein from diet.
   (2) Intestinal antibiotics—neomycin, kanamycin, chlortetracycline.
2 Its production by metabolizing *kidney* tissue (deamination of various amino acids, especially glutamine).
   a. Increases with:
   (1) Diuretics (steroids, chlorothiazide).
   (2) Restriction of dietary sodium (hyponatremia).
   (3) Potassium depletion (hypokalaemia).
   (4) Alkalosis.
3 Its liberation from contracting *muscle* cells.
   Increases during exercise.

Treatment

1 Begin early to control coma and eliminate precipitating causes.
2 Arrest gastrointestinal bleeding.
   a. If upper gastrointestinal bleeding, constant gastric aspiration may be required.
   b. If bleeding has ceased, administer a laxative or enema to clear blood from intestine.
3 Cancel orders for ammonium products, sedatives, tranquillizers and narcotics.
4 Greatly reduce dietary protein—if patient begins to improve, gradually increase protein intake; provide sufficient calories in absorbable form such as intravenous glucose or oral lipid emulsion.
5 Administer antibiotics to reduce intestinal flora of organisms; neomycin is preferred.
6 Correct electrolyte abnormalities, especially hypokalaemia.
7 Correct pre-existing complicating diseases—cardiovascular, renal and pulmonary.
8 Treat any infections which can be severe in this patient.
9 Administer antacids to reduce gastric acid and to protect against peptic ulceration.

Nursing Management

1 Observe patient's neurologic status (for example, his ability to perform simple arithmetic calculations and his handwriting). Keep a daily record and note differences.
   a. Observe and record the extent and magnitude of characteristic tremor.
   b. Note and record state of consciousness to include slight drowsiness, slight confusion, drowsy, confused or disoriented.
   c. Note presence of a 'far-away' look.
   d. When patient does not respond, note sucking and grasping abilities; check corneal reflex.
2 Weigh him daily and keep an accurate intake and output record; record quantity of faeces.
3 Take and record vital signs frequently.
4 Be alert for any signs of infection, including infections of upper respiratory tract.

5 If hepatic coma is anticipated, reduce the patient's protein intake and administer antibiotics as prescribed for control of enteric flora.
6 Administer sedatives and analgesics only if doctor is informed.
7 Cleanse the intestinal tract of nitrogenous substrates by administering a 'high' enema as prescribed using maximum amount of fluid.
8 See caring for the unconscious patient (Volume 3, Chapter 1).

HEPATIC CIRRHOSIS

Cirrhosis of the liver is a chronic disease in which there has been diffuse destruction of parenchymal cells followed by liver cell regeneration and an increase in connective tissue. These processes result in disorganization of the lobular architecture and obstruction of the hepatic venous and sinusoidal channels, causing portal hypertension.

Classification of Hepatic Cirrhosis

1 Alcoholic cirrhosis of the liver (micronodular).
   a. Fibrosis—mainly around central veins and portal areas.
   b. Most commonly due to chronic alcoholism.
2 Postnecrotic (macronodular).
   a. Broad bands of scar tissue—due to collapse of necrotic lobules and confluence of portal areas.
   b. Due to previous acute virtal hepatitis or drug-induced massive hepatic necrosis.
3 Biliary.
   a. Scarring around bile ducts and lobes of liver.
   b. Results from chronic biliary obstruction (with or without infection).
   c. Much more rare than alcoholic and postnecrotic cirrhosis.
4 Posthepatic.
   a. Fine bands of scar tissue extend from portal areas whipsawing the lobules.
   b. Usually due to chronic viral hepatitis.

Aetiology and Clinical Manifestations

1 Cirrhosis of the liver is characterized by repeated occurrences of death of the liver cells, replacement with scar tissue and regeneration of liver cells.
2 Onset is insidious; it may be developing and progressing over many years.
3 Major causes are excessive consumption of alcohol and chronic viral hepatitis.
4 Anorexia, weight loss, weakness and fatigability occur; jaundice and fever may be present in the active stage. There are signs of portal hypertension and oestrogen–androgen imbalance.
5 Twice as many men as women are affected; age group most often affected is from 40–60 years.

Altered Physiology

1 Early in disease—gastrointestinal disturbances, fever and liver enlargement due to cells being loaded with fat; as tissue is replaced, scars contract and become smaller, the surface becomes rough and has a hobnail effect.

2   Later—chronic failure of liver function and obstruction of portal circulation.
    a. Obstruction of portal circulation, causing portal hypertension with congestion of spleen, pancreas and gastrointestinal tract.
    (1) Chronic dyspepsia, change in bowel habits—diarrhoea, constipation.
    (2) Oesophageal varices, dilated cutaneous veins around the umbilicus, internal haemorrhoids, ascites, splenomegaly, pancytopenia and caput medusae.
    b. Chronic failure of liver function.
    (1) Plasma albumin is reduced, thereby leading to oedema and contributing to ascites.
    (2) Weakness increases, leading to depression, wasting, delirium, coma and eventually death.
    (3) Oestrogen–androgen imbalance, causing spider angiomata and palmar erythema; amenorrhoea develops in females; testicular and prostatic atrophy, gynecomastia, loss of libido and impotence develops in males.

Diagnosis

1   Liver biopsy.
2   Oesophagoscopy.
3   Barium-contrast oesophagography (only about 50% accurate) to check for oesophageal varices.
4   Arteriography or umbilical venous catheterization to visualize portal collaterals; by placement of a catheter in the portal vein via recanalized umbilical vein, direct venous pressure and portovenography can be done in 75% of cases.
5   Radioisotopic liver scans—increased splenic and vertebral uptake of ^{99}Tc (radioactive technetium) sulphur colloid.
6   Paracentesis to examine ascitic fluid, for cell count, for protein content and for bacterial count.

Treatment

May be slow and tedious.

1   Prevent further damage to the liver by withdrawing toxic substances, alcohol and drugs.
2   Offer supportive care of the patient.
3   Maintain adequate nutritional levels.
    a. Provide protein within ability of liver to handle it. Normal nutritious diet with vitamin supplements, especially B, C and K and folate.
    b. Restrict alcohol consumption.
4   Restrict salt intake when fluid retention occurs.
5   Protect patient from infections and toxic agents.
6   Treat ascites with diuretics gently and only when acute activity of liver damage has subsided.
7   Treat hepatic coma as necessary (see p. 490).
8   Provide vitamins A, B complex, D and K to compensate for liver's inability to store or activate them.

9 Give folic acid to correct folic acid deficiency anaemia.
10 Control or reduce pruritus in patients with liver disease.

Nursing Management

1 Instruct and prepare patient for the very many laboratory and x-ray studies needed.
   a. Diagnosis and nursing implications (see p. 494).
   b. Liver studies and nursing significance (see p. 484).
2 Evaluate nutritional status and needs.
   a. Offer small frequent meals rather than three large meals.
   b. Consider patient preferences in food.
   c. If patient is severely anorexic or nauseated and eating poorly, tube feeding may be necessary; include milk and starch hydrolysate (Dextri-maltose).
   d. Give pancreatin (if diarrhoea and steatorrhoea) to permit better tolerance of diet.
3 Adjust nutritional offerings if the patient has ascites or oedema.
   a. Restrict sodium intake to 200–500 mg daily.
   b. Maintain caloric and vitamin intake; give protein as tolerated.
   c. Avoid table salt, salty foods, salted margarine and butter as well as all ordinary frozen and canned foods, mouthwash, baking soda and all other products containing large quantities of salt.
   d. Use 'salt' substitutes such as lemon juice, oregan, thyme to enhance flavour; commercial salt substitute should be cleared by doctor.
   e. Encourage use of powdered low-sodium milk and milk products.
   f. If water accumulation is not controlled on above regime, resort to the following:
     (1) Limit sodium allowance to 200 mg daily.
     (2) Restrict fluids if serum sodium is low.
     (3) Administer oral diuretics: hydrochlorothiazide (Hydrosaluric) frusemide (Lasix).
     (4) Administer spironolactone (Aldactone) if prescribed—this is an aldosterone-blocking agent used to reinforce the actions of diuretics and prevent undue potassium loss.
     (5) Promote diuresis slowly. Give no more than 1 kg daily to avoid renal failure.
   g. Abdominal paracentesis is to be avoided as long as possible (if necessary, see Procedure, p. 496.
4 Assist the patient in overcoming anorexia, weight loss and fatigue.
   a. Encourage him to eat all meals and supplementary feedings by serving them with eye-catching appeal, in small servings and in small frequent meals.
   b. Recognize the effect of aesthetic factors—control odours, disturbing conversations, unpleasant situations.
   c. Eliminate alcohol but encourage high calorie intake.
   d. Give supplementary vitamins (A, B complex, C and K) and folate.
   e. Conserve patient's energy so that total food intake is not expended to replace energy requirements.
5 Observe skin and control pruritus.

    a. Provide good skin care; bathe without soap; apply soothing lotions.
    b. Keep patient's fingernails short to prevent him from scratching his skin.
6 Be aware of signs of haematemesis and melaena.
    a. Assess for anxiety, weakness, restlessness and epigastric fullness as possibly heralding haemorrhage.
    b. Take and record vital signs frequently.
    c. Administer vitamin C as prescribed.
    d. Observe each stool for colour, consistency and amount. Test for occult blood with Haemoccult.
    e. Record nature, amount and time of vomiting.
    f. Note patient's reaction frequently if he receives a blood transfusion.
7 Anticipate manifestations of haemorrhage such as ecchymosis, petechiae, epistaxis and nose bleeds; initiate preventive measures.
    a. Maintain a safe environment to prevent injury.
    b. Avoid trauma such as forceful nose blowing, use of hard toothbrush, large gauge needles for injection.
    c. Apply pressure to small bleeding sites; record their nature and location.
    d. Encourage intake of foods high in Vitamin C.
8 Recognize signs of increasing stupor, notify doctor and initiate nursing measures as follows:
    a. Be alert for evidences of mental changes, lethargy, hallucinations.
    b. Avoid giving patient narcotics and barbiturates.
    c. Restrict dietary protein; offer small high caloric feedings frequently.
    d. Protect patient by keeping him in bed; pad side-rails.
    e. Arouse patient at intervals.
    f. Limit visitors.
    g. Provide constant nursing surveillance and emphasize sensitivity to patients's changes and needs.

Health Teaching

Instruct patient regarding precautions and regime to follow upon his discharge from the hospital.

1 Stress the necessity of giving up alcohol completely; urge acceptance of skilful assistance from psychiatrist. Alcoholics Anonymous or the alcohol treatment unit in the hospital.
2 Provide written dietary instructions, emphasizing the restriction of sodium (and protein, if necessary).
3 Emphasize the significance of rest, a sensible way of life and an adequate well-balanced diet.
4 Involve the person closest to him (usually spouse), because recovery often is not easy and relapses are common; a close trusted helper can help patient over the rough spots.
5 See items, 4, 5, 7 above, for nutrition, hygiene and safety aspects.

GUIDELINES: Assisting With Abdominal Paracentesis

Paracentesis (abdominal) is the withdrawal of fluid from the abdominal cavity.

Purposes

1   To remove no more than 1 litre at a time of accumulated fluid from the abdominal cavity to relieve pressure on the following:
   a. Diaphragm, which impairs breathing.
   b. Stomach, which aggravates anorexia.
   c. Umbilical hernia.
2   For diagnostic purposes, especially in patient with unexplained fever, abdominal pain and change in bowel habits.

Danger and Complications

1   In chronic liver disease, paracentesis may precipitate hepatic coma.
2   Shock and hypovolaemia can occur if fluid from general circulation shifts to abdomen to replace withdrawn fluid; this can be minimised if no more than one litre of paracentesis fluid is withdrawn or if lost fluid is replaced in kind by parenteral administration of human albumin (salt poor).

Equipment

Sterile paracentesis pack and gloves
Lignocaine 1%
Drape or cotton blankets
Many tailed bandage

Gate clip
Sterile drainage jar (e.q., Winchester)
Skin preparation tray with antiseptic
Specimen bottles and laboratory forms

Procedure

Nursing Action	Reason
Preparatory Phase	
1 Have patient pass urine before treatment is begun.	1 This will lessen the danger of accidentally piercing the bladder with the needle.
2 Position patient in upright position with back, arms and feet supported (sitting on the side of the bed is frequently used position).	2 Patient is more comfortable and a steady position can be maintained.
3 Drape patient with sheet exposing abdomen.	3 Minimizes exposure of patient and keeps him warm
Performance Phase	
1 Assist doctor in preparing skin with antiseptic solution.	1 This is considered a minor surgical procedure requiring aseptic precautions.
2 Open sterile pack and package or sterile gloves; provide anaesthetic solution.	
3 Position drainage jar and be prepared to place end of rubber tubing into drainage jar.	

Nursing Action	Reason
4 Assess pulse and respiratory status frequently during procedure; watch for pallor, cyanosis or syncope (dizziness).	4 Preliminary indications of shock must be watched for. Keep emergency stimulants available.
5 Doctor administers local anaesthesia and introduces trocar and cannula into abdomen.	
6 Withdraw trocar seal, rubber tubing and apply gate clip.	6 Fluid withdrawn slowly by adjusting gate clip.
7 Apply dressing when cannula is withdrawn.	7 This allows for slight pressure to be exerted in a downward direction to help drainage. As ascites is reduced, apply bandage as required.

Follow-up Phase

1 Assist patient to be comfortable after treatment.	
2 Record amount and kind of fluid removed, number of specimens sent to laboratory, patient's condition throughout treatment.	
3 Check blood pressure and vital signs every half hour for 2 hours, every hour for 4 hours, and every 4 hours for 24 hours.	3 Close observation will detect poor circulation adjustment and possible development of shock.
4 Usually a dressing is sufficient.	
5 Watch for leakage or scrotal oedema after paracentesis.	5 If seen, notify doctor at once.

BLEEDING OESOPHAGEAL VARICES

Oesophageal varices are dilated tortuous veins found in the submucosa of the lower oesophagus; they may extend up in the oesophagus and down into the stomach.

Causes

1 Nearly always due to portal hypertension which may result from obstruction of the portal venous circulation and cirrhosis of the liver.
2 Abnormalities of the circulation in splenic vein or superior vena cava.

Altered Physiology and Symptoms

1 Increasing portal vein obstruction—venous blood returning to right atrium from intestinal tract and spleen seeks new pathways, through enlarging collateral oesophageal veins.
2 Usually no symptoms are produced by dilated veins unless mucosa becomes ulcerated.
3 Haematemesis and melaena plus a history of alcoholism tend to point toward

oesophageal varices; however, bleeding may result from associated gastritis or duodenal ulcer in 25% of patients with varices.

4   The strain of coughing or vomiting may precipitate variceal rupture, haemorrhage and death.

5   Irritation of vessels by gastro-oesophageal reflux may cause oesophagitis, oesophageal rupture, haemorrhage and death.

Diagnosis

1   Fibreoptic endoscopy may be used if bleeding is controlled. It is essential to exclude other causes of bleeding.

2   Arteriography may be substituted if bleeding is massive.

3   Splenoportography using contrast dye can be effective when studied as a series of x-ray plates or done as a segmental x-ray; extensive collateral circulation of oesophageal vessels may be indicative of varices.

4   Portal vein pressure above 250 mm of water is abnormal; this can be measured in the operating room by introducing a needle into spleen or via umbilical vein catheter.

5   Liver function tests include bromsulphalein retention, serum transaminase, bilirubin, serum proteins, alkaline phosphatase.

Treatment and Nursing Management

1   Initiate measures to overcome blood loss.
   a. Replace blood with *fresh* whole blood.
      (1) Ammonia content is lower than in stored blood.
      (2) Coagulation effect is greater, particularly if the patient has severe liver disease.
   b. Administer vitamin K intramuscularly.

2   Recognise the importance of controlling haemorrhage.
   a. Purpose:
      (1) To lessen transfusion requirements.
      (2) To reduce large amounts of blood in gastrointestinal tract.
      (3) To avoid hepatic coma.
   b. Methods:
      (1) Administer Vasopressin systemically to reduce portal pressure and to initiate haemostasis. Intra-arterial infusion into the superior mesenteric artery may be used after angiography, but offers no definitive advantage.
      (2) Ice-water lavage of stomach (gastric hypothermia) may temporarily control bleeding.
      (3) Aspirate blood from the stomach if necessary.
      (4) Oesophageal tamponade—pressure is exerted on the cardiac portion of the stomach and against the bleeding varices by a double balloon tamponade (Sengstaken–Blakemore tube). (See below.)
      (5) Treat bleeding by complete rest of the oesophagus (parenteral feedings); avoid straining and vomiting and continue gastric suction.
      (6) Initiate vitamin-K therapy; administer multiple blood transfusions.
      (7) Avoid sedation, since it may lead to coma.
      (8) Administer laxatives plus enemata to remove blood.

GUIDELINES: Using the Sengstaken–Blakemore Tube to Control Oesophageal Bleeding

Purposes

1 To exert pressure on the cardiac portion of the stomach and against bleeding varices by a double balloon tamponade.
2 To reduce transfusion requirements.
3 To prevent blood accumulation in the gastrointestinal tract which could precipitate hepatic coma.

Equipment

Sengstaken–Blakemore tube
Basin with cracked ice
Clamp for tubing

Towel and vomit bowl
Glass of water and straw
Flashlight

Procedure (Fig. 4.17).

Preparatory Phase

1 Provide nursing support by reassuring patient that this procedure will help to control his bleeding.
2 Explain procedure to patient and tell him how breathing through the mouth and swallowing can help in passing the tube.
3 Elevate head of bed slightly unless patient is in shock.

Nursing Action	Reason
Performance Phase	
1 Check balloon by trial inflation to detect leaks.	1 This is best done under water because it is easier to see escaping air bubbles.
2 Chill the tube then lubricate it before doctor passes it via mouth or nose (preferable).	2 Chilling will make the tube more firm and lubrication will lessen friction.
3 After the tube has entered the stomach, wash out stomach and aspirate all clots.	
4 After obtaining x-ray of the lower chest and upper abdomen to check position of the balloon, it is fully inflated (200–250 ml) with air and then pulled back gently.	4 This is to exert force against cardia. The triple-lumen tube provides two channels to inflate each compression bag, one in the stomach and one in the oesophagus. Balloons are inflated using a manometer to measure pressure to 25 or 30 mmHg; position of balloons is verified by fluoroscope.
5 Traction is placed on tubing where it enters the nose of the patient. Then	5 This keeps balloons in position and assists in exerting proper pressure.

Nursing Action	Reason
the oesophageal bag is inflated to 35–40 mmHg. This is tied with double ties to prevent leakage (Fig. 4.17).	
6 Gastric suction may be attached to the third outlet of the catheter.	6 By using suction and irrigating the tubing hourly, it is possible to tell how well the bleeding is controlled by the appearance of the drainage.
7 A second nasogastric (Levin) tube is passed into the lower oesophagus.	7 To aspirate saliva and to check for bleeding *above* the oesophageal balloon.

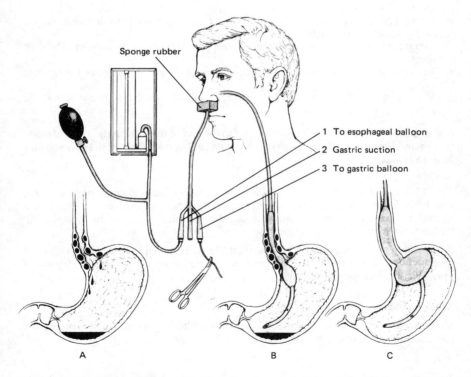

Figure 4.17.   Diagram showing oesophageal varices and their treatment by a compressing balloon tube (Sengstaken–Blakemore). a. Dilated veins of the lower oesophagus. b. The tube is in place in the stomach and the lower oesophagus but is not inflated. c. Inflation of the tube and the compression of the veins which can be obtained by inflation of the balloon. In some instances, it may be necessary to pass an additional tube through the other nostril for the purpose of aspirating secretions.

Nursing Action	Reason
8 Deflate tube for 5 min at 8- or 12-hour intervals.	8 To prevent erosion and necrosis of the oesophagus or stomach.
9 Pressure on tubes and traction is released in 2–4 days.	9 If bleeding remains controlled, the tubing is removed in 24 hours.

Nursing Resposibilities

1   Maintain *constant* vigilance while balloons are inflated in the patient.
2   Keep balloon pressures at required level to control bleeding.
3   Observe and record vital signs frequently—bleeding, shock, etc.
4   Be alert for chest pain—may indicate injury or rupture of oesophagus.
5   Irrigate suction tube as ordered; observe and record nature and colour of aspirated material.
6   Keep head of bed elevated to avoid gastric regurgitation and to diminish nausea and a sensation of retching.
7   Maintain nutritional and electrolyte levels parenterally or by feedings through the tube.
8   Maintain nasogastric suction to aspirate saliva through an accessory nasogastric tube.
9   Note nature of breathing: if counterweight pulls the tube into oropharynx, the patient may be asphyxiated.

Nursing Alert: Keep a pair of scissors taped to the end of the bed. In the event of *acute respiratory distress*, use the scissors to cut across tubing (to deflate both balloons) and remove tubing.

CHIEF HAZARD: Vomiting with an inflated oesophageal balloon tamponade in place, which results in massive pulmonary aspiration. Manage this problem by inserting a nasogastric tube in the free nostril to drain the oesophagus above the oesophageal balloon, thereby preventing aspiration.

NOTE: This procedure should be reserved for patients who are known without a doubt to be bleeding from oesophageal varices, and in whom all forms of conservative therapy failed.

Surgical Intervention

If bleeding of oesophageal varices is not controlled by conservative measures, surgical procedures may be employed:

Surgical Procedures

1   Direct ligation of varices.
2   Surgical bypass (*portacaval anastomosis*). By shunting portal blood into the vena cava, pressure in the portal system is reduced.
3   Splenorenal shunt. A shunt is made between the splenic vein and the left renal vein; this is done when the portal vein cannot be used because of thrombosis or for other reasons.

Evaluation of Surgery

1   Varying degrees of success are reported with shunting procedures.
2   The success depends mainly on the condition of the patient; it is used as an emergency procedure following bleeding. Most common use is to prevent recurrence after the patient recovers from an initial variceal bleed.
3   Complications are acute hepatic failure and chronic portal systemic encephalopathy.
4   Postoperative care is similar to postabdominal surgery complicated by care required for a patient with cirrhotic liver.

DISEASE OF THE BILIARY (GALLBLADDER) SYSTEM

Incidence

1   Women acquire the disease more frequently than men: 4:1.
2   Patients are most often past 40, multiparous and overweight; however, the condition is common also in younger patients.

Types of Gallbladder Disease

(Chole—gallbladder)
Cholecystitis—inflammation of the gallbladder.
Cholelithiasis—stones in the gallbladder.
Choledocholithiasis—stones in the common duct.

Chronic Cholecystitis with Cholelithiasis

1   Clinical manifestations:
    a. History of episodic, usually colicky epigastric or right upper quadrant pain often associated with nausea and vomiting.
    b. Jaundice due to choledocholithiasis.
2   Treatment:
    a. Surgery is advised if gallstones are present with typical pain attacks and/or jaundice. Whether asymptomatic stones should be removed surgically is still open to debate.
    b. In the older patient, the risk of surgery must be evaluated in relation to other disease conditions present.
    c. Chenodeoxycholic acid, an experimental drug, can dissolve cholesterol gallstones, which are usually radiolucent.
        (1) The only adverse effects appear to be mild diarrhoea and cramps and SGOT elevation; with dose regulation these disappear.
        (2) Stones are likely to recur; therefore, long-term therapy may be required.
        (3) Studies continue to evaluate this drug for its proper place in the management of the patient with cholelithiasis.

Acute Cholecystitis

1   Clinical manifestations and features:
    a. Right upper quadrant pain, fever, nausea and vomiting.

    b. The condition may occur at any age, but it is most common in patients over the age of 40.
    c. The chief hazard is perforation with local or generalized peritonitis.
2 Treatment:
    a. Provide hospitalization, bedrest, withholding of oral fluids and insertion of nasogastric tube with suction.
    b. Administer intravenous fluids to correct electrolyte imbalance, to maintain adequate urinary output and to provide nutritional needs.
    c. Administer medication for pain and antibiotics for infection control.
    d. Prepare patient for laboratory studies, chest x-ray, ECG and possibly intravenous cholangiogram.
    e. Record vital signs every 4 hours and prepare patient for surgery.

Diagnosis of Biliary Conditions

Overall assessment of the patient should include detection of associated disease processes (cardiovascular, pulmonary and renal); diabetes status; and realization of increased surgical risk if patient is over age 65.

Flat Plate of Abdomen

Used to visualize the 25% of stones that are radiopaque.

Cholecystography

Used to visualize the shape and position of the gallbladder.

NOTE: This test is effective only if the liver cells are functioning properly and are capable of excreting the radiopaque dye into the bile.

1 *Purpose:*
    a. To detect gallstones.
    b. To estimate ability of gallbladder to fill, concentrate its contents, contract and empty in a normal manner.
2 *Method:*
    a. Because gallstones are usually radiolucent, it is necessary to fill the gallbladder with a radiopaque dye which permits stones to show up as clear areas.
    b. Iodide-containing dye is excreted into bile by the liver and concentrated in the gallbladder.
        (1) Orally:
            (a) Contrast media may be given by mouth (e.g., Biloptin, Telepaque, Priodax, Oragrafin, Teridax, Monophen).
            (b) Iodide preparation is usually given in oral doses of 3.6 g approximately 10–12 hours before x-ray. If there is no visualization the next morning, repeat dose of 3.6 g the following evening.
            (c) Administer nothing by mouth from the time of iodide administration to the time of x-ray to prevent contraction of gallbladder and expulsion of contrast medium.
        (2) Intravenously:
        Intravenous cholecystography involves giving an iodide preparation (e.g., Biliodyl) about 10 min before x-ray.

3   *Patient preparation:*
   a. At least 1 hour after the evening meal, the patient takes the prescribed tablets or capsules of iodide preparation by mouth.
   b. These tablets are taken one at a time at 3- to 5-min intervals with at least 250 ml of water.
   c. From this time to bedtime, nothing is taken by mouth except water; from midnight on, water is also excluded. (If nausea, vomiting or diarrhoea occurs notify doctor; test may be postponed.)
   d. No laxatives are given during this time; however, a saline enema may be required on the morning of the x-ray.
   e. Breakfast is withheld and patient goes to x-ray.
   f. Right upper abdominal quadrant is x-rayed.
   g. The patient is fed a fatty meal containing cream, butter or eggs to test contractility of the gallbladder.
   h. X-ray examination is repeated at intervals until gallbladder has expelled dye.

Cholangiography

Dye is injected directly into biliary tree.

1   Advantages:
   a. Procedure is best way to visualize biliary tree in patient after cholecystectomy.
   b. All components of the biliary tree can be observed: hepatic ducts within liver, common hepatic duct and cystic duct, but the gallbladder is often not well visualized.
2   Clinical usefulness:
   a. In differentiating hepatocellular jaundice from jaundice due to biliary obstruction. Note that the dye is rarely excreted enough to visualize if serum bilirubin is less than 4 mg/dl.
   b. In locating stones within bile ducts.
   c. In detecting and diagnosing cancer of the biliary system.
   d. In investigating gastrointestinal symptoms of patients who had cholecystectomy.
3   Patient preparation:
   a. The patient is dehydrated by restricting his fluid intake.
   b. Enema is given early in morning of test.
   c. A sedative is given at least 1 hour before the x-ray.
   d. Dye (e.g., Biligrafin) is injected either intravenously (results not as conclusive) or directly into the common duct.
      (1) Operatively; this can be done during surgery.
      (2) Postoperatively; by injecting dye into the common duct drain.
      (3) Via retrograde endoscopic cannulation of duct via duodenum.
   e. Following the x-ray, regardless of method of dye injection, as much as possible of the dye and bile are aspirated to prevent leakage into the peritoneal cavity, thus avoiding a possible bile peritonitis.

NOTE: Operative cholangiography may be done during gallbladder surgery in the operating room.

Ultrasound Examination

B scanner and transducer.

This test can be used to demonstrate gallbladder distension, bile duct distension and calculi.

Liver Scan

1   In the jaundiced patient, this scan may show evidence of hepatocellular disease or metastatic lesions.
2   With radioactive rose bengal, which is excreted by the liver-like gallbladder dyes, obstructive pathology of the biliary tree may be revealed.

Endoscopic Retrograde Pancreatico-cholecystography (ERPC)

See Guidelines, p. 508.

Types of Gallbladder Surgery

1   *Cholecystostomy*—simple opening of gallbladder to remove stones, bile or pus; a tube is then sutured into the gallbladder for drainage.

NOTE: When patient returns to the recovery unit, this drainage tube is connected to a drainage bottle.

2   *Cholecystectomy*—removal of the gallbladder after ligation of the cystic duct and vessels; done in most situations of acute or chronic cholecystitis. A drain (penrose type) may be inserted in the gallbladder bed to permit drainage into dressings.
3   *Choledochostomy* (Cholecystectomy and exploration of common bile duct)—an opening into the common duct for the purpose of removing obstructing stones; a drainage T-tube is inserted into the duct which needs to be connected to a drainage bottle. Usually a cholecystectomy is done at this time because the gallbladder often contains stones also.

Preoperative Nursing Management

1   Diagnostic evaluation:
    a. Gallbladder x-rays (p. 504).
    b. Chest x-ray.
    c. Examination of urine and stool.
    d. Blood studies including liver function tests (p. 484).
2   It may be necessary to administer vitamin K and fresh frozen plasma to correct a low prothrombin.
3   Proper nutritional levels may require supplements of protein to aid in wound healing and to prevent liver damage.
4   Adequate instruction regarding immediate postoperative requirements such as turning and deep breathing to prevent hypostatic pneumonia, a common postoperative complication.

Postoperative Nursing Objectives and Management

1   To prevent respiratory complications which are common in obese patients and in those having upper abdominal incisions.
    a. Encourage the patient to take 10 deep breaths hourly and to turn frequently.

b. Administer analgesics as ordered to permit patient to take deep breaths comfortably (may be painful otherwise).

c. Place patient in semirecumbent position to facilitate lung expansion.

d. Activate and ambulate as early as permissible; apply a many tailed bandage if it will make the patient more comfortable.

e. Since he may still have a drainage bottle, place it in a below-the-waist pocket or fasten so that it is at desired level.

2 To promote drainage from T-tube or cholecystostomy tube until normal flow of bile is established.

a. Place patient in semirecumbent position and later in upright position as tolerated to facilitate drainage.

b. Connect drainage tube to drainage bottle at side of bed; observe for kinking, twisting and blockage of tubes.

c. Check postoperative orders regarding positioning of drainage bottle; often the bottle or tubing is elevated so that bile drains through the apparatus only if pressure develops in the system. This is done purposely to prevent total bile loss and to promote normal bile flow through the common bile duct.

d. Allow enough tubing leeway to permit the patient to be turned without dislodging tubes.

e. Observe, describe and record amount and character of drainage frequently.

f. After 5 or 6 days of drainage, the T-tube may be clamped 1 hour before and after each meal to allow bile to flow into duodenum to aid in digestion. (Done with doctor's permission.)

g. T-tube drain may be removed in 10 days. Cholecystostomy tube is removed in 6 weeks to 6 months. Drainage tube from gallbladder bed may be removed in 5–6 days.

3 To maintain fluid and nutritional needs of the postoperative biliary patient.

a. Intravenous fluids are usually initiated; fluids by mouth are given in 24 hours.

b. Insert nasogastric tube to relieve distension and promote normal peristalsis.

c. An enema or suppositories are usually given after 72 hours after which the patient is offered a soft, low fat diet.

d. If necessary to feed the patient his own bile (in chronic biliary drainage) it may be best not to tell the patient what the liquid is other than it is to stimulate his appetite; bile may be chilled, strained and diluted with grape or other fruit juice.

e. Provide diets which are low in fats and high in carbohydrate and proteins (fatty foods are usually avoided because they cause nausea).

f. It may be necessary to continue to give vitamin K.

4 To observe colour changes in skin, sclerae and stool which will indicate whether bile pigment is disappearing from blood and draining again into the duodenum.

a. Note colour and consistency of all stools; chart an accurate description.

b. Send specimens of urine and stool to the laboratory at frequent intervals for examination of bile pigments.

c. Observe skin and sclerae for yellowish colour which would indicate bile-flow obstruction.

5 To protect skin around incision site due to bile seepage.

a. Change the outer dressings frequently to provide for absorption of drainage; Montgomery straps may facilitate dressing changes.

b. Apply skin pastes of zinc oxide or petroleum jelly to prevent the bile drainage from attacking and digesting the skin.

Health Teaching and Discharge Planning

Objective

To stress elements in posthospital care that will assist patient in his convalescence.

1   It is not unusual after cholecystectomy for patient to have 'looseness of the bowel', consisting of one to three movements a day. This diminishes over a period of a few weeks to several months; within a year, the bowel habit is normal.
2   Emphasize the importance of follow-up visits to the doctor.

GUIDELINES: Endoscopic Retrograde Pancreatico-cholecystography (ERPC)

A fibreoptic endoscope (a side-viewing instrument) is placed in the descending duodenum so that the ampulla of Vater can be located and cannulated (Fig. 4.18).

In this examination, both the common and pancreatic ducts may be injected with contrast media to visualize the hepatobiliary tree and pancreatic ducts radiologically.

The clinician is able to diagnose abnormalities of the ductal system, detect disease processes and obtain direct secretory information as well as cells for cytologic examination

Indications

1   Biliary disease.
2   Pancreatic disease.
3   To diagnose:
    a. Cancer of the papilla.
    b. Obstructive jaundice.
    c. Calculus disease, pre- and postcholecystectomy.
    d. Carcinoma of biliary ducts.
    e. Carcinoma of pancreas.
    f. Pancreatitis.

Contraindications

1   Acute cardiorespiratory disease.
2   Acute recent attack of pancreatitis (within 3 weeks) because of risk of inducing another attack.
3   Stricture or obstruction of oesophagus or duodenum.
4   Acute cholangitis.

Equipment

A side-viewing duodenoscope* (to be sterilized after use with suspected infectious patients)
Sterilized cannula
This duodenoscope is 125 cm long and 1 cm in diameter

* Olympus Corporation.

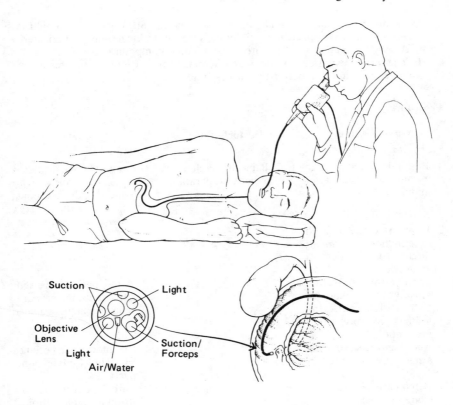

Figure 4.18. Endoscopic retrograde cholangiopancreatography (ERCP). The patient is moved from left lateral to prone position as the flexible scope is passed. The circle on the left shows the tip of the scope: the objective lens is the viewing section assisted by two side lights. Air or water may be directed to an area and suction is available. The right diagram shows the scope nearing the ampulla of Vater; the scope is in the duodenum; gallbladder is the topmost sac—from which note the biliary and common bile ducts.

Visual fields are oriented 90° to its long axis
It includes a channel through which a cannula or biopsy forceps can be passed under
    direct vision

Considerations

1   ERPC is not a simple endoscopic procedure; it must be done by a skilful well-trained doctor.
2   There are certain risks, described below:
    a. After ERPC a very small percentage of patients develop clinical pancreatitis which may last 1–3 days.
    b. The patient may retain contrast material injected proximal to an obstructed

duct; this may result in cholangitis or pancreatitis. Such a patient should be covered with broad-spectrum antibiotics; surgical drainage may be indicated.

c. A very few patients are sensitive to iodinated compounds.

d. The more experienced the team in performing ERPC's, the fewer the complications and the better the success rate.

Procedure

Nursing Action	Doctor's Role	Reason
Preparatory Phase		
1 Remind patient to take nothing by mouth after midnight.	1 Collaborate with nurse in patient preparation.	1 Limited intake produces a basal condition with reduced body secretions; this permits better visualization of tissues.
2 Explain contemplated examination to patient; discuss possibilities of after-effects.		
3 Determine patient's sensitivity to iodine (or fish which contains iodine) or any other medication.		3 A few patients are sensitive to iodine preparations (Hypaque sodium).
4 Take and record vital signs.		4 This information becomes a baseline for later comparison.
5 Offer patient Amethocaine lozenges to suck.		Amethocaine is an oropharyngeal topical anaesthetic.
	6 Start an intravenous infusion with normal saline.	6 This becomes the avenue for direct intravenous medications such as diazepam (Valium) and meperidine (Demerol) to promote relaxation prior to insertion of duodenoscope.
7 Instruct patient to remove dentures; a mouthpiece is inserted.		7 To facilitate insertion of scope.
Performance Phase		
1 Place patient in left lateral position.	1 Scope is passed through patient's mouth into oesophagus and stomach.	1 Anatomy is carefully examined as the scope advances.

Nursing Action	Doctor's Role	Reason
2 Place patient in prone position. (This provides the radiologist with a better position for fluoroscopy and radiography.)	2 Administer intravenous medication, which may include Demerol, Valium, atropine or glucagon.	2 Atropine will produce a hypotonic duodenum and relaxed sphincter at ampulla of Vater; secretion will be reduced.
3 Prepare a special radiopaque Teflon cannulation tube by filling it with contrast medium (to eliminate air).	3 Gently, advance tip through pyloric ring into duodenal bulb into descending duodenum.	
	4 Minimal air insufflation used to search for the ampulla of Vater.	4 Unless this is obstructed by tumour, is can usually be identified with careful search
	5 Administer glucagon.	5 Glucagon is given to further reduce duodenal motility
	6 When cannulation tubing is in correct position, dye is slowly injected: 3–5 ml for pancreatic ductal system; 15–20 ml for biliary ductal system.	6 Cannulation tube is passed through biopsy channel of scope. Contrast medium is warmed to body temperature. Tube is advanced under fluoroscopy. X-ray pictures are taken while patient is in prone position following injection of contrast media.
7 Upon completion of film-taking, turn patient to lateral position. Use suction to remove oropharyngeal secretions	7 Draw blood sample for amylase determination. Keep scope and cannula in place and patient in prone position until films are completed. If films are satisfactory, scope is carefully removed.	7 Await return and reading of films.

Follow-up Phase

1 Check vital signs every 4 hours. Notify family as to when patient will return to his room.		1 Postcannulation patient may experience a temperature rise, chills, abdominal pain. Report these responses to doctor.

Nursing Action	Doctor's Role	Reason
2 In the absence of complications, permit the patient to eat in 2–4 hours (light diet); permit a full diet the next day.		2 A mild rise in serum amylase is observed in a high percentage of the patients.
3 Watch for palpitations related to atropine sulphate injection. Also watch for respiratory depression and transient hypotension.		3 Some patients experience mild to severe epigastric pain, nausea, and vomiting. These discomforts are usually transitory.

4. Conditions of the Pancreas*

ACUTE PANCREATITIS

Acute pancreatitis is an inflammation of the pancreas brought about by the digestion of this organ by enzymes, particularly trypsin, an enzyme it produces.

Aetiology

1 Unknown.
2 Associated with excessive intake of alcohol—this is the most common cause.
3 Associated with blockage of ampulla of Vater by gallstones, causing activation of pancreatic enzymes.
4 Associated with spasm and oedema of ampulla of Vater following duodenitis or after treatment with opiates.
5 May occur as a complication of mumps or bacterial disease.
6 Some congenital hyperlipidaemias appear to be related to acute pancreatitis.

Clinical Manifestations

Acute Interstitial Pancreatitis

1 Pancreatic oedema and escape of enzyme into nearby tissues and peritoneal cavity.
2 Fat necrosis of omentum caused by pancreatic lipase.
3 Increase in peritoneal fluid.
4 Abdominal and back pain.
5 Nausea, vomiting.
6 Tenderness across upper abdomen—often minimal.
7 Elevated blood lipase and amylase.

Acute Haemorrhagic Pancreatitis

1 A more advanced form of acute pancreatitis.

* For discussion of diabetes mellitus see Chapter 5, Metabolic and Endocrine Disorders.

2   Enzymatic digestion of gland more widespread.
3   Tissue becomes necrotic—blood escapes into pancreas and retroperitoneally.
4   Severe abdominal and back pain; tenderness is often present in epigastrium, but rigidity is often absent.
5   Symptoms similar to acute interstitial pancreatitis, only more severe.
6   Blood lipase and amylase are elevated.
7   Respiratory distress may occur.
8   With severe pancreatitis, there is often psychic disturbance manifested in restlessness, hallucinations, coarse tremor.
9   Severe leakage of exudate from plasma into peritoneum (large third-space loss).
10 Shock, due to activation of kinins.
11 Hypokalaemic alkalosis and hypocalcaemia usually present.

Diagnosis

1   Determination of serum amylase. If serum amylase is elevated, and there is clinical evidence, pancreatitis is likely.
2   An elevated serum lipase may also be present and persists longer than elevation of amylase.

Treatment and Nursing Managmenet

Objectives

To halt the progress of the illness.
To treat the haemodynamic abnormality.
To treat systemic and local complications.

1   Relieve discomfort and pain to control restlessness which increases body metabolism causing stimulation of enzyme secretions.
    a. Give meperidine (Demerol); this is preferred because it depresses the central nervous system. (Opiates on the other hand may produce spasm of biliary-pancreatic ducts).
    b. Encourage patient to assume position of comfort. Turn frequently to prevent pulmonary-vascular complications.
2   Decrease pancreatic secretions by reducing stimulation.
    a. Give nothing by mouth to eliminate chief stimulus to enzyme secretion.
    b. Offer anticholinergic medications as ordered to assist in reducing pancreatic secretions by suppressing vagal mechanisms.
    c. Initiate nasogastric suction to remove hydrochloric acid from stomach thus preventing release of secretin; adynamic ileus is also treated.
       (1) Record colour and nature of gastric secretions.
       (2) Measure secretions at periodic intervals.
    d. Maintain the comfort of the intubated patient.
       (1) Assist patient in cleansing and refreshing mouth care.
       (2) Apply lubricant to external nares to prevent irritation of mucous membrane and skin.
       (3) Alternate side-positioning to prevent oesophageal and gastric irritation by tube.

(4) Provide cool mist vapour therapy to increase humidity and control drying of mucous membrane.
3 Monitor blood gases to detect early signs of respiratory failure.
  Administer oxygen therapy if necessary.
4 Provide medications to correct deficiencies and prevent complications.
  a. Give parenteral fluids: electrolytes, blood and plasma to meet body's nutritional needs, replace losses and combat shock. Keep accurate intake and output record.
  b. Administer antibiotics to ward off secondary infection or abscess formation. (Use of antibiotics remains controversial. Some doctors suggest intravenous administration of cephalothin every 6 hours.)
  c. If marked hyperglycaemia occurs, give insulin in small doses (soluble insulin at 6-hour intervals) rather than long-acting insulin.
5 Support cardiopulmonary system in patients with acute haemorrhagic pancreatitis.
  a. Monitor haematocrit (if it rises in first 24–48 hours, volume replacement was inadequate);
    Monitor central venous pressure (keep to 8–10 cm of water above baseline);
    Monitor urinary output (keep to 50–100 ml/hour).
  b. Provide blood, plasma and balanced electrolytes to maintain blood volume; limit solutions containing glucose, because this patient is often hyperglycaemic.
  c. Maintain surveillance of vital signs.
  d. Monitor blood sugar every 4 hours; administer intravenous insulin to keep blood sugar levels under 200 mg/100 ml.
  e. Monitor serum calcium; it may be necessary to administer calcium gluconate if calcium falls low enough to produce symptoms.
  f. Keep the body metabolism of the patient low.
    (1) Administer oxygen therapy if breathing is laboured.
    (2) Keep patient in bed to control overexertion.
    (3) Turn on air-conditioning to keep body heat under control.
6 Surgical intervention:
  a. There is considerable disagreement about the place of surgery in treating acute pancreatitis. It is considered only if all other therapy has failed.
  b. Laparotomy may reveal an alternate problem which can be corrected:
    (1) Tense gallbladder—cholecystostomy.
    (2) Stones in ductal system—establish common duct patency.
    (3) Removal of necrotic material and fluid—peritoneal lavage.

Health Teaching and Discharge Planning

Manage recovery phase and offer guidelines to the patient to prevent future attacks of pancreatitis.

1 By the fifth or sixth day, offer the following:
  a. Small amounts of clear-fat liquids.
  b. Anticholinergics parenterally or orally
  c. Nonabsorbable antacids hourly.
2 Instruct the patient as follows:
  a. Gradually resume normal diet.

b. Prohibit the use of alcohol and excessive use of coffee, since they increase pancreatic secretion.
3   Urge follow-up visits with doctor. (Biliary tract studies and surveillance may uncover the cause of the pancreatitis).

CHRONIC PANCREATITIS

Chronic pancreatitis is a chronic fibrosis and calcification of the pancreas with obstruction of its ducts and destruction of its secreting acinar cells.

Incidence

1   Occurs most in men between 45 and 60.
2   Follows repeated attacks of acute interstitial pancreatitis.
3   Usually occurs in patients having a history of prolonged use of alcohol.
4   Gallstones, hyperparathyroidism and hyperlipidaemia are occasionally associated with chronic pancreatitis.

Clinical Manifestations

1   Recurrent episodes of severe upper abdominal and back pain (morphine often does not relieve pain), vomiting and low-grade fever. Drug addiction is often a secondary problem.
2   Protein and fat digestion is disturbed because of deficient pancreatic secretion.
3   Steatorrhoea; stools that are frequent, frothy and foul-smelling with high fat content because of faulty fat digestion.
4   Later formation of calcium stones in the duct as calcification develops.
5   Weight loss.
6   Jaundice may occur because of constriction of common bile duct as it passes through head of pancreas.

Diagnosis

1   Determine whether levels of serum amylase and lipase are elevated. Levels often are not elevated in chronic pancreatitis.
2   Examine stool to measure faecal fat and trypsin content.
3   Arteriography and x-ray may show fibrous tissue and calcification.
4   Diabetes or abnormal glucose tolerance may be detectable.

Treatment and Nursing Management

1   Offer patient bland, low-fat diet in six feedings daily.
2   Give antacids and anticholinergic medication to reduce acid which would stimulate the release of secretin and enhance pancreatic activity.
3   Pancreatic insufficiency is controlled by giving medication containing amylase, lipase and trypsin—Pancreatin, Cotazyme, Viokase.
      Medication may need to be administered with antacids or bicarbonates.

NOTE: Steatorrhoea should be present before initiating enzyme replacement therapy.

4   Since these patients often develop diabetes, be alert for symptoms such as polydipsia, polyuria, weakness, polyphagia (excessive eating) or weight loss and report these to doctor.
5   The use of alcohol should be discouraged, since this will aggravate the pancreatitis; treatment of alcoholism must be done if this is a problem as it usually is.
6   If hyperparathyroidism or hyperlipaemia is diagnosed, these certainly must be treated.
7   Surgical aspects are similar to biliary tract surgery (see p. 506).
8   Nature of surgery is determined by identifying the cause; surgery usually fails if alcoholism or drug addiction persists.
   a. With gallbladder disease—biliary tract surgery to explore common bile duct, choledocholithotomy (removing stones in duct) and cholecystectomy (removing gallbladder).
   b. Sphincteroplasty or sphincterotomy—dividing sphincter of Oddi to improve drainage of common bile duct *or*
   c. Selective or generalized drainage of dilated ducts via pancreatico-jejunostomy.
   d. Pancreatectomy may be done when pancreas is severely diseased or when persistent pain is a major problem.

PSEUDOCYSTS AND PANCREATIC ABSCESSES

Pseudocysts of the pancreas are collections of inflammatory fluid walled off by fibrous tissue in the pancreas, usually resulting from local necrosis at the time of acute pancreatitis.

Clinical Manifestations and Diagnosis

1   Cysts may attain considerable size; they develop rapidly or slowly (within 72 hours or over several weeks or months).
2   Because they occur in the posterior peritoneum, they may exert pressure against the stomach or colon, visible on barium studies.
3   Persistent elevation of amylase (serum or urine) is the most common finding. Pain and vomiting may occur.
4   Leucocytosis and fever are common but are usually mild with pseudocysts; these responses are more striking with abscess formation.
5   Sonography has been found useful in confirming diagnosis.

Treatment

1   Pseudocysts may occasionally subside spontaneously.
2   Symptoms of secondary infection may require surgery for drainage.
3   Drainage may be established into gastrointestinal tract (internal) or through skin surface (external); this latter method is frowned upon, because it presents the risk of the patient's developing pancreatic fistulae.

Nursing Management

1 Should external drainage be done, recognize the irritating qualities of the pancreatic enzyme; meticulous skin care is required.
2 Maintain adequate drainage, avoiding tube dislodgment.

PANCREATIC CANCER

Cancer may arise in the head, body or tail of the pancreas; insulin-secreting pancreatic islet cells may or may not be involved.

Clinical Manifestations

The 'big three' are *weight loss, pain* and *jaundice.*

1 Initial symptoms of cancer of the pancreas are often vague, thereby accounting for a reported 4–9 months' delay from onset of symptoms to diagnosis.
2 Disease usually occurs in older men; alcoholism may be a contributing cause.
3 Weight loss, anorexia, dyspepsia, nausea, some bowel disturbance and occasionally chills and fever develop.
4 Intermittent, dull-to-severe, vague, epigastric, or back pain, often aggravated by eating or associated with fullness and bloating occurs.
   a. Right upper quadrant pain suggests involvement of the head of pancreas.
   b. Left upper quadrant pain suggests involvement of the body or tail of pancreas.
   c. Pain often radiates to back or is exclusively in back.
   d. Pain is often worse at night, aggravated in lying-down position and relieved by lying with legs drawn up or by walking bent over.
   e. Fear of eating may take place.
5 The patient may experience depression and loss of ambition combined with a feeling of anxiety and premonition of serious illness.
6 Obstruction of the common bile duct produces jaundice, clay-coloured stools, dark urine and itching (due to cancer of head of pancreas).
     Differentiation must be made between jaundice due to biliary obstruction (due to a stone in the common duct) and jaundice due to hepatic metastases.

Diagnosis

1 Blood studies including serum bilirubin, alkaline phosphates, SGOT and prothrombin time.
2 Secretin studies and radiologic procedures: gallbladder studies, and possibly fibreoptic duodenoscopy with cannulation of papilla and pancreatic ductography, or transhepatic cholangiography.
3 Scanning.
4 Angiography.
5 Ultrasonography.
6 Computed tomography.

Treatment

Surgical only: although surgical cures are possible, 5-year survival is about 25%. Tumour is removed if it has not invaded important surrounding structures.

1   Whipple Resection—removal of head (and sometimes neck) of pancreas; removal of adjacent stomach, distal portion of common duct and duodenum. Patient has severe malabsorption afterward.
2   If Whipple procedure cannot be done, jaundice should be relieved by diverting bile from gallbladder into jejunum (cholecystojejunostomy). If duodenum is invaded, gastrojejunostomy should be done to bypass duodenal obstruction.
3   For cancer of the body and tail of the pancreas, distal pancreatectomy and splenectomy are the most commonly employed procedures.
4   Total pancreatectomy—en bloc resection of the common bile duct, stomach, duodenum, pancreas and spleen.

Nursing Management

1   Because of the patient's poor nutritional state, it is a challenge to maintain adequate caloric levels. A bland, low fat diet is recommended plus whatever he can tolerate without overeating.
2   Medium-chain triglycerides are better tolerated causing less fat excretion.
3   Alcohol to be avoided.
4   Anticholinergics used.
5   See management of the patient undergoing major gastrointestinal surgery (p. 441) and biliary surgery (p. 506).

FURTHER READING

Books

Angell, J C (1978) The Acute Abdomen for the Man on the Spot, 3rd edition, Pitman
Bloom, A (1981) Toohey's Medicine for Nurses, 13th edition, Churchill Livingstone
Bodley Scott, R (1978) Price's Textbook for the Practice of Medicine, Oxford Medical Publications
Chilman, A and Thomas, M (1981) Understanding Nursing Care, Churchill Livingstone
Evans, D M D (1979) Special Tests and Thier Meaning, 12th edition, Faber

Henderson, M A (1980) Essential Surgery for Nurses, Churchill Livingstone

Hollanders, D (1979) Gastro Intestinal Endoscopy, Baillière Tindall
MacLeod, J (1981) Davidson's Principles and Practice of Medicine, 13th edition, Churchill Livingstone
Nash, D E (1980) The Principles and Practice of Surgery for Nurses and the Applied Professions, 7th edition, W Arnold
Rains and Ritchie, (1977) Short Practice of Surgery, 17th edition, Lewis
Shafer, et al. (1975) Medical-Surgical Nursing, 6th edition, Mosby

Sykes, M (1981) Aspects of Gastroenterology for Nurses, Pitman
Tiffany, R (1980) Cancer Nursing, Update Baillière Tindall
Tiffany, R (1978) Oncology for Nurses and Health Care Professionals, volume 2, Allen and Unwin
Tinker, J and Porter, S (1980) A Course in Intensive Therapy Nursing, Edwards Arnold
Todd, I P (1978) Intestinal Stomas, William Heinemann Medical
Triger, D (1981) Practical Management of Liver Disease, Blackwell Scientific Publications
Wright, L (1974) Bowel Function in Hospital Patients, R.C.N.

Articles

Beck, M L (1981) Diagnostic tests: three common gastro-intestinal tests—and how to help your patient through each, Nursing, 11: 34–35
Breckman, B (1981) Stoma care—and radiotherapy, Journal of Community Nursing, 5: 26–30
Breckman, B (1981) Nursing care study—Abdomino-perineal excision of rectum, Nursing Times, 77: 1701–1703
British Medical Journal (1981) Prognosis of Crohn's Disease, British Medical Journal: 1415–1416
Foulkes, B (1981) Stoma care—tell it like it is, Journal of Community Nursing, 4: 4–6
Graham, P (1981) Reflection on the role of a stoma care nurse, Nursing Times, 77: 1107–1109
McCrea, J and Cherry F M (1981) Massive small bowel ressection, Nursing Times, 77: 592–594
McConnell, E A (1981) Curtailing a life threatening crisis—GI bleeding, Nursing 11: 70–73
Motson, R (1981) Ileal reservoir—side stepping the stoma, Nursing Mirror, 152: 36–40
Stuchfield, B (1981) Nursing care study—ileal reservoir: reserving their strength, Nursing Mirror, 152:
Tedder, R S (1980) Hepatitis B in hospitals, British Journal of Hospital Medicine, 23: 266
The Practitioner (1981) The symposium, liver, gall bladder and pancreas, Practitioner, 225: 447–506
Thomson, A D (1981) Cirrhosis of the liver, Practitioner, 225: 449–450, 453–455, 457–459
Wilson, D (1981) Colostomy—changing the body image, Nursing Mirror, 152: 38–40

Chapter 5

METABOLIC AND ENDOCRINE DISORDERS

1. Disorders of the Thyroid Gland

THE THYROID GLAND AND TESTS OF THYROID FUNCTION

Physiology

1   The thyroid gland affects the rate at which all tissues metabolize.
    a. Speed of chemical reactions.
    b. Volume of oxygen consumed.
    c. Amount of heat produced.
2   The stimulating effect is through the production and distribution of two
    hormones:

a. Levothyroxine (T_4)—contains four iodine atoms; maintains body's metabolism in a steady state; it is believed that T_4 serves as a precursor of T_3.
b. Triiodothyronine (T_3)—contains three iodine atoms; is approximately five times as potent as thyroxine; has a more rapid metabolic action and utilization than thyroxine. Most conversion of T_4 to T_3 occurs at the cellular level in the periphery. Some T_3 is produced in the thyroid gland.

Diagnosis

Radioiodine (^{131}I) (^{99m}Tc)

1   ^{131}I *uptake.*
   a. A solution of sodium iodide-131 is administered orally to the fasting patient.
   b. After a prescribed interval (anywhere from 2 to 48 hours, but frequently by 24 hours), measurements are taken with a scintillator of radioactive counts per minute that are detected above the isthmus of the thyroid gland.
   c. Normal thyroid will remove 15–50% of the iodine from the bloodstream.
   d. Hyperthyroidism may result in the removal of as much as 90% of the iodine from the bloodstream.
2   *Thyroidal iodide clearance.*
   a. Radioiodine clearance test measures the amount of circulating blood that is completely cleared of iodide per unit of time.
   b. Radioiodine is injected intravenously; radioactivity over the thyroid gland is measured continuously for 30–60 min—total amount of ^{131}I concentrated in the gland per minute is computed.
   c. Also, plasma ^{131}I content is measured in samples of blood collected 45–70 min after injection; these values are averaged.
   d. Thyroid ^{131}I divided by the mean plasma ^{131}I equals thyroid clearance, i.e., millilitres of plasma cleared of iodide per minute.
   e. Normal, 25 ml/min; hyperthyroidism, 250 ml/min; hypothyroidism, 1.6 ml/min.
3   ^{131}I *excretion.*
   a. Urinary output of radioiodine is measured during 6- and 24-hour periods after ingestion.
   b. Normal, 40–80% of ingested iodine in 24 hours; hyperthyroidism, less than 40%; hypothyroidism, greater than 80%.
4   *Thyroid 'scan' ^{131}I.*
   a. Patient ingests sodium iodide-131 and is scanned the next day; if medium is given intravenously, patient may be scanned within 30–60 min.
   b. Patient is supine; the detector head of the scintillation camera with a pinhole colimeter is centred over the patient's neck.
   c. The thyroid images from the oscilloscope of the camera are recorded on film; colour adds dimension.
   d. A decrease in ^{132}I uptake in a particular area of the thyroid is considered suggestive of malignancy.
5   *Thyroid 'scan' ^{99m}Tc*
   a. Patient is given an intravenous injection of sodium pertechnetate.
   b. A scintillator electromechanically maps the activity in the scanned area to produce a scintogram.

c. This simple procedure facilitates the diagnosis of goitrous changes, cold and hot nodules, cystic degeneration and thyroid malignancy.

6 *Triiodothyronine (T_3) suppression test.*
   a. Measure 24-hour radioactive iodine uptake.
   b. Place patient on T_3 for 7 days.
   c. Again measure 24-hour radioactive iodine uptake.
   d. Normal: Suppression to a radioactive iodine uptake below 20% at 24 hours (half original value). Graves disease: No suppression.

Serum Thyroxine (T_4)

1 Normal values: 3.5–8.5 μg
2 Elevated values found with oestrogens and pregnancy.

T_s Resin Uptake

1 Is an indirect measure of thyroid function based on the available protein-binding sites in a serum sample which can bind to radioactive T_3.
2 The radioactive triiodothyronine is added to the serum sample in the test tube.
3 The effect of oestrogen and pregnancy is to produce an increase in binding sites, causing a lowered percentage of binding by the available thyroid hormones.
4 Rates:
   a. Normal binding: 25–35%.
   b. High T_3 is associated with hyperthyroidism.
   c. Low T_3 is associated with hypothyroidism.
5 This test is often used in conjunction with serum thyroxine (T_4).

Thyrotropin-releasing hormone (TRH)

1 Prior to TRH injection, draw a blood specimen.
2 Doctor injects into venous system 0.2 mg synthetic TRH; draw blood specimen for TSH (thyroid-stimulating hormone).
3 Draw blood specimens.

HYPOTHYROIDISM

Hypothyroidism may be classified as primary, secondary or tertiary. *Primary hypothyroidism* is a condition resulting from the inability of the thyroid gland to secrete a sufficient amount of hormone. *Secondary hypothyroidism* is caused by a failure of the pituitary gland to secrete an adequate amount of TSH (thyroid-stimulating hormone). *Tertiary hypothyroidism* results from failure of the hypothalamus to release thyroid-releasing hormone (TRH).

Cretinism is a condition in which a person is born with a thyroid deficiency. The mother may have a similar deficiency.

Causes

Of primary hypothyroidism:

1 Prior surgery or radioactive iodine therapy.
2 Idiopathic.
3 Hashimoto's thyroiditis.

Clinical Manifestations

1 Temperature and pulse become subnormal.
2 Patient begins to gain weight.
3 Skin becomes thickened and dry.
4 The hair thins and falls out.
5 Menorrhagia may develop.
6 Blood pressure is low; feet are cold.
7 Facial expression becomes stolid and mask-like.
8 Complaint of fatigue is most common.
9 Mental processes become dulled.
10 Neurological signs are manifested (polyneuropathy, cerebellar ataxia).
11 There may be a tendency to rapid development of arteriosclerosis.

Diagnosis

1 Total serum thyroxine level; low levels are indicative of hypothyroidism.
2 T_3 (radioactive triiodothyronine uptake); low value suggests hypothyroidism.
3 Thyroid-stimulating hormone; elevated level is suggestive of hypothyroidism.
4 Slow reflex return suggests hypothyroidism.
5 Complete physical examination.

Treatment

Objective

To restore a normal metabolic state.

1 Administer thyroid hormone: thyroxine (Eltroxin).
   Give once a day.
2 Anticipate such effects of treatment as:
   a. Diuresis, decreased puffiness.
   b. Improved reflexes and muscle tone.
   c. Accelerated pulse rate.
   d. A slightly higher level of total serum thyroxine.

Advanced Hypothyroidism

Effects

1 May lead to myxoedema coma.
2 Causes increased susceptibility to all hypnotic and sedative drugs.
3 Survival rate is 50%.

Clinical Manifestations

Hypotension, unresponsiveness, bradycardia, hypoventilation, hyponatraemia, possible convulsions, hypothermia (cerebral hypoxia).

Objectives of Treatment and Nursing Management

1 *To maintain vital functions with supportive therapy.*
   a. Measure arterial blood gases to determine CO_2 retention.
   b. Provide assisted ventilation if needed to combat hypoventilation.

c. Even though hypothermia exists, do not apply external heat, since the resulting increased oxygen requirements and decreased peripheral vascular tone may compound the existing cardiac failure.

d. Administer fluids cautiously even though hyponatraemia is present.

e. Give glucose in concentrated amounts to prevent fluid overload if hypoglycaemia is in evidence.

2 *To replace thyroid hormone in order to assist in achieving a euthyroid state.*

a. Because triiodothyronine acts more quickly than thyroxine, give this initially; if patient is unconscious, give via stomach tube.

b. Administer thyroxine (Eltroxin) parenterally (until consciousness is restored) to restore thyroxine level; continue daily.

c. Later, continue patient on oral thyroid hormone therapy.

d. Recognize that with rapid administration of thyroid hormone, plasma thyroxine levels may initiate adrenal insufficiency—hence, steroid therapy may be initiated.

3 *To recognize precipitating factors and avoid them so that further cardiovascular damage is prevented.*

a. Treat initiating factors such as infection, stress from trauma.

b. Prevent chilling to avoid increasing metabolic rate, which in turn places strain on the heart.

Provide bed socks, bed jacket, warm environment.

c. Recognize sensitivity of patient to hypnotics and tranquillizers; use in small doses and provide effective observation.

d. Note that patient is usually disturbed by his mental and physical changes; be alert for signs of depression. Be compassionate and understanding.

4 *To initiate comfort measures and promote good care.*

a. Apply lubricant to the skin since it is usually dry and scaly.

b. Observe for pressure areas and initiate measures to stimulate circulation to these areas.

c. Arrange furniture to prevent patient's bumping into it, since he bruises easily because of increased capillary fragility.

5 *To encourage proper fluid and nutritional intake.*

a. Offer fluids frequently and include dietary roughage to prevent constipation.

b. Administer stool softeners if necessary.

c. Discourage straining at stool because of increased strain on the heart.

d. Serve attractive low calorie meals; this patient is usually overweight, although his appetite is poor.

HYPERTHYROIDISM

Hyperthyroidism (diffuse toxic goitre) is excessive activity of the thyroid gland.

Incidence

More common in women than in men.

Aetiology

1 Unknown.

2   Possible causes.
   a. LATS (long-acting thyroid stimulator) and/or LATS protector may be found in serum; it is capable of inducing iodine accumulation and thyroid hyperplasia independent of the pituitary.
   b. May appear after an emotional shock, infection or emotional stress.
   c. Genetic predisposition, female sex.
   d. B and T lymphocytes (immunological factors).

Clinical Manifestations

1   Single or multiple adenomas.
2   Nervousness, emotional hyperexcitability, irritability, apprehension.
3   Difficulty in sitting quietly.
4   Rapid pulse, at rest as well as on exertion (ranges between 90 and 160); palpitation is evident.
5   Low heat tolerance; profuse perspiration; flushed skin (warm, soft, moist).
6   Fine tremor of hands; change in bowel habits—constipation or diarrhoea.
7   Bulging eyes (exophthalmos)—startled expression.
8   Increased appetite—progressive weight loss.
9   Muscle fatigue and weakness; *amenorrhoea*.
10   Atrial fibrillation possible. (Cardiac decompensation is common in elderly patients.)

Diagnosis

1   Serum thyroxine   ⎫
2   T_3 resin uptake. ⎬ if elevated—hyperthyroidism is suspected.

Clinical Course

1   Mild, characterized by remissions and exacerbations.
2   In rare instances, it may progress relentlessly—leading to emaciation, extreme nervousness, delirium, disorientation and eventual death.

Immediate Treatment

1   Admit patient to hospital only if 'thyroid crisis' (see p. 531) or other complications, such as heart failure, are impending.
2   Administer sedatives such as phenobarbitone or diazepam (Valium) or tranquillizers such as chlordiazepoxide (Librium) to combat nervousness, hyperactivity and irritability.
3   Give vitamin supplements to offset demands of appetite which may continue after hyperthyroidism is controlled.
4   Administer digitalis if heart failure or atrial fibrillation occurs.
5   Give propranolol for sinus tachycardia and other supraventricular arrhythmias.

Other Forms of Treatment

1   General considerations.
   a. Types of treatment—pharmacology, radiation and surgery.

   b. Treatment depends on causes, age of patient, severity of disease and complications.
2 *According to causes.*
   a. Remission of hyperthyroidism (Graves' Disease) occurs spontaneously within 1–2 years; however, relapse can be expected in half of the patients.
   All three forms of therapy are appropriate.
   b. Nodular toxic goitre—excessive amounts of thyroid hormone secreted.
   Surgery or radioiodine is preferred.
   c. Thyroid carcinoma.
   Surgery or radiation.
3 *According to age of patient.*
   a. Radioiodine therapy may be used in all patients, regardless of age, when other forms of therapy are contraindicated.
   b. Use radioiodine in older patients for whom surgery is contraindicated.
4 *According to severity.*
   Administer drug therapy before proceeding with radioiodine or surgery.
5 *According to patient preference.*
   a. Radioiodine or surgery is suggested to patient who does not take medication regularly.
   b. Surgery is recommended to those who prefer it.

Pharmacotherapy—Drugs that Inhibit Hormone Formation

Objective

To bring the metabolic rate to normal as soon as possible and maintain it at this level.

Anticipated Results

1 Diagnosis can be confirmed if patient responds to antithyroid therapy.
2 Autonomic nervous system is brought into balance and patient is more comfortable.
3 Opportunity is provided for getting to know the patient.

Thiourea Derivatives

1 Most commonly used.
2 Act by interfering with the formation of thyroid hormone.
3 Administered orally.
   a. Detectable in blood in 15 min.
   b. 80% absorbed within 2 hours
   c. Because half-life is short, must be given every 6–8 hours.
4 Preparations.
   Propylthiouracil.
5 Assessment and duration of treatment determined by clinical criteria.
   a. Observe clinical course—thyroid gland usually gets smaller.
   b. Measure T_4 and T_3 uptake to determine adequacy of dose.
   c. Continue treatment for 1–2 years; if euthyroidism cannot be maintained without therapy, then another form of therapy (i.e, radioactive iodine (RAI) or surgery) should be recommended.
   d. Gradually withdraw therapy to prevent exacerbation.

  e. For relapses, recommend radioiodine or surgery.
6 Toxicity.
  a. Agranulocytosis is a most serious toxic condition, occurring with a sudden onset—therefore, patient should be informed of this possibility and urged to report any signs of infection such as fever, sore throat, upper respiratory infection.
  b. Skin rashes, fever, urticaria, granulocytopaenia, inflammation of the salivary glands are other possible side effects.
  c. Substitute an alternate drug if there are toxic manifestations.

Pharmacotherapy–Drugs that Control Peripheral Symptoms of Hyperthyroidism

Propranolol (Inderal)

1 Acts as a beta-adrenoceptor blocking agent.
2 Abolishes tachycardia, tremor, excess sweating, nervousness.
3 Controls hyperthyroid symptoms until antithyroid drugs or radioiodine can take effect.

Radioactive Iodine

1 Action.
  a. Limits secretion of thyroid hormone by damaging and destroying thyroid tissue.
  b. Control dosage so that hypothyroidism does not occur.
2 Considerations in use.
  a. Radiation thyroiditis, a transient exacerbation of hyperthyroidism, may occur as a result of leakage of thyroid hormone into the circulation from damaged follicles.
  b. Iodide should not be given prior to radioiodine since it interferes with the uptake of ^{131}I.
  c. Vigilance is required during treatment to detect occurrence of hypothyroidism.

Psychotherapy

1 Greater emphasis is being placed on the effect that psychogenic factors have on the severity of this disease.
2 A determination needs to be made in caring for each patient about whether psychotherapy would be of value in preventing exacerbations.

Surgery

Subtotal Thyroidectomy

Effective in treating hyperthyroidism; involves removal of most of the thyroid gland.

Preparation for Surgery

1 Patient must be euthyroid at time of surgery.
2 Administer thiourea derivatives to control hyperthyroidism.
3 Give iodide to increase firmness of thyroid gland and reduce its vascularity.

Nursing Alert: Observe patient for evidence of iodine toxicity–swelling of buccal mucosa, excessive salivation, coryza, skin eruptions. If these occur, discontinue iodides.

Complications

1 Damage to recurrent laryngeal nerve may occur (1–4%).
   a. Unilateral damage—results in minimal voice change.
   b. Bilateral damage—serious airway obstruction develops.
2 Hypothyroidism.
      Occurs in 5% of patients in first postoperative year; increases at rate of 2–3%/year.
3 Hypoparathyroidism.
   a. About 4% occurrence.
   b. Usually is mild and transient.
   c. Requires calcium supplements intravenously and orally when more severe.

Nursing Management

See p. 533.

Exophthalmos in Hyperthyroidism

Exophthalmos is abnormal protrusion of the eyeball, probably due to an auto-immune phenomenon.

Treatment

Objective

To protect eyes from irritation.

Mild

1 Recommend wearing sunglasses.
2 Instil methylcellulose eyedrops 0.5–1% for comfort.
3 Advise the patient to elevate his head while sleeping to improve drainage.

Rapidly Progressive or Severe (chemosis, conjunctivitis, proptosis, visual impairment)

1 Tarsorrhaphy (suturing eyelids together) may be required—to extend lid when proptosis is so marked that lid does not close during sleep.
2 Administer corticosteroids in high doses to help arrest rapid progression of exophthalmos; with improvement, reduce dose.

Orbital Decompression Procedures

1 Decompression of orbit into ethmoid sinus and maxillary antrum.
2 Removal of lateral orbital wall.
3 Decompression of orbit into cranial cavity.

Muscle Surgery

1 Correction of imbalance of extraocular muscles.
2 Lysis of adhesions.

Experimental Study

Research continues into supravoltage orbital irradiation and use of azathioprine.

Thyroid Crisis

Thyroid crisis is characterized by tachycardia, vasomotor activity, agitation and, at times, delirium and heart failure. It is assumed to result from an increase in thyroid hormone.

Predisposing Factors

1 Decompensation of hyperthyroid state occurs spontaneously.
2 May be precipitated by infection (pneumonia, appendicitis, pharyngitis, cystitis); surgical procedures (thyroidectomy, caesarean section, appendicectomy); minor procedures (dental extractions, forceps delivery); insulin reaction; pulmonary embolism; palpation of thyroid gland; and even fear.
3 Crisis may also be precipitated by inadequate surgical preoperative preparation (unrecognized hyperthyroidism).

Clinical Manifestations

1 Hyperpyrexia, diarrhoea, dehydration, tachycardia, arrhythmias, (Fig. 5.1).
2 Coma, leading to shock and death.

Objectives of Treatment and Nursing Management

To Control Synthesis and Release of Thyroid Hormone

1 Administer sodium iodide intravenously—inhibits release of hormone from thyroid.
2 Give propylthiouracil orally or by nasogastric tube to prevent accumulation of hormone stores.

To Diminish Metabolic Effects of Thyroid Agents and to Reverse Peripheral Effects of Hyperthyroidism

Administer propranolol, reserpine or guanethidine.

To Restore and Maintain Vital Functions.

1 Give steroids because of possibility of a relative adrenal insufficiency state.
2 Administer fluids, electrolytes and vasopressor agents to treat dehydration, electrolyte imbalance and hypotension.
3 Control agitation with intravenous barbiturates.
4 Lower the temperature with electric fans and salicylates.
5 Try phenothiazines in large doses for hyperpyrexia, but watch for hypotension.

CLINICAL PICTURE OF THYROTOXIC CRISIS

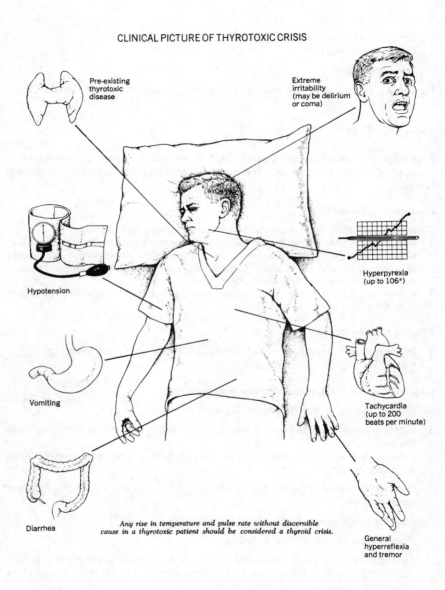

Figure 5.1.   Thyrotoxic crisis. (From: Hospital Medicine, 3: 39, Jan. 1967 by permission. Copyright 1967 Hospital Publications, Inc.)

6   Sustain nutritional requirements with glucose intravenously; administer vitamin B.
7   Guard against infection; treat if infection is likely.

Medical and Nursing Management of the Patient Undergoing Thyroidectomy

Preoperative Objectives

To Provide a Restful and Therapeutic Environment

1   Place the patient in a unit which is away from disturbing sights, very ill patients and noisy lifts or kitchens.
2   Provide, if possible, a pleasant window view.
3   Suggest radio music programmes rather than exciting soap operas or films.
4   Restrict visitors who may upset the patient with disturbing conversation or boisterous tendencies.
5   Administer soothing back massage at prescribed rest times during the day; draw the blinds for rest times.
6   Be selective in placing the patient near other suitable patients.
7   Gain the confidence of the patient and attempt to uncover anything that might cause aggravation or unhappiness; if a disturbance exists, it could thwart treatment efforts.

To Regulate His Nutritional Intake

Order an ample diet of carbohydrate and protein foods.

To Study the Exact Nature of the Endocrine Problem by Supporting the Patient Undergoing Various Diagnostic Tests

1   Explain the purpose and requirements of each prescribed test.
2   Inform the patient and visitors of safeguards required during radioisotope tests.
3   Remind the patient that he must remain in his room until tests are completed.

To Prepare the Patient for Surgery

1   Shave the upper chest, neck, up to chin edge.
2   Make a special effort to ensure that this patient has a good night's rest preceding surgery.
3   Explain to the patient that speaking is to be minimized immediately postoperatively and that oxygen may be administered to facilitate breathing.
4   Tell the patient that postoperatively, fluids may be given intravenously to maintain fluid, electrolyte and nutritional needs; glucose may also be given intravenously in the hours before the administration of anaesthesia.
5   Proceed with usual preoperative preparation.

Postoperative Objectives

To Provide Optimum Immediate Postoperative Care in Order to Avoid Complications

1   Move the patient carefully; provide adequate support to the head, so that no tension is placed on the sutures.

2   Place the patient in an upright position with the head elevated and supported by pillows; avoid flexion of neck.
3   Administer oxygen for a few hours if breathing is laboured; check the infusion for prescribed flow rate and smooth flow into patient.
4   Avoid administration of adrenaline, noradrenaline, anticholinergic (atropine) because of patient's sensitivity to these drugs.
5   Discontinue antithyroid drugs as a metabolic rate closer to normal is attained (to continue such medication might cause a hypometabolism—hypothyroidism).

To Assess the Patient's Condition as He Emerges From Anaesthesia

1   *Damage of laryngeal nerve.*
    a. Observe for hoarseness or 'whispery' voice suggesting possible nerve damage.
    b. Recognize that a bilateral flaccid paralysis may lead to cord paralysis→closure of glottis→suffocation, months after operation.
2   *Haemorrhage*
    a. Be alert for this possibility between 12 to 24 hours postoperatively.
    b. Watch for signs of irregular breathing, swelling and choking—signs pointing to the possibility of haemorrhage and tracheal compression.
    c. Keep a tracheostomy set in the patient's room for 48 hours for emergency use.
3   *Tetany.*
    a. The likelihood that tetany may develop depends on the number of parathyroid glands that have been removed or disturbed:
    1—no clinical tetany.
    2—tetany mild and transient.
    4—tetany within 24 hours and worsening within the next 24 hours.
    b. Progression of signs.
    (1) *First*—tingling of toes and fingers and around the mouth; apprehension.
    (2) *Second*—positive Chvostek's sign (tapping the cheek over the facial nerve causes a twitch of the lip or facial muscles).
    (3) *Third*—Trousseau's sign (carpopedal spasm induced by occluding circulation in the arm with a blood pressure cuff).

Medical and Nursing Management

1   Position patient for optimal ventilation; pillow may be removed to prevent head from bending forward and compressing trachea.
2   Keep siderails in position and position patient to prevent injury if a convulsion occurs; do not use restraints since they only aggravate patient and may result in muscle strain or fractures.
3   Have equipment available to treat respiratory difficulties; provide tracheostomy and cardiac arrest equipment.
4   Determine calcium levels: If in 48 hours levels are low (normal range 2.25–2.55 mmol/l) replacement of calcium (gluconate, lactate) is done intravenously.
5   Exert caution in intravenous administration of calcium to the patient who has renal disease or who is receiving digitalis preparations.

OTHER THYROID-RELATED CONDITIONS

Subacute Thyroiditis

Thyroiditis is inflammation of the thyroid gland.

Incidence

Affects younger women predominantly.

Clinical Manifestations

1   Pain, swelling, thyroid tenderness which lasts weeks or months, then disappears.
2   Pain referred to the ear, making swallowing difficult and uncomfortable.
3   Fever, malaise, chills.
4   Irritability, nervousness, insomnia and weight loss.

Treatment

1   Patient may be placed on thyroid medications to maintain a normal level of circulating thyroid hormone.
2   Steroids may be administered in active inflammatory stage.

Hashimoto's Thyroiditis (Chronic Thyroiditis)

Hashimoto's thyroiditis is a progressive disease of the thyroid gland caused by infiltration of lymphocytes and resulting in progressive destruction of the parenchyma and hypothyroidism.

Cause

Unknown. Believed to be autoimmune disease, genetically transmitted and perhaps related to Graves' disease.

Incidence

1   Predominantly affects women (95%) in their 40s and 50s.
2   Possibly the most common cause of adult hyperthyroidism.
3   Appears to be increasing since it was described in 1912.

Clinical Manifestations

1   Marked by slowly developing firm enlargement of the thyroid gland.
2   Usually no gross nodules.
3   Basal metabolic rate usually low.
4   Normal or high concentration of protein-bound iodine.
5   Hyperthyroidism develops in the later stages of the disease.

Diagnostic Testing

1   Antibody test—agglutination of tanned red cells.

2 Thyroxine and resin T_3 uptake determination.
3 Thyroid needle biopsy.

Treatment

1 Patient should be placed on thyroid medications to maintain a normal level of circulating thyroid hormone; this is done to suppress production of thyrotropin, to prevent enlargement of the thyroid and/or to maintain a euthyroid state.
2 Firm nodular thyroid enlargement may at times be associated with tracheal compression, cough, hoarseness. Resection of isthmus can produce relief of symptoms.

Cancer of the Thyroid

Incidence

1 It has been estimated that of the thyroid lumps which occur in 40 000 out of 1 000 000 persons in any one year, only 25 will be cancerous; this is a relatively rare disease.
2 It occurs twice as frequently in females as in males and more frequently in whites than in blacks; incidence increases with age.
3 It appears well established that an association exists between external radiation to the head and neck in infancy and childhood and subsequent development of thyroid carcinoma. (Between 1940–1960 radiation therapy was often given to shrink enlarged tonsil and adenoid tissue, to treat acne or to reduce an enlarged thymus.)
   It is advised that these individuals should:
   a. Consult a doctor.
   b. Request an isotope thyroid scan as part of the evaluation.
   c. Submit to surgical thyroidectomy or take thyroid hormones if abnormalities of the gland are present.
   d. Continue with annual checkups if all is normal.

Types

1 Papillary and well-differentiated adenocarcinoma.
   a. Growth is slow and spread is confined to lymph nodes that surround thyroid area.
   b. Cure rate is excellent after removal of involved areas.
2 Rapidly growing, widely metastasizing type.
   a. Occurs predominantly in middle-aged and elderly persons.
   b. Brief encouraging response may occur with x-ray irradiation.
   c. Progression of disease is rapid; high mortality rate.

Diagnosis

1 History and physical examination are important.
2 If a scan is to be done, ^{99m}Tc is preferred since it delivers a much lower radiation than ^{131}I.

3   ^{123}I, when purified (and when it becomes available), will probably be preferred over ^{131}I and ^{99m}Tc because of even lower radiation.
4   Needle biopsy is recommended only for the very skilled performer and for the experienced pathologist.
5   Surgical exploration.

Treatment

1   Surgical removal is extensive, as required.
2   Thyroid replacement.
   a. Thyroid hormone is administered to suppress secretion of TSH.
   b. Such treatment is continued indefinitely and requires annual checkups.
3   For unresectable cancer, patient is referred to a thyroid specialist for consideration of treatment with ^{131}I, chemotherapy or radiation therapy.

2. Disorders of the Parathyroid Glands

THE PARATHYROID GLANDS

The *parathyroid glands* are small, bean-sized structures embedded in the posterior section of the thyroid gland.

Functions

1   Produce, store and secrete parathormone.
2   Increase plasma calcium ions by acting on:
   a. The kidney—to decrease elimination of calcium ions in the urine.
   b. The gastrointestinal tract—to increase absorption of calcium ions from chyme.
   c. Bone—to increase its contributions of calcium ions to the plasma.

HYPERPARATHYROIDISM

Hyperparathyroidism is overactivity of the parathyroids.

Cause

An overgrowth of parathyroid glands.

Clinical Manifestations

1   Decalcification of bones.
   a. Skeletal pain, backache, pain on weight-bearing, pathologic fractures, deformities, formation of bony cysts.
   b. Formation of bone tumours—overgrowth of osteoclasts.
2   Formation of calcium containing stones in the kidneys.

3 Depression of neuromuscular apparatus.
   a. The patient may trip, drop objects, show general fatigue and experience blurring of the mind.
   b. Cardiac standstill may result.

Diagnosis

1 Persistently elevated serum calcium (Normal range 2.25–2.55 mmol/l; test must be taken three times to determine consistency of results.
2 Exclusion of all other causes of hypercalcaemia—malignancy, vitamin D excess, multiple myeloma, sarcoidosis, milk-alkali syndrome, drugs such as thiazides, Cushing's disease, hyperthyroidism.
3 Skeletal changes—revealed by x-ray.
4 Diagnosis often extremely difficult (complications may occur before this condition is diagnosed).
5 Cineradiography will disclose parathyroid tumours more readily than x-ray.

Complications

1 Kidney disturbances.
   a. Formation of renal stones.
   b. Calcification of kidney parenchyma.
   c. Renal shutdown.
2 Gastrointestinal complications.
   Ulceration of upper gastrointestinal tract (stomach, duodenum) leading to haemorrhage and perforation.
3 Skeletal problems.
   a. Simple demineralization.
   b. Cysts and fibrosis of marrow—leading to fractures.
   c. Collapse of vertebral bodies and fractures of the ribs.

Objective of Treatment and Nursing Management

To Offset the Likelihood of Impending Complications

1 Provide adequate hydration—administer water, glucose and electrolytes by mouth or intravenously.

Nursing Alert: A low specific gravity for urine does not necessarily mean adequate hydration.

2 Avoid calcium and alkalies in the diet to prevent stone formation and renal calcification. Daily serum calcium and urea estimations are taken.
3 Administer diuretic—frusemide (Lasix).

Nursing Alert: Thiazide diuretics should not be used in the patient with hyperparathyroidism since they decrease the renal excretion of calcium, thereby causing hypercalcaemia.

4 Administer phosphate therapy as prescribed to control hypercalcaemia
   Daily serum calcium, urea and electrolyte estimations are taken.
5 Limit operative procedures until primary metabolic disorder is treated.

    a. A rising serum calcium level may indicate increasing dehydration—impending crisis.

    b. A falling serum calcium indicates dehydration is being corrected.

To Treat Complications as They Arise

1 For ureteral stone—cystoscopic manipulation.
2 For urinary tract infection—antibiotics, high fluid input.
3 For upper gastrointestinal ulceration—aluminium hydroxide and proteins other than milk.
4 For ulcer haemorrhage not stopped by conservative measures—surgical plication.
5 For fractures—treatment for vertebral body fractures.
                —strapping for broken ribs.
                —fixation of other long bones.
                —continued hydration of patient.
                —earliest mobilization of fracture areas.

To Operate and Remove Parathyroid Tissue

This is resorted to when diagnosis is established and clinical condition warrants definitive treatment.

To Develop Priorities of Care in the Postoperative Phase that will Control Possible Concomitant Complications

1 Assess fluid input and output.
2 Recognize that the patient will retain some fluid.
    a. This will be shown by a low urinary output.
    b. Therefore, avoid overhydration for first day or two.
3 Avoid giving calcium until nature of the patient's calcium level is determined.
    a. To verify success of operation.
    b. To observe level to which calcium falls and the rate at which it falls.
        (1) If calcium level fails to fall, surgery was inadequate.
        (2) If calcium levels falls somewhat but not to normal and then rises, surgery was inadequate.
    c. To determine patient's skeletal deficit and need for additional calcium.
4 Evaluate signs and symptoms which may lead to tetany.
    a. Observe calcium levels—if well below normal and if decline continues into the second week, the skeletal system is absorbing calcium.
    If some involvement was noted preoperatively (elevated alkaline phosphatase level), calcium should be administered.
    b. Administer calcium—usually lactate or gluconate.
    When gastrointestinal tract cannot absorb large amount, administer intramuscularly as gluconate, or intravenously in emergency.
    c. Give vitamin D to increase absorption of calcium.
5 Reassure patient about skeletal recovery.
    a. Bone pain diminishes fairly quickly.
    b. Cysts, brown tumours and osteoporosis resolve themselves.
    c. Fractures are cared for by usual orthopaedic procedures.

HYPOPARATHYROIDISM

Hypoparathyroidism is a condition brought about by a diminution or absence of the secretion of the parathyroid gland.

Cause

1   Decrease in gland function (idiopathic hypoparathyroidism).
2   Surgical or radiation trauma to parathyroid glands.
3   Malignancy or metastasis from a cancer to the parathyroid glands.
4   Resistance to parathyroid hormone action.

Altered Physiology

1   Blood calcium falls to a low level—causing symptoms of muscular hyperirritability, uncontrolled spasms and hypocalcaemic tetany.
2   Blood phosphate level is elevated. Phosphate excretion by renal tubules is decreased.

Clinical Manifestations

1   Due to deficiency of parathormone.
    a. Accumulation of phosphorus in blood.
    b. Decrease in amount of blood calcium.
2   Tetany.
    a. General muscular hypertonia; attempts at voluntary movement result in tremors and spasmodic or unco-ordinated movements; fingers assume classic position.
    b. Chvostek sign—a spasm of facial muscles that occurs when muscles or branches of facial nerve are tapped.
    c. Trousseau sign—carpopedal spasm induced by occluding circulation in the arm with a blood pressure cuff.
    d. Reduced blood calcium level—to a low level (normal range 2.25–2.55 mmol/l).
    e. Laryngeal spasm.
3   Anxiety and apprehension are very marked.
4   Renal colic is often present if the patient has had stones; pre-existing stones loosen and fall down into the ureter.

Treatment and Nursing Management

1   Administer calcium.
    a. A syringe and an ampoule of a calcium solution are to be kept at the bedside at all times.
    b. Most rapidly effective calcium solution is ionized calcium chloride (10%).
    c. For rapid use to relieve severe tetany, infuse every 10 min.
        (1) Administer ionized calcium chloride (10%) slowly. It is highly irritating, stings and causes thrombosis; patient experiences unpleasant burning flush of skin and, more particularly, of the tongue. Too rapid calcium administration may cause cardiac arrest.

(2) Give calcium intravenously; calcium carbohydrate combination may also be used—gluconate (10%) is not irritating.

d. Continue a slow drip of intravenous saline containing calcium gluconate until control of tetany is assured; then switch to intramuscular or oral administration of calcium.

e. Later, add vitamin D to calcium intake—increases absorption of calcium and also induces a high level of calcium in the bloodstream.

2 Control anxiety.

a. It is difficult to reassure this patient since he has a strong feeling of impending disaster.

b. Administration of intravenous calcium seems to bring about rapid relief of anxiety.

3 Relieve renal colic.

Stone may have to be removed cystoscopically or by surgery.

4 Monitor for hypercalciuria. Recommended periodic 24-hour urinary calcium determinations.

5 Blood calcium is monitored periodically; variations in vitamin D may affect calcium levels.

6 Inform patient about symptoms of hypocalcaemia and hypercalcaemia; should these occur, he is to notify his doctor.

3. Diabetes Mellitus (Pancreatic Disorders)

DIABETES MELLITUS

Diabetes mellitus is a disease characterized by abnormalities of the endocrine secretions of the pancreas resulting in disordered metabolism of carbohydrate, fat and protein and, in time, structural abnormalities in a variety of tissues.

Altered Physiology

1 Insulin reduces the release of glucose from the liver by both inhibiting glycogenolysis and gluconeogenesis.

2 Insulin also promotes the storage of glycogen in the liver, the ulitization of glucose in the muscles and the storage of fat in adipose tissue by enhancing the transport of glucose across the cell wall. In nondiabetics, the rate of insulin-release from the pancreas is proportional to the amount of glucose in the blood.

3 In diabetes, insulin is not proportional to blood sugar levels because of several possible factors:

a. Insufficient numbers of islet cells (juvenile diabetes).

b. Delayed or insufficient release (adult-onset diabetes).

c. Excessive inactivation by chemical inhibitors of 'binders' in the circulation and at the cell membrane.

4 Glucose in the blood comes from ingested carbohydrates or from conversion of amino acids and fatty acids to glucose by the liver (gluconeogenesis). An elevated fasting blood glucose level in diabetes reflects the presence of

decreased utilization of glucose and increased gluconeogenesis. If the concentration of glucose in the blood is sufficiently high, the kidney does not reabsorb all of the filtered glucose; glucose then appears in the urine (glucosuria).

5   With increased gluconeogenesis (in part under the control of the adrenocortical hormones), protein and fats are mobilized rather than stored or deposited in the cells. Persistently elevated levels of fats in the blood may damage blood vessels.

6   When there is a deficiency of insulin, muscles cannot utilize glucose, and free fatty acids are mobilized from adipose tissue cells and broken down by the liver into ketone bodies for energy.

7   Diabetic ketoacidosis is characterized by excessive amounts of ketone bodies in the blood.

8   Patients with diabetic ketoacidosis exhibit hyperventilation and the loss of sodium, potassium, chloride and water from the body.

9   The net metabolic result of diabetes mellitus is loss of fat stores, liver glycogen, cellular protein, electrolytes and water.

10   The sequelae of long-term diabetes lead to involvement of large vessels in the brain, heart, kidneys and extremities and of the small vessels in the eyes and kidneys, and to neuropathy. The mechanism is not precisely determined.

Types of Diabetes

Differ in prognosis, treatment, causative mechanisms.

Growth-onset or Juvenile Type

1   Patient usually lacks insulin and requires exogenous insulin therapy.
2   Onset abrupt.
3   Stable or labile.
4   Uusally begins in childhood, but may occur at any age.
5   Patient more prone to ketoacidosis and is *dependent upon insulin*.

Maturity-onset (Adult Diabetes)

1   Usually occurs after 40; about three-quarters of adult-onset patients are obese.
2   Patient usually retains a capacity for endogenous insulin production.
3   Patient not usually ketosis-prone.
4   Usually stable.

Secondary or Nonhereditary

1   Damage to or removal of pancreatic islet tissue—tumours of pancreas, surgical removal of pancreas, pancreatitis.
2   Factors that increase peripheral resistance to insulin—acromegaly or obesity.
3   Disorders of endocrine glands other than pancreas.

Incidence

1   Approximately 5% of world population has diabetes mellitus—estimated that 25% of persons are carriers.

2 About 2% of British population has diabetes.
3 One-third of all patients have a known relative with the disease.

Individuals at Risk for Diabetes Mellitus

1 Relatives of known diabetics (heredity).
2 Overweight individuals.
3 Mothers of large babies or those who have had an abnormal obstetrical history.
4 Persons with early onset of arteriosclerosis.
   a. Premenopausal women with myocardial infarction.
   b. Men having myocardial infarctions before the age of 40.
5 Persons with frequent or chronic infections (gallbladder disease, pyelonephritis, pancreatitis).
6 Patients exhibiting temporary reduction in glucose tolerance during stress (myocardial infarction, infection, trauma, surgery).
7 Patients developing glucose intolerance during drug therapy (thiazides, glucocorticoids, ovulatory suppressants).
8 Persons with retinopathy, nephropathy, neuropathy or other vascular manifestations.

Clinical Manifestations

Growth-onset or Juvenile Diabetes

1 May occur in adults as well as children.
2 Abrupt onset—weight loss, weakness, polyuria (excessive excretion of urine), polydipsia (excessive thirst), polyphagia (excessive ingestion of food). (Polyphagia may be shortlived as the metabolic imbalance worsens.)
3 Patient prone to develop ketosis—may be brought into hospital with acidosis or in coma.

Maturity-onset

1 Early adult diabetes exhibits postprandial hypoglycaemia.
2 Insidious onset—fatigue, tendency to be drowsy after a meal, irritability, nocturia, pruritus (especially of vulva in the female), poorly healing skin wounds, blurring of vision, loss of weight, muscle cramps.
3 Symptoms may be absent in mild cases.
4 Stress (surgery, febrile illness, etc.) will induce hyperglycaemia.

Clinical Course

1 Intensity of diabetes mellitus, as measured by blood sugar levels, tends to wax and wane—depends on patient's general state of health, life stresses, dietary control, weight control, physical activity and other factors.
2 Lifelong care is mandatory—poorly controlled diabetes leads to accelerated development of neuropathy, nephropathy, retinopathy, generalized atherosclerosis and decreased resistance to infection. *The threat of complications always exists.*
3 Meticulous control of diabetes may postpone but does not necessarily prevent the development of complications.

Diagnosis

1   Suspiciousness of diabetes mellitus (signs and symptoms; family history).
2   *Urine testing for glucose (sugar).*
   a. Negative finding does not always rule out diabetes.
   b. Instruct patient to micturate and discard urine.
   c. Micturate 30–45 min later and check this specimen; the second urine specimen gives an indication of the blood sugar at the *time of testing.*
3   *Postprandial blood glucose.*
   a. Blood sample taken 2 hours after a high carbohydrate meal (75–100 g).
   b. Values over 10 mmol/l (50 mg/100 ml) of blood are diagnostic of diabetes. Values under 6.7 mmol/l (100 mg/100 ml) rule out diabetes.
   Values within this range indicate a glucose tolerance test should be done.
4   *Glucose tolerance test* (most sensitive test).
   a. Blood samples are drawn after an overnight fast.
   b. Glucose load (50–100 g) is given (usually in form of a carbonated sugar beverage).
   c. Specimens of blood for glucose determination are taken 1, 2 and 3 hours after glucose ingestion.
      (1) Patient fasts for 8 hours prior to test.
      (2) During test the patient is to avoid exercise, emotional stress, tobacco or any oral intake except water.
5   The following glucose tolerance curve is considered within the upper limits of normal:

Serum Glucose	*True Blood Glucose*
Fasting value 7.0 mmol/l (125 mg/100 ml)	6.0 mmol/l (110 mg/100 ml)
1-hour value of 10.5 mmol/l (190 mg/100 ml)	9.0 mmol/l (170 mg/100 ml)
2-hour value of 8.0 mmol/l (140 mg/100 ml)	6.5 mmol/l (120 mg/100 ml)
3-hour value of 7.0 mmol/l (125 mg/100 ml)	6.0 mmol/l (110 mg/100 ml)

Treatment and Nursing Management

Objectives

To correct biochemical and metabolic abnormalities.
To attain and maintain optimal body weight.
To prevent the progression of the disease and complications.
To promote patient education.

Means of Accomplishing Objectives

1   Diet and weight control—the essential foundation of diabetic management, or
2   Diet and insulin injections, or
3   Diet and oral hypoglycaemic drugs and
4   Exercise.
5   Continuing programme of patient education.

Principles of Dietary Treatment

Objective

To meet the basic nutritional requirements of the individual so that he may lead a normal life in comfort and good health.

1   The diet is planned according to patient's weight and activities and is adequate in all nutritional elements.
2   Dietary principles are different in the two main types of diabetes:
    a. Maturity-onset diabetes.
    (1) Limitation of calories is the goal of therapy in overweight diabetics—obese individuals are more resistant to both endogenous and exogenous insulin.
    (2) Weight loss tends to restore insulin sensitivity.
    (3) Diet helps control diabetes and reduces severity of disease.
    b. Growth-onset or juvenile diabetes.
    (1) Calories are not restricted below normal levels.
    (2) Smaller meals with one to three between-meal snacks are provided, to match the time-action pattern of administered insulin—to prevent after-meal surges of hyperglycaemia and protect against hypoglycaemia.
    (3) There should be consistency in the distribution, amount and characteristics of meals.
    (4) These patients need continuing instruction in dietary adjustment to adapt to unavoidable delay in meals, unusual exercise, intercurrent illness, prevention and management of hypoglycaemia, etc.
3   To find patient's calorie requirements:
    a. The basic calorie requirement is assessed.
    b. May be increased depending on patients activity.
    c. Basic calorie requirements are reduced if the patient is obese, elderly or inactive.
4   Most dietitians now advise patient to follow some form of carbohydrate-exchange groups from which he may make selections for his diet.
    a. Further advice on diet may be obtained from the British Diabetic Association or hospital dietitian.
    b. Patient modifies his prescribed diet by exchanging one item for another item on the same exchange list.
    c. Carbohydrate, fat and/or protein values of each food item on the list are essentially the same.
5   The diabetic diet should fit the patient's food preferences and economic status, and *emphasis should be on what the patient is allowed* rather than on what is forbidden.
6   Patient is not to omit meals or between-meal and bedtime snacks if prescribed.
7   The patient should test his urine or blood glucose before each meal and at bedtime while control is being attained. Daily urine or blood glucose testing thereafter is carried out as directed by doctor.

Exercise

1   Exercise promotes metabolism and utilization of carbohydrates and thus diminishes insulin requirements of the body.

2   Exercise enhances the effects of insulin and helps regulate blood glucose levels.
3   Encourage the patient to engage in *daily* exercise.

Insulin Therapy

1   Insulin is the active principle of secretion of beta calls in the islets of Langerhans. It is given to persons who do not have adequate endogenous insulin.
2   Physiological effect of insulin—lowers the blood sugar by facilitating the uptake and utilization of glucose by muscle and fat cells by decreasing release of glucose from the liver.
3   One or more insulin injections each day is usually required by:
     a. Persons whose diabetes is characterized by polydipsia, polyuria, weight loss and ketonuria.
     b. Hyperglycaemic pregnant patients.
     c. Patients with acute infections, febrile illness; those undergoing major surgery, or those with acutely decompensated diabetes. These may include those patients who are normally controlled on diet alone or diet and tablets.

Nursing Alert: There is a narrow margin between the therapeutic and toxic (hypoglycaemic) effects of insulin. Exercise, illness and emotional stress can alter needs for insulin.

Insulin Preparations

1   Insulin preparations are prescribed in units/ml (units 40 and units 80 strengths) and each type has its own specific colour coded label.
2   There are a number of available insulin preparations; each varies in onset of action, time of peak effect and duration of action (Table 5.1). The patient and nurse should know when insulin is having its effect—will help in assessing patient's behaviour and problems.

Insulin Syringes and Needles

1   The insulin syringe is a British standard 1 ml or 2 ml.
2   Needles are numbered according to diameter; the higher the number the thinner the needle.
3   No. 25 or No. 26 needles are usually used; 1.2 cm (0.5 in) long.

Regulation of Insulin Dosage

1   The dosage of insulin is adjusted according to the presence (or absence) of glucosuria; the degree in which it is present; and its time of appearance in relation to insulin injections and meals. The dosage of insulin is also adjusted according to determinations of blood glucose levels.
2   In the absence of complications, treatment may be started with 10 to 20 units of Lente or NPH insulin given subcutaneously before breakfast.
     a. Dosage is increased as indicated by patient's response to the previous dose until glucosuria is absent and the blood sugar before each meal is normal.

Table 5.1   Insulin Preparations

Agent	Duration of Action
Short action insulin Insulin injection (soluble) Neutral insulin injection	These have a relatively rapid action and when injected subcutaneously, their effect is maximal in 2–4 hours and last up to 12 hours
Intermediate acting insulin Biphasic insulin injection Globin zinc insulin injection Insulin zinc suspension Isophane insulin injection	These are usually given twice daily, producing much smoother blood glucose control than twice daily soluble insulin. They may be combined with soluble insulin.
Long acting insulin Insulin zinc suspension (mixed) Insulin zinc suspension (crystalline) Protamine zinc insulin injection	Peak activity occurs about 6 hours after injection and its action lasts up to 24 hours

Insulin preparations are available in concentrations of 20, 40 and 80 units/ml.

    b. During initial regulation and when insulin requirements are changing rapidly, supplemental injections of soluble insulin may be given before each meal, depending on results of urine testing and response of patient.
3   Instruct the patient to test his urine for sugar before each meal and at bedtime while insulin is being regulated (use the second of two specimens micturated 30 min apart for greater accuracy) or blood glucose may be estimated.
4   Ask the patient to keep a record of results in a notebook—to facilitate subsequent insulin adjustments.

Insulin Administration (see p. 558)

Hypoglycaemia as a Complication of Insulin Treatment

1   *Hypoglycaemic reaction* is an abnormally low level of glucose (sugar) in the blood; likely to occur when for any reason the blood sugar falls below 2.5 mmol/l (50 mg/100 ml) of blood; it may occur at a higher level if glucose has fallen rapidly.
2   Hypoglycaemia occurs as a result of too much insulin, not enough food (delayed or missed meal) and/or unusual vigorous activity.
3   Reactions begin 5–20 min following injection of regular insulin but not for several hours after NPH insulin—majority of attacks occur in morning and in early evening.

Signs and Symptoms of Hypoglycaemia

1   Nervousness, weakness, sweating, trembling.
2   Faintness, hunger pangs in epigastrium.
3   Headache, numbness or tingling of tongue or lips.
4   Tachycardia, palpitation.
5   Confusion, aggressive or erratic behaviour, change in mood.
6   Double vision; unsteady gait.
7   Pallor, chilling sensation.

Nursing Alert: Some patients experience hypoglycaemia so rapidly that the symptoms progress to convulsions almost without warning. Severe and prolonged hypoglycaemia may cause brain damage and sometimes death.

Treatment of Hypoglycaemia

1   Give some form of glucose orally if patient is conscious—orange juice, sweets, sugar lump.
2   Give glucagon (subcutaneously or intramuscularly) if patient cannot take anything by mouth—causes glycogenolysis in the liver, which raises blood glucose level.
3   Give patient orange juice or milk as soon as he regains consciousness—glucose level may fall faster than the transient rise produced by glucagon.
4   If patient is unconscious for period of time:
    a. Give 50% glucose solution intravenously—to restore normal blood glucose level quickly.
    b. Follow this with intravenous infusion of 5–10% glucose solution in water.
    c. Administer mannitol to combat cerebral oedema if necessary—cerebral function may be compromised when patient has low level of blood glucose.
5   Once rapidly-absorbed carbohydrate is given, give a feeding with protein or fat.

Preventing Hypoglycaemic Reactions Due to Insulin

Instruct the patient as follows:

1   Prevent hypoglycaemia with uniformity and timing of diet, insulin and daily exercise.
2   Recognize the early symptoms of hypoglycaemia—hunger, nausea, faintness, sweating, headache, rapid heart rate, double vision, inability to concentrate.
3   Take between-meal and bedtime snacks—to distribute the carbohydrate load over period of maximum insulin effect.
4   Test the urine so that changing insulin requirements can be anticipated.
5   Check urine for glucose before and after unusual physical exertion and consume extra food if needed.
6   Carry rapidly-absorbed carbohydrate (sugar/sweets) and take at first warning of a reaction.
7   Carry an identification card or wear an identification bracelet—hypoglycaemic symptoms can imitate intoxication with alcohol or drugs.
    a. Card—British Diabetic Association, 10 Queen Anne Street, London W1N 0BD.

b. Identification Bracelet—Medic Alert Foundation, 9 Hanover Street, London W1R 9HF.

Other Complications of Insulin Therapy

Insulin Allergy

1 Local reaction associated with stinging, redness and induration at injection site.
2 The reaction may be immediate (within an hour) or delayed (within 6–24 hours).
3 These reactions usually occur at beginning stages of therapy and do not last longer than a few weeks.
4 If local reactions continue, the more highly purified crystalline insulin or pork insulin may be tried.
5 Patients with severe insulin resistance or hypersensitivity should be referred to a hospital for antibody testing and regulation of insulin therapy.

Insulin Lipodystrophy

1 Two forms of lipodystrophy:
   a. Hypertrophy (bumps that may progress to thickened patches in the skin) at site of injection.
   Reinforce patient teaching about changing sites of insulin injection so that same site will not be used more than once in 1 month (see p. 561).
2 Fatty atrophy (sunken areas at site of injection).
   a. Incidence higher in girls and older patients.
   b. The newer, highly purified forms of insulin appear to have a lower incidence of fat atrophy.

Insulin Oedema

1 Characterized by generalized retention of fluid.
2 Usually appears with sudden restoration of diabetic control in a patient with uncontrolled diabetes over a period of time.

Insulin Resistance

Term applied to a patient whose insulin requirement is at least 200 units daily over a period of weeks to months in the absence of infection.

Oral Hypoglycaemic Agents

1 Oral hypoglycaemic agents (Table 5.2) may be given to maturity-onset nonketotic diabetics who cannot be treated by diet alone and who are unable or unwilling to take insulin (aged, infirm, blind, unable to follow a diet).
2 Serious questions have been raised about the effectiveness and safety of long-term use of oral hypoglycaemic agents—increase in cardiovascular mortality during treatment with sulphonylureas.
3 Patient should be placed on an effective dietary and weight control programme before trying oral hypoglycaemia agents.
4 Insulin is preferable to oral agents if dietary treatment fails to control diabetes.
5 Insulin is *required* when infection, trauma, major surgery or gangrene are present since these conditions usually produce temporary insulin resistance.

Table 5.2. Oral Hypoglycaemic Agents

Agent	Duration of Action
Sulphonylurea group—stimulates release of insulin from the pancreatic beta cells. These drugs depend on a functioning pancreas.	
Tolbutamide (Rastinon)	6–12 hours
Chlorpropamide (Diabinese)	Up to 60 hours
Glibenclamide (Daonil Euglocon)	12–24 hours
Tolazamide (Tolanase)	12–24 hours
Biguanides—act in a different way from the sulphonylureas. They are effective only in the presence of functioning pancreatic islet cells, and inhibit glucose absorption from the intestine and glucose oxidation. They should not be regarded as interchangeable with sulphonylureas.	
Metformin	8–12 hours
Phenformin (Dibotin)	Tablet 4–6 hours Slow release capsule 8–12 hours

6   Side effects of sulphonylureas—nausea and skin rash.
7   Side effects of biguanides—anorexia, nausea, vomiting, diarrhoea, loss of weight.

COMPLICATIONS OF DIABETES

Ketoacidosis and Coma

Ketoacidosis is caused by the absence or by an inadequate amount of insulin. This lack results in decreased utilization of carbohydrate and increased breakdown of fat and protein and, consequently, in dehydration and loss of sodium, potassium, chloride and bicarbonate. The number of ketone bodies (organic acids) increases as a result of rapid breakdown of fat.

Precipitating Causes

1   Failure to take insulin, insufficient insulin intake or resistance to insulin.
2   Infections (respiratory tract, urinary, gastrointestinal or skin).
3   Physiological stresses—pregnancy, injury, shock, surgery, emotional stress—make available insulin less effective.

Clinical Manifestations

Early Manifestations

1   Polyuria, thirst, malaise, drowsiness.
2   Abdominal pain.
3   Headache, weakness, shortness of breath.
4   Fever.
5   Hot, dry skin.

Later Manifestations

1 Kussmaul breathing—very deep but not laboured respiratory movements; a symptom of profound acidosis.
2 Sweetish odour of breath—due to acetone.
3 Lowered blood pressure.
4 Drowsiness; coma.

Laboratory Tests

Blood

1 Blood glucose elevated.
2 Serum bicarbonate decreased.
3 Blood pH decreased.
4 Blood urea increased.
5 Plasma ketone is strongly positive.

Urine

Strongly positive for sugar, ketones; also contains protein.

Treatment

Objective

To restore carbohydrate utilization and correct electrolyte imbalance.

1 Secure blood and urine samples immediately.
   a. Insert indwelling catheter in comatose patient to obtain urine specimens at prescribed times.
   b. Obtain full blood count, blood glucose, urea and serum, electrolytes and blood pH.
2 Carry out rapid physical examination.
   a. Look for evidence of infection.
   b. Look specifically at vital signs, state of hydration, skin colour, cardiac status.
3 Start intravenous infusion of isotonic saline—to establish urine flow and improve hydration and circulation.
4 Simultaneously administer insulin (intravenous or subcutaneous route).
   a. A continuous infusion of small amounts of insulin may be given or a low, medium or high dose regime may be administered.
   b. Subsequent insulin is given depending on the response to the previous dose, changes in the blood and urine chemistry, and condition of the patient.
   c. If intravenous insulin is given, administer it in intravenous tubing.
5 Carry out frequent determinations of blood glucose, serum ketone, serum bicarbonate and serum potassium; use other tests as needed.
6 Administer potassium as directed—hyperkalaemia may occur owing to rapid migration of potassium ions into the cells.
7 Give glucose infusion to prevent hypoglycaemia when blood glucose reaches desired level, since carbohydrate metabolism will be accelerated by insulin and blood glucose will begin to decrease.
8 Treat for circulatory collapse if present—diabetic patients in ketoacidosis may also be hypovolaemic.

    a. Give intravenous fluids, plasma expanders and vasopressors as needed.

    b. Elevate the lower extremities.

9 Prepare for gastric lavage if ordered—to relieve vomiting or acute dilatation of stomach.

10 Obtain serial electrocardiogram tracings—used to determine potassium need.

11 Keep a flow sheet giving patient's vital signs, urine test, blood chemistries, mental state and treatment.

12 Prevent the recurrence of diabetic ketoacidosis; *the precipitating cause of coma should be determined.*

    a. Avoid and treat infection.

    b. Make insulin and dietary adjustments during the period of illness.

    c. Teach and reteach the fundamentals of insulin administration, urine testing and home management (see p. 555).

Infection

Underlying Considerations

1 Infections are more serious in the diabetic for the following reasons:

    a. Resistance to infection is decreased because of hyperglycaemia.

    b. Diabetes becomes temporarily more severe.

    c. Insulin deficiency may impair ability of granulocytes to carry out a number of vital functions.

    d. Several important steps in normal host defence are impaired in poorly controlled diabetic patient.

    e. May precipitate ketoacidosis.

2 Infection increases the need for insulin.

Types of Infection

1 Infections of urinary tract—probably from increased frequency of catheterization; aggravated by incomplete emptying of bladder due to bladder paresis that may result from diabetic neuropathy.

2 Gram negative bacteraemia.

3 Furunculosis and other staphylococcal infections.

4 Tuberculosis—diabetics more susceptible to tuberculosis than the general population.

5 Fungal infections.

    Candidiasis

    (1) Due to *Candida albicans* normally found on skin, oral cavity, gastrointestinal tract and vagina.

    (2) Local infection of these areas (particularly vagina and skin) may occur in poorly controlled diabetes.

6 Yeast infections—Monilia infections of intertriginous (where folds of skin rub together) areas.

7 Gas gangrene—by nonclostridial organisms (*Aerobacter* or other coliform organisms) which are part of normal faecal flora; lower extremities usual site for these infections, which often lead to gangrene and amputation.

Treatment

1   The dosage of insulin is increased—due to elevation of blood glucose and the inability of leucocytes to effectively destroy bacteria.
2   Test the urine for sugar and acetone frequently and carry out frequent blood glucose determinations—to ascertain and compensate for rapidly changing insulin requirements.
3   Carry out cultures so that appropriate antibiotic may be given.

Long-Term Complications of Diabetes

Underlying Considerations

1   Diabetes is the number one cause of blindness in people aged between 35–64 years; heart attacks and strokes may also be related to diabetes. The majority of amputations performed for gangrene are the result of diabetes; diabetic nephropathy and neuropathic complications are significant factors.
2   The life expectancy among people with diabetes is approximately one-third less than that of the general population.
3   Current clinical and experimental data demonstrate that optimal regulation of glucose levels should be achieved, since microvascular complications occur less frequently when blood glucose concentrations are reduced.

Vascular Complications

1   The specific pathological lesion (microangiopathy) of long-standing diabetes is characterized by thickening of the capillary basement membrane in every organ.
2   The prevalence of microangiopathy parallels the duration and rate of progression of diabetes; it is probably associated with poor control.
3   Intracapillary glomerulosclerosis (Kimmelstiel–Wilson syndrome) is the specific renal disease of diabetes and is related to the thickening of the capillary basement membrane in the glomeruli.
4   Microangiopathy of the vessels supplying the skin, peripheral nerves and walls of large arteries may be a factor in skin diseases, diabetic neuropathy and the increased prevalence of atherosclerosis.
5   Major vessel occlusion (macroangiopathy) due to atherosclerosis causes strokes, myocardial infarction, intermittent claudication and gangrene; often occurs before the diabetes is recognized.

Diabetic Retinopathy

Diabetic retinopathy is a progressive impairment of retinal circulation that causes vitreous haemorrhage and sudden loss of vision.

1   Incidence and severity of retinopathy are generally proportional to the duration of the disease; half of the persons who have diabetes of more than 10 years' duration will have some evidence of retinopathy.

2 Impaired vision (and blindness) are caused by haemorrhages into the vitreous, formation of scar tissue and detachment of retina.
3 *Treatment:*
   a. Photocoagulation—produced when a narrow, intensive beam of light is directed into the eye and focused on the retina; the absorption of light produces heat which coagulates the treated vessel and prevents it from bleeding.
     (1) Used when there are localized areas of newly formed blood vessels and proliferative retinopathy, to prevent the events that lead to blindness.
     (2) Photocoagulation must be done when proliferative changes first occur.
   b. *Health teaching:*
   Patient should have yearly funduscopy (examination of the fundus of the eye) by an ophthalmologist.

Neuropathy

Neuropathy is a disease of the nervous system that occurs primarily as a consequence of diabetes mellitus; peripheral nerves are most frequently involved.

1 An exacerbation of neuropathy usually follows prolonged hyperglycaemia and weight loss due to inadequate diabetic control.
2 There are a wide variety of manifestations—numbness, tingling, burning of feet, pain and loss of deep tendon reflexes.
3 Involvement of the autonomic nervous system causes orthostatic hypotension, sexual impotency, pupillary changes, abnormal sweating, bladder paralysis, gastric paralysis and nocturnal diarrhoea.
4 *Treatment:*
   a. Ensure meticulous dietary control.
   b. Give supplementary vitamins if there is indication of dietary deficiency; evidence is accumulating that thiamine may have importance as a factor in peripheral nerve function.

MANAGEMENT OF THE DIABETIC PATIENT UNDERGOING SURGERY

Underlying Considerations

The diabetic patient must be followed very closely at the time of surgery because of the incidence of generalized vascular disease, diabetic neuropathy, decreased resistance to infection and changing insulin requirements due to stress and infection.

1 Surgical stress may increase hyperglycaemia because of increased secretion of adrenaline and glucocorticoids.
2 Infection may cause insulin antagonism.
3 Diabetic ketoacidosis may simulate an acute surgical abdomen.
4 Metabolic stress of anaesthesia also accentuates problems of hyperglycaemia and ketosis.
5 Surgical trauma produces further metabolic derangements, depending on degree and duration of surgery.

Treatment and Nursing Management

Objective

To achieve the best nutritional balance and best possible metabolic control of diabetes preoperatively.

Preoperative Preparation

1 Essential evaluation studies are done preoperatively—urinalysis for sugar and acetone, blood sugar levels, blood urea and other essential tests.
2 Give an adequate diet; the insulin dose may be reduced the day before surgery.

Day of Surgery

1 Give intravenous infusion of 5% dextrose instead of breakfast.
2 Give subcutaneous injection of insulin at the time the intravenous infusion is first started; usually one-half of patient's regular dose is given.
3 Continue the intravenous infusions during and following surgery (5% dextrose in either water or salt solution according to the patient's needs).
4 Give subcutaneous insulin as required on patient's return to recovery room.
5 Obtain a blood glucose determination in midafternoon on the day of surgery—to assess diabetic condition and to determine the need for more insulin or more dextrose.

Postoperative Management

1 Maintain nutrition with intravenous dextrose until patient is able to tolerate food by mouth.
2 Check urine for glucose and ketone and blood glucose several times daily as guideline for therapy.
3 Give insulin as directed each morning; supplemental doses of regular insulin may be given before each meal depending on results of urine tests.
4 Watch for signs and symptoms of ketoacidosis (p. 550).

PRINCIPLES OF HEALTH TEACHING FOR DIABETES MELLITUS

The person with diabetes mellitus must accept a major role in the management of his disease. His education must be amplified, reinforced and updated continuously, since diabetes is a life-long disease.

Objective

To maintain the best possible control of diabetes.

Patient's Objectives

To Become Familiar with Diabetes and How it Affects the Body

1 Visit the doctor on a regular basis.
2 Study and review available literature from reputable sources.
3 Secure booklets and pamphlets from the British Diabetic Association, 10 Queen Anne Street, London, W1N 0BD.
4 Attend available classes.

To Maintain Health at an Optimal Level

1   Maintain a consistent daily routine.
2   Get adequate rest and sleep.
3   Exercise regularly and consistently.
    a. Avoid 'spurts' of arduous exercise before meals.
    b. Exercise 1½ hours after meals.
    c. Keep some form of carbohydrate (sugar or sweets) available during exercise periods.
4   Seek employment with regular hours.
5   Have an annual test for tuberculosis.

To Follow the Prescribed Dietary Regimen

1   Eat three or more regular meals each day.
2   Become thoroughly familiar with the carbohydrate exchange lists.
3   Avoid concentrated carbohydrates.
4   Keep weight at optimal level; correct body weight.
5   If taking insulin, eat extra calories when unusual physical activity is anticipated.
6   Eat a bedtime snack when taking insulin (if permissible).

To be Aware of the Degree of Diabetic Control

1   Test urine for both sugar and acetone at each testing or test blood glucose.
2   Test urine or blood glucose before each meal and at bedtime while control is being attained or during periods of illness.
3   Test urine or blood glucose at least once daily.
4   Keep a daily record of urine and blood sugar tests (date, hour, colour reaction).
5   Test only freshly micturated urine using the second specimen (micturated 30 min after the first specimen).
6   Take the record of urine tests to doctor at appointed times.
7   Know that acetone in the urine indicates need for *more insulin.*
8   Protect all testing equipment from light, moisture and heat (to prevent false interpretation due to deterioration of test materials).

To Become Familiar With All Aspects of Insulin Usage (see p. 558 for guidelines for teaching self-injection of insulin).

1   Know when the prescribed insulin is having its peak action.
2   Adjust insulin dosage according to urine and blood sugar tests as prescribed.
3   Rotate the sites of insulin injections in a systematic manner.
4   Keep the syringe and needle in one particular place.
5   Keep a reserve supply of insulin in the refrigerator.
    a. Keep bottle in current use at *room temperature.*
    b. Avoid injecting cold insulin because it may contribute to tissue reaction.
6   Have an extra insulin syringe available.
7   Know the conditions that produce insulin reactions.
    a. Omission of a meal.
    b. Unaccustomed or strenuous exercise.
    c. Too much insulin.

8 Know the symptoms of an insulin reaction.
   a. Any unfamiliar or peculiar sensation.
   b. Hunger, perspiration, palpitation, tachycardia, weakness, tremor, pallor.
9 Know how to combat an impending insulin reaction.
   a. Eat carbohydrates (sugar, sweets) when symptoms first occur.
   b. Test urine.
   c. Carry extra carbohydrate at all times (sugar lumps, sweets).
   d. Eat extra carbohydrate before strenuous exercise and during periods of prolonged exercise, or reduce insulin dosage.
   e. Eat a snack at bedtime.
10 Keep a check-off system to ensure taking insulin.
11 Carry diabetic identification card or wear identification bracelet.

To Take Prescribed Oral Hypoglycaemic Medication

1 Adhere faithfully to the prescribed diet.
2 Test urine daily.
3 Take the medication exactly as directed.

To Appreciate the Importance of Proper Foot Care to Prevent Infection, Ischaemia and Neuropathy Which May Lead to Amputation and Death.

1 Inspect the feet carefully and routinely for calluses, corns, blisters, abrasions, redness and nail abnormalities.
   a. Use a small mirror to check bottom of each foot.
   b. Use a magnifying glass under good light if eyesight is poor, or ask someone else to check feet.
2 Bathe the feet daily in warm (never hot) water.
   a. Do not soak the feet for prolonged periods.
   b. Dry feet carefully, especially between the toes.
3 Massage the feet with a lubricating lotion, except between the toes.
4 Prevent moisture between the toes to avert maceration of the skin.
   a. Insert sheepskin between overlapping toes.
   b. Use powder in the web spaces, especially if feet perspire.
5 Wear well-fitting, noncompressive shoes and socks—long enough, wide enough, soft, supple and low-heeled.
   a. Buy shoes in the afternoon—feet are larger in the afternoon than in the morning.
   b. Have each foot measured before buying shoes—feet enlarge with age.
   c. Have the measurement taken while standing, since foot is larger in the standing position.
   d. Do not 'break in' shoes all at one time.
   e. Avoid working in bedroom slippers or other casual footwear.
6 Go to a chiropodist on a regular basis if corns, calluses and ingrown toenails are present.
   a. Cut toenails straight across to prevent ingrown toenails.
   b. See Volume 1, Chapter 3, The Ageing Person for instructions for cutting toenails.
7 Avoid heat, chemicals and injuries to the feet—do not go barefoot or expose feet to hot water bottles, heating pads, caustic solutions, etc.

8   If an injury occurs to the foot:
    a. Wash the area with mild soap and water.
    b. Cover with a dry sterile dressing *without* adhesive.
    c. Consult the doctor.

To Maintain Diabetic Control During Periods of Illness

1   Call doctor immediately when any unusual symptoms become evident; *do not allow diabetes to get out of control.*
2   Make dietary adjustments during illness according to doctor's directions.
3   Continue taking insulin; doctor may increase dosage during illness.
4   Test urine for sugar and acetone or blood glucose more frequently; keep records.
5   Know the conditions that bring about diabetic acidosis.
    a. Nausea and vomiting.
    b. Failure to increase insulin when urine sugar is increasing.
    c. Failure to take insulin.
    d. Dietary excesses.
    e. Infections.
6   Know how to combat impending diabetic acidosis.
    a. Examine urine for sugar and acetone and report results to doctor.
    b. Take additional insulin as advised by doctor.
    c. Go to bed and keep warm.
    d. Alert someone to be in attendance.
    e. Drink a glass of liquid hourly if possible.

To Follow Other Health Directives

1   Avoid tobacco—nicotine constricts blood vessels, causing reduction in blood flow to feet.
2   Report excessive itching—may indicate elevated blood sugar.
3   Take only medications prescribed by doctor—many drugs enhance effect on insulin and oral antidiabetic agents.

GUIDELINES: Teaching Self-Injection of Insulin

Underlying Considerations

1   Insulin injection should be taught as soon as the need for insulin treatment has been established.
2   A member of the patient's family should also be taught how to administer insulin.
3   An optimistic approach will offer the patient encouragement.
4   Teach insulin injection *first* since this is the patient's major concern; then include loading the syringe and sterilizing equipment as the patient is able to grasp these concepts.

Equipment

Prescribed bottle of insulin
Insulin syringe and needles (may be disposable) usually bought by patient
Carrying case
Methylated spirit

Procedure

Teaching Action	Reason
1 Give the patient the prepared syringe containing the prescribed dose of insulin.	
2 Instruct the patient to hold the syringe as he would a pencil.	
3 Show the patient how to spread the skin taut on the anterior thigh (Fig. 5.2a). or Form a skin fold by picking up subcutaneous tissue between the thumb and forefinger if the patient is thin (Fig. 5.2b).	3 Either of the techniques ensures that the needle tip is inserted into subcutaneous tissue and outside the muscle. Avoid pressing the skin *tightly* between the fingers since this is a common cause of local induration and infection.
4 Select areas of upper arms, thighs, flanks and upper buttocks or abdomen for injection after patient becomes proficient with needle insertion (Fig. 5.2a).	4 The skin is loose and there is more subcutaneous fat in these areas. The skin of the abdominal wall is a good site for women who develop atrophy of subcutaneous fat at sites of insulin injection.
5 Assist the patient to insert needle with a quick thrust to the hub at a right angle to the skin surface (Fig. 5.2c)	5 The insulin is injected into deep subcutaneous tissue.
6 Instruct the patient to release the skin fold and pull back on the plunger. If no blood is seen, push in the plunger.	6 Pulling back on the plunger and checking for blood ensures that the needle is not in a blood vessel.
7 Gently withdraw the needle. Wipe area with paper tissue if necessary.	7 This manoeuvre prevents painful pulling of the skin as the needle is withdrawn.
8 Put syringe and needle into carrying case. Carrying case is half filled with methylated spirit which is changed weekly.	
9 Remove all traces of spirit before loading syringe, by pushing plunger back and forth. Spirit may alter the effect of insulin and is also irritating when introduced under the skin.	
10 Develop a systematic plan for insulin administration; e.g., rotation of sites in a clockwise fashion (Fig. 5.3).	10 Systematic rotation of sites will keep the skin supple, will favour uniform absorption of insulin and will prevent scar formation.

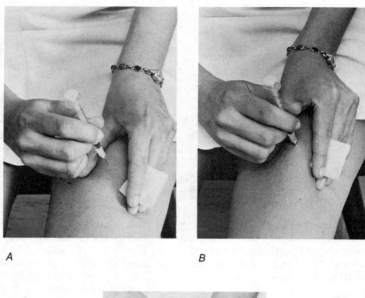

A   B

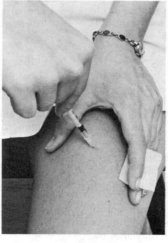

C

Figure 5.2. Self-injection of insulin. a. The insulin syringe is held perpendicular to the stretched skin before the needle is thrust into the subcutaneous tissues. b. Alternate method: If the patient has only a thin layer of subcutaneous fat, a fold of skin is pinched between the fingers to keep the needle from penetrating into the muscle. c. The patient exerts slight traction on the plunger before the insulin is injected.

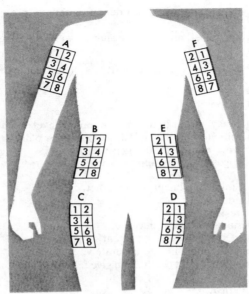

Figure 5.3. Setting up a rotation circle. The sketch shows that the right arm is marked A, the right side of the abdomen is B, and the right thigh is C. The left side of the body going upwards is marked D, E and F counter-clockwise. Each of these areas can be marked as a rectangle and divided into eight squares more than 1 in on each side. These squares are numbered starting from the upper and outside corner (number 1) to the lowest corner (number 8). All even numbers are towards the body. If you take the number 1 square and inject into it at each of the six areas through F, it will take you six days to reach area A again. Then you take square number 2 and inject each time on the squares so numbered in the areas A through F and so on. This provides 48 different places for an injection (6 × 8). At one injection daily, it will take 48 days or 7 weeks to cover each of the squares. (From: A. D. A. Forecast—the Diabetics' Own Magazine, 4: O, Jan. 1951. Courtesy: Becton, Dickenson.)

Teaching Action	**Reason**

To Load the Syringe

1 Roll the bottle of insulin between the palms of the hands.	1 The rolling action mixes the insulin.
2 Wipe off the top of the insulin vial with an alcohol sponge.	
3 Inject approximately the same volume of air into the insulin vital as the volume of insulin to be withdrawn.	3 Air is injected into the vial to keep its contents under slight positive pressure and to make it easier to withdrawn the insulin.

To Fill a Syringe With Long- and Short-acting Insulin

1 Wipe off the vial tops with an alcohol swab.
2 Inject air into long-acting insulin first; withdraw needle.

3   Inject air into short-acting insulin bottle and withdraw prescribed amount of insulin.
4   Then withdraw prescribed amount of insulin from long-acting insulin bottle.

Rapid Methods of Urine Testing for Glucose (Sugar) and Ketones (Acetone)

Underlying Considerations

1   In diabetes, sugar may appear in the urine when the level of glucose in the blood rises above 9 mmol/l (160 mg/100 ml) as patients grow older the renal threshold tends to rise above 9 mmol/l (160 mg/100 ml).
2   Urinary sugar (glucosuria) may appear when:
    a. Treatment is inadequate.
    b. Patient is not following his prescribed diet.
    c. Exercise is inadequate.
    d. Infection is present.
3   Incorrect test results may occur because:
    a. Deteriorated reagent tablets or reagent strips are used.
    b. The directions are not followed accurately.
    c. Certain medications affect results; can give false positive or negative results.

Instructions to the Patient

Use the second-micturition technique to collect the urine specimen.

1   Micturate and discard the urine.
2   Drink several glasses of liquid.
3   Micturate into a clean container 30–45 min later—the second specimen reflects the status of glucose spillover into the urine more accurately.
4   Test this specimen.

Tests for Sugar (Glucose)

*Clinitest** (uses a reagent tablet)

1   *Two-drop method*—allows estimation of concentration of sugar up to 5%.
    a. Hold dropper vertically and place 2 drops (0.1 ml) of urine in test tube.
    b. Rinse dropper. Add 10 drops (0.5 ml) of water to test tube.
    c. Add 1 Clinitest reagent tablet. *Do not shake test tube.*
    d. Wait 15 s after boiling stops.
    e. Compare colour of urine with appropriate colour chart.
    (Use only the two-drop method colour scale which has seven colours ranging in value from 0–5%).
2   *Five-drop method*
    a. Hold dropper vertically and place 5 drops of urine in test tube.
    b. Rinse dropper. Add 10 drops of water to test tube.

---

* Clinitest is a product of Ames Company, Division of Miles Laboratories, Inc., Stoke Poges, Slough SL2 4LY.

c. Put 1 Clinitest tablet in test tube.

    (1) Watch while reaction takes place.

    (2) Do not shake test tube during reaction or for 15 s after boiling inside test tube has stopped.

d. Observe the solution in the test tube *while the reaction takes place and during the 15-s waiting period to detect pass-through colour changes caused by glucosuria over 2%.*

    (1) If the solution passes through orange and dark shades of green-brown it indicates more than 2% (4+) urine sugar is present.

    (2) Record as such without reference to colour scale.

e. After 15-s waiting period, shake test tube gently and compare with the colour scale.

f. Record results.

*Diastix** (reagent strip)

1   Dip reagent end of strip in urine specimen for 2 s and remove (or wet end of strip for 2 s by passing through urine stream).

2   Tap edge of strip against side of urine container to remove excess urine.

3   Exactly 30 s after removing from urine, compare reagent side of strip to closest matching colour block on package label.

Tests for Acetone (Ketone Bodies)

*Acetest** (reagent tablets)

1   Use freshly micturated specimen—prolonged standing of urine specimen encourages bacterial growth which can lead to changes in the number of ketone bodies.

2   Place tablet on a piece of white paper.

3   Place 1 drop of urine on tablet.

4   Compare urine ketone test results to colour chart after 30 s.

*Ketostix** (reagent strips)

1   Dip test area in freshly micturated specimen or pass if briefly through the urinary stream.

2   Remove immediately.

3   Wait 15 s. Compare colour of test strip with the colour chart.

Combined (Ketone-Glucose) Reagent Strip

*Keto-Diastix** (combined ketone-glucose reagent strip)

1   Dip reagent end of strip in urine specimen for 2 s and remove (or wet the end of strip for 2 s by passing through urine stream).

2   Tap edge of strip against side of urine container to remove excess urine.

3   Exactly 15 s after removing from urine, compare ketone test area on reagent side of strip to closest matching colour block on package label; exactly 30 s after

---

* Diastix, Acetest, Ketostix, Keto-Diastix and Dextrostix are products of Ames Company, Division of Miles Laboratories, Inc., Stoke Poges, Slough SL2 4LY

removing from urine, compare glucose test area on reagent side of strip to closest matching colour block on the glucose section of the package label.

Rapid Methods of Blood Testing for Glucose

Normal blood glucose level between 3–7 mmol/l and no greater than 10 mmol/1 after a meal.

Patient is taught to use a lancet to obtain blood from finger tip.

*Dextrostix**

1   Compare test area on strip closely with 'o' block on colour chart. If reagent area on strip does not closely match the 'o' block discard strip.
2   Freely apply a large drop of capillary or venous blood sufficient to cover entire reagent area on printed side of strip.
3   Wait exactly 60 s (use sweep second hand or stop watch for timing).
4   Quickly wash off blood (within 1 or 2 s) with a sharp stream of water using a wash bottle.
5   Read result within 1 or 2 s after washing. Hold the strip close to the colour chart. Interpolate if necessary.

BM Test

1   Drop blood onto BM test strip, after 1 min wipe excess blood.
2   After 2 min match colour with chart.
3   When more than 13.3 mmol/l (240 mg/100 ml) compare colours after 3 min.

A selection of glucose meters is available for the patient to use at home, e.g., Glucocheck, Hypocount, Ames Eyetone Meter.

4. Disorders of the Adrenal Glands

THE ADRENAL GLANDS

Composition

Medulla

1   Is not necessary to maintain life but enables a person to cope with stress.
2   Secretes two hormones:
   a. Adrenaline
     (1) Acts on alpha and beta receptors.
     (2) Increases contractility and excitability of heart muscle, leading to increased cardiac output.
     (3) Facilitates blood flow to muscles, brain and viscera.
     (4) Enhances blood sugar—by stimulating conversion of glycogen to glucose in liver.
     (5) Inhibits smooth muscle contraction.
   b. Noradrenaline
     (1) Acts primarily on alpha receptors.

(2) Increases peripheral vascular resistance leading to increases in diastolic and systolic blood pressure.

Cortex

1   Is essential of life.
2   Secretes adrenocortical hormones—synthesized from cholesterol.
    a. Glucocorticoids: cortisone and hydrocortisone.
        (1) Enhance protein catabolism and inhibit protein synthesis.
        (2) Antagonize action of insulin.
        (3) Increase synthesis of glucose by liver.
        (4) Influence defence mechanism of body and its reaction to stress.
        (5) Influence emotional reaction.
    b. Mineralocorticoids.
        (1) Aldosterone—supplied by adrenal cortex.
        (2) Desoxycorticosterone—usually not present in significant amounts.
        (3) Regulate reabsorption of sodium cation.
        (4) Regulate excretion of potassium cation by renal tubules.
    c. Sex hormones.

HYPERFUNCTION OF THE ADRENAL MEDULLA

Phaeochromocytoma

Phaeochromocytoma is a neoplasm associated with hyperfunction of the adrenal medulla.

Clinical Manifestations

1   Variable symptoms depend upon whether the tumour secretes adrenaline or noradrenaline.
    Symptoms are often triggered by allergic reactions, physical exertion, emotional upset; they can also occur without identifiable stimulus.
2   Hypertension may be paroxysmal or chronic.
    Chronic form may be difficult to diffentiate from 'essential hypertension'.
3   Tachycardia, excessive perspiration, tremor, pallor or face flushing, nervousness and hyperglycaemia.
4   Polyuria, nausea, vomiting, diarrhoea and abdominal pain, paresthesia in extremities.

Diagnosis

1   If there is sympathetic overactivity along with marked elevation of blood pressure phaeochromocytoma is strongly suspected.
2   Administration of certain drugs produces certain changes in arterial pressure.
    a. Provocative drugs—stimulate a sharp rise in arterial pressure (histamine, tyramine).
    b. Adrenergic blocking drugs—produce a sharp fall in arterial pressure—phentolamine (Rogitine).

3   Intravenous pyelogram (IVP) on x-ray examination may help in identifying the location of tumour.
4   Tests:
   a. Vanillylmandelic acid (VMA) determination in urine.
   b. Normal urinary value: VMA up to 35 mmol/24 hours (0.7–6.8 mg/24 hours).

Treatment and Nursing Management

Objective

To remove the cause.

Preoperative Preparation

1   This requires effective control of blood pressure and blood volume. Often may take 1 or 2 weeks.
2   To accomplish blood pressure control, administer alpha-adrenergic blocking agents such as phentolamine (Rogitine) or phenoxybenzamine hydrochloride (Dibenyline) to inhibit the effects of catecholamines.
3   Catecholamine synthesis inhibitors may also be used.
4   Propranolol is helpful in controlling cardiac arrhythmias, if present.

Postoperative Care (see p. 571).

Of particular concern is the evaluation and documentation of 24-hour urine specimens. The patient is considered surgically cured when 24-hour urine specimens are evaluated as 'normal' when tested for previously 'abnormal' substances.

Cushing's Syndrome

Cushing's syndrome is a disease produced by hyperactivity of the adrenal cortex.

Aetiology

1   Cushing's syndrome results mainly from the hypersecretion of cortisol and corticosterone.
2   The disorder may be caused by:
   a. A neoplasm of the adrenal cortex: adenoma or carcinoma.
   b. Hyperplasia of both glands due to overstimulation of the adrenal cortex by ACTH.
   c. Pituitary tumours.
   d. Tumours elsewhere in body producing excess ACTH.

Diagnosis

1   Excessive plasma cortisol levels.
2   An increase in blood sugar—diabetes.
3   A decrease in concentration of potassium in the blood.
4   A reduction in the number of blood eosinophils.
5   Elevation in the urine level of 17-hydroxycorticoids and 17-ketogenic steroids.
6   Elevation of plasma ACTH in patients with pituitary tumours.

Clinical Manifestations

In Children

1 Precocious puberty.
2 Affected growth rate.

Females

Cushing's syndrome occurs 10 times more frequently in females than in males.

1 'Virilism' or masculinization.
   a. Hirsutism—excessive growth of hair on the face and midline of trunk.
   b. Breasts—atrophy.
   c. Clitoris—enlarges.
   d. Voice—musculine.
2 In utero—possible hermaphrodite.
3 Menses—irregular and scanty; libido lost.

Adult ('central type obesity')

1 'Buffalo hump' in neck and supraclavicular area.
2 Heavy trunk; thin extremities.
3 Skin—fragile and thin; striae and ecchymosis, acne.
4 Face—rounded, plethoric, oily.
5 Muscles—wasted due to excessive catabolism.
6 Osteoporosis—characteristic kyphosis, backache.
7 Mental disturbances—mood changes, psychosis.
8 Increased suspectibility to infections.
9 Hypertension oedema.

Objectives of Treatment and Nursing Management

To Establish the Diagnosis

1 Overnight dexamethasone suppression test.
   a. Dexamethasone is administered orally the night before in the amount equivalent to amount of cortisol normally produced by the patient in a day.
   b. Dexamethasone will normally suppress ACTH secretion and stop cortisol production.
   c. The next day, blood studies will be done; patients with Cushing's syndrome will not show suppression below a certain level.
2 If above test does not rule out the possibility of Cushing's syndrome, specific urinary excretion tests are performed with dexamethasone suppression.
3 Additional tests are done to determine whether the problem is due to hyperplasia or adrenocortical tumour.
4 Explain to the patient the necessity for the many blood and urine studies.
5 Recognize the need for accurately recording intake of food and fluid as well as output of urine.
6 Record all pertinent observations that may assist the doctor in making the diagnosis.

To Consider Medical Treatment in Patients Unable to Face Surgery (e.g., myocardial infarction)

1   Consider mitotane, an agent toxic to the adrenal cortex (DDT derivative)—'medical andrenalectomy'.
    Serious side effects accompany this drug.
2   Try metyrapone (Metopirone) to inhibit steroid biosynthesis; this is used for temporary control.

To Encourage the Patient to Eat the Prescribed Diet

1   Explain to the patient that his diet (low sodium and high potassium) is as significant to his treatment as his medications.
    a. Foods high in potassium—meats, fish, most vegetables and fruits, legumes.
    b. Foods low in sodium—cereal, fruits, squash, potatoes, lettuce, honey, unsalted butter.

To Be Aware of the Psychological Manifestations of This Syndrome

1   Identify those situations which are disturbing to the patient; record these on the nursing care plan as situations to be avoided.
2   Be alert for evidence of depression; in some instances this has progressed to suicide; therefore, mood changes are most important.
3   Report when depression continues after surgery.
4   Understand the emotional stress in female patients who manifest masculinization tendencies.
5   Reassure the patient who has benign adenoma or hyperplasia that, with proper treatment, evidence of masculinization can be reversed.
6   Note that weakness is a frustrating experience in a patient who heretofore has been active.

To Remove the Cause via Surgery

1   Tumour (adrenal or pituitary)—should be removed or treated with irradiation.
2   Hyperplasia of adrenals—calls for an adrenalectomy.

To Administer Replacement Therapy Postoperatively.

This is a lifelong corticosteroid maintenance therapeutic programme.

1   Adrenalectomy patients require replacement therapy with the following:
    a. A glucocorticoid—cortisone.
    b. A mineralocorticoid—fludrocortisone (Florinef).
    c. Extra salt.
2   Following pituitary irradiation or hypophysectomy, patients may require adrenal replacement plus thyroid and gonadal replacement therapy.
3   Protein anabolic steroids may facilitate protein replacement; potassium stores are usually depleted rapidly and may require replacement.

ADDISON'S DISEASE

Addison's Disease is a condition due to deficiency of the adrenal glands.

Cause

A deficiency of cortical hormones due to:

1 Destruction of adrenal cortex.
2 Atrophy—following prolonged steroid therapy or secondary to pituitary deficiency.

Clinical Manifestations

Due to (1) disturbance of sodium and potassium metabolism and (2) depletion of sodium and water—urine loss, severe chronic dehydration.

1 Muscular weakness, fatigue, weight loss.
2 Gastrointestinal problems—anorexia, nausea, vomiting, diarrhoea, constipation, abdominal pain.
3 Low blood pressure, low blood sugar, low basal metabolic rate, low blood sodium.
4 High potassium.
5 After a while, symptoms worsen and the patient is forced to go to bed.
   a. Skin colour changes to tan, bronze or brown—diffuse or patchy, freckling.
   b. Mucous membranes also discolour—bluish black or grey.
   c. Mental changes occur—depression, irritability, anxiety, apprehension.
6 Normal responses to stress are lacking.

Diagnosis

Blood Studies

1 Hypoglycaemia—decrease in sugar concentration.
2 Hyponatraemia—decrease in sodium concentration.
3 Hyperkalaemia—increase in potassium concentration.
4 Lymphoid hyperplasia.
5 Low fasting plasma cortisol levels.

Urine Studies

24-hour specimen for 17-ketosteroids, 17-hydroxycorticoids and 17-ketogenic steroids—all values decreased.

Injection of a Potent Pituitary Adrenocorticotropic Hormone to Artificially Stimulate Adrenals

1 Normal response—normal rise in plasma cortisol and urinary 17-ketosteroids.
2 In Addison's disease:
   a. Decrease in circulating eosinophils.
   b. Increase in uric acid excretion in about 4 hours.
   c. No rise in plasma cortisol and urinary 17-ketosteroids.

Treatment and Nursing Management

1 Attempt to restore normal electrolyte balance.
   a. Administer high sodium, low potassium diet and fluids.

   b. Give hydrocortisone (17-hydroxycorticosterone).
   (1) Addisonian crisis—inject hydrocortisone 21-sodium succinate (Solu-Cortef) or hydrocortisone phosphate, 50–100 mg intravenously and follow with an infusion of Solu-Cortef intravenously over 8 hours.
   (2) Long-term basis—hydrocortisone in doses of 20–30 mg plus deoxycortone (DOCA) or Florinef.
2 Detect early signs of *Addisonian crisis.*
   a. Nausea, vomiting, cyanosis.
   b. Sudden drop in blood pressure.
   c. Very high temperature.
3 Recognize that circulatory collapse may result from the following:
   a. Overexertion.
   b. Exposure to cold.
   c. Acute infection.
   d. Decrease in salt intake.
   e. Excessive diarrhoea.
4 Be on guard for later signs of Addisonian crisis.
   a. Fall in systolic pressure to 40–50 mmHg.
   b. Weak pulse and cold clammy skin.
5 Initiate treatment immediately.
   a. Administer blood transfusions to replace blood volume.
   b. Start intravenous flow of sodium chloride solution to replace sodium ions.
   c. Give hydrocortisone.
   d. Inject circulatory stimulants.
6 Assess vital signs frequently for deviation.
   a. Monitor vital signs and blood pressure; a drop in blood pressure may suggest impending crisis.
   b. Record the temperature hourly since an elevation may easily be precipitated.
7 Observe carefully the emotional state of the patient.
   a. Encourage rest periods to avoid overexertion.
   b. Control the temperature of the room to avoid sharp deviations in patient's temperature.
   c. Maintain a quiet, peaceful environment; avoid loud talking and noisy radios.
8 Record conscientiously the salt intake and urine output.
     Inform the patient's family as well as all nursing staff who come in contact with this patient that all urine must be saved for a 24-hour urine specimen.
9 Give total nursing care.
   a. Do not allow the patient who is in adrenal crisis to do anything for himself.
   b. Assist him in moving and turning, in feeding and in providing mouth care.
   c. Limit conversation to what is essential to his care.
10 Protect the patient from infection.
   a. Control his contacts so that infectious organisms are not transmitted.
   b. Protect him from draughts, dampness, etc.
11 Be familiar with the nature of hormonal replacement required by the individual patient.
   a. Some require cortisol.

b. Other patients require additional electrolyte-type medications to maintain homoeostasis.

c. Determine the method of administration of drug for the particular patient: most are taken by mouth, but some are administered intramuscularly.

d. Note whether there is an effect on fluid retention—weigh patient frequently and record weight.

12 Inform the patient of the nature of long-term therapy for adrenocortical insufficiency

   a. Inform the patient that therapy must be continued for the rest of his life.

   b. Emphasize the importance of taking more hormones when he is under stress.

   c. Suggest that he carry an identification card on which are indicated the type of medication he is receiving and the phone number of his doctor.

PRIMARY ALDOSTERONISM

Primary Aldosteronism is a disorder caused by hypersecretion of the adrenal cortex.

Diagnosis and Clinical Manifestations

1 A profound decline in blood levels of potassium (hypokalaemia) and hydrogen ions (alkalosis)—results in muscle weakness and inability of kidneys to acidify or concentrate urine, leading to excess volume of urine (polyuria).

   a. Increase in pH.

   b. Increase in CO_2-combining power.

2 A decline in hydrogen ions (alkalosis)—results in tetany, paraesthesias.

3 An elevation in blood sodium (hypernatraemia)—results in excessive thirst (polydipsia) and arterial hypertension.

4 Hypertension.

Treatment

Removal of adrenal tumour—adrenalectomy (see p. 571).

MANAGEMENT OF THE PATIENT HAVING AN ADRENALECTOMY

Preoperative Care

1 Correct hyperglycaemia by proper diet and insulin.

2 Administer high protein diet to correct protein deficiency.

3 See Volume 1, Chapter 4, Care of the Surgical Patient—care of patient is similar to that for general surgery of abdomen.

Postoperative Care

1 Similar to that for an abdominal operation.

2 Will require administration of hydrocortisone or similar compounds in large amounts; this should begin prior to surgery. If bilateral adrenalectomy is performed, lifetime replacement is necessary.

3   For removal of phaechromocytoma:
    a. Because of manipulation of tumour during surgery, there may be extreme fluctuations of blood pressure.
    b. Upon ligation of vessels from tumour an abrupt fall of blood pressure may result. Large amounts of adrenaline are given intravenously.

Nursing Alert: Be prepared to monitor blood pressure frequently for 24–48 hours and alter the dose of vasopressor intravenous medications in order to stabilize the blood pressure.

4   Monitor vital signs, including blood pressure and central venous pressure, up to 48 hours—to detect early changes which may lead to cardiovascular collapse.
5   Anticipate stressful situations for the patient and avoid them; provide rest periods, anticipate his needs, provide comfort measures.

STEROID THERAPY*

Classification of Steroids

By major metabolic effects on body.

1   Mineralocorticoids.
    a. Concerned with sodium and water retention and potassium excretion.
    b. Example—aldosterone and 11-desoxycorticosterone.
2   Glucocorticoids.
    a. Concerned with metabolic effects, including carbohydrate metabolism.
    b. Example—cortisol.
3   Sex hormones
    a. Important when secreted in large amounts or when the growth of hormone-sensitive cancers is stimulated.
    b. Examples:
    Androgens—dehydroepiandrosterone, testosterone.
    Oestrogens—oestradiol.
    Progestins—progesterone

Effects of Glucocorticoids (corticosteroids, steroids)

1   Antagonize action of insulin—promote gluconeogenesis, which provides glucose.
2   Increase breakdown of protein (inhibit protein synthesis).
3   Increase breakdown of fatty acids.
4   Suppress inflammation, inhibit scar formation, block allergic responses.
5   Decrease number of circulating eosinophils and leucocytes; decrease size of lymphatic tissue.
6   Exert a permissive action (allow full expression of effects of another hormone) on all effects caused by catecholamines.
7   Exert a permissive action on functioning of central nervous system.
8   Inhibit release of adrenocorticotropin.

* Source acknowledgement: Melick, M E : Nursing intervention for patients receiving corticosteroid therapy. In Kintzel (1977) Advanced Concepts in Nursing, 2nd edition, Philadelphia, J B Lippincott.

IN SUMMARY: Glucocorticoids give an organism the capacity to resist all types of noxious stimuli and environmental change.

Uses of Steroids

1 Physiologically—to correct deficiencies or malfunction of a particular endocrine organ or system, e.g., Addison's disease.
2 Diagnostically—to determine proper functioning of the endocrine system.
3 Pharmacologically—to treat the following:
   a. Rheumatoid arthritis.
   b. Acute rheumatic fever.
   c. Blood conditions.
      (1) Idiopathic thrombocytopenic purpura.
      (2) Leukaemia.
      (3) Haemolytic anaemia.
   d. Allergic conditions—bronchial asthma, allergic rhinitis.
   e. Dermatologic problems—drug rashes, atopic dermatitis.
   f. Ocular diseases—conjunctivitis, uveitis.
   g. Collagen diseases—lupus erythematosus, polyarteritis nodosa.
   h. Gastrointestinal problems—ulcerative colitis.
   i. Organ-transplant recipients—as an immunosuppressive.
   j. Neurological—cerebral oedema.
   k. Other conditions—gout, multiple sclerosis.
4 Emergency conditions.
   a. Status asthmaticus.
   b. Acute adrenal insufficiency.
   c. Anaphylactic reaction (only after adrenaline has been given).

Preparing the Patient to Receive Steroid Therapy

1 Require a thorough physical examination and medical history.
2 Determine contraindications for such therapy.
   a. Peptic ulcer
   b. Diabetes mellitus.
   c. Viral infections.
3 Take a tuberculin test to determine need for antituberculin drugs.
   If this is not done prior to steroid therapy, the patient's hypersensitivity to tuberculin may be suppressed.
4 Assess the patient's own level of steroid secretion, if possible.
5 Explain the nature of the therapy, what is required of the patient, how long he is to be on steroid medications, what adverse signs to watch for, etc.

Choice of Steroid and Method of Administration (see Table 5.3)

1 Determined on an individual basis by the doctor.
2 May be given for local effects or systemic effects.
3 May be given by a wide variety of methods: orally, parenterally, sublingually, rectally, by inhalation, or by direct application to skin or mucous membrane.
4 Combinations of steroids with other drugs should be avoided.
5 To help avoid steroid side effects, alternate-day therapy should be used if at all possible; this is not always feasible.

Table 5.3. Characteristics of Pharmaceutical Derivatives of Adrenocorticosteroids

Oral Preparations		Topical Preparations	
BP Name	Trade Name(s)	BP Name	Trade Names(s)
Dexamethasone	Decadron	Triamcinolone acetate	Adcortyl, Ledercort
Betamethasone	Betnelan		
Triamcinolone	Adcortyl, Ledercort	Fluocinolone acetonide	Synalar
Methylprednisolone	Medrone		
Prednisone	Decortisyl, Cortelan, Deltacortone	Slow Release Preparations	
Cortisone	Cortelan, Cortistab, Cortisyl	Hydrocortisone acetate	Hydrocortistab
Hydrocortisone (cortisol)	Cortril, Hydrocortone	Methylprednisole	Medrone
Fludrocrotisone	Florinef	Intravenous Preparations	
Prednisone	Delortisyl, Delta Cortelan, Deltacortone	Hydrocortisone sodiumsuccinate	Solu-Cortef
		Hydrocortisone sodiumphosphate	Efcortesol
		Dexamethasone sodiumphosphate	Decadron
		Prednisolone sodiumphosphate	Codelsol, Parisolon, Prednesol

* In addition to these topical preparations, most of the anti-inflammatory steroids are supplied in the form of creams, aerosols, eye drops, etc., for special topical use.

6   Sometimes steroids are given in extremely high doses, then sharply reduced; if patient has been taking steroids for a while, doses must be tapered gradually.

Potential Side Effects of Steroid Therapy

Classification

1   Mineralocorticoid.
    a. Sodium and water retention.
        Oedema, weight gain, elevated blood pressure.
    b. Potassium depletion.
        Weakness, tiredness, alkalosis.
2   Glucocorticoid.
    a. Masking of infections.
    b. Osteoporosis.
    c. Steroid diabetes.
    d. Exacerbation of tuberculosis.

Control or Avoidance of Side-Effects

1 Mineralocorticoid.
   Use triamcinolone or newer synthetic steroids. (Some of the newer synthetics cause less sodium retention but have other side effects).
2 Glucocorticoid.
   Difficult to separate anti-inflammatory effects from sodium-retaining effects.

Acceptable and Expected Side-Effects

Nature of Effect	**Action**
Facial mooning (Cushing's Syndrome)	May be minimized by restricted calorie intake
Weight gain	Restrict calorie intake; may require a change in steroid medication; may require a diuretic
Oedema	May require diuretics and potassium
Potassium loss	Prescribe diuretics and potassium
	May require addition of a fluorinated synthetic
Acne	Administer potassium supplement
	Treat with topical medications
Increase frequency and nocturia	Check for evidence of genitourinary infection or diabetes mellitus; urinalysis
Insomnia, headache, fatigue, euphoria	
Glycosuria leucocytosis.	Treat symptomatically

Undesirable and Unacceptable Side-Effects

Nature of Effect	**Action (Report to Doctor)**
Allergic reaction to ACTH or steroid	Withdraw drug promptly
	Substitute steroid or synthetic ACTH
Cardiovascular system effect:	
Hypertension	Suggest reduction in dosage of steroids.
Thromboembolic complications	
Arteritis	
Infection	Suggest antibiotic medications as indicated
Eye complications:	
Glaucoma	Refer to ophthalmologist
Corneal lesions	
Subcapsular cataract	
Musculoskeletal effects:	
Osteoporosis	Suggest sex hormones—synthetic oestrogens and/or androgens
Pathologic fractures	
Growth suppression	
Myopathies	Suggest calcium supplement
Central nervous system:	
Seizures	Refer to neurologist

Nursing Action	Reason
Neuritis	
Psychotic reactions	
Adrenal insufficiency (after steroid withdrawal) manifested by peripheral circulatory collapse—in upright position.	Administer hydrocortisone promptly (intravenously). The following day give steroid replacement.

Advice and Admonitions for Patients on Long-term Steroids

1   Recognize that steroids are valuable and useful medications but if taken longer than 2 weeks, they may produce certain side-effects.
2   'Acceptable' side-effects may include weight gain (perhaps due to water retention), acne, headaches, fatigue and increased urinary frequency (see above).
3   'Unacceptable' side-effects which are to be reported to the doctor: dizziness when rising from chair or bed (postural hypotension indicative of adrenal insufficiency), nausea, vomiting, thirst, abdominal pain or pain of any type (see above).
4   Additional side-effects which are reportable are: convulsive seizures, feelings of depression or nervousness or development of an infection (see above).
5   If the patient has a fall or is in a road traffic accident, his condition may precipitate adrenal failure. He requires an immediate injection of hydrocortisone phosphate. (Long-term patients should wear an identification bracelet and carry hydrocortisone).
6   See doctor on a regular follow-up basis.

Nursing Management of Patients Receiving Steroid Therapy

1   Know the routes by which steroids are given.
   a. Ascertain advantages of the method chosen for the particular patient.
   b. Determine what is expected of the medication in a particular situation.
   c. Be informed about side effects and untoward manifestations.
   d. Note:
      (1) Local application of steroid medications to the skin (to a large area, over a prolonged period, using occlusive dressings) leads to adrenal suppression.
      (2) Local administration to the eye over a prolonged period leads to increased eye pressure, corneal ulceration.
   e. Recognize that it is necessary to understand pharmacological action of a particular steroid before planning the scheduled doses. Be aware of the following:
      (1) How frequently it can be given.
      (2) How late in the day it may be administered.
      (3) Whether every other day is sufficient, etc.
      Patients on intermittent therapy have few side-effects.
2   Be aware of the problems encountered during periods when steroids are being withdrawn or lowered in dosage.
   a. Associate symptoms of tiredness, muscular weakness and lethargy with drug withdrawal.
   b. Report any stress situations during this time, such as surgery, a family crisis, etc.

c. Instruct the patient why it may be necessary to save all urine for 24 hours (for determination of 11-hydroxycorticosteroid level).
3   Monitor carefully the patient who is on intravenous corticosteroid therapy.
   a. Determine the flow rate of fluids necessary to give a precise amount of medication.
   b. Observe the tissues, catheter site, flow rate, fluid level and patient's response at frequent intervals to be sure the system is functioning well.
   c. Note signs and symptoms indicative of adrenal crisis—restlessness, weakness, headache, nausea, vomiting, diarrhoea and falling blood pressure.

Health Teaching

1   Be sure the patient or a responsible member of his family knows that he is taking a steroid medication; explain why he is receiving it and what effects are desired.
2   The patient must also know what complications can occur, how to prevent them, and what to do should they occur.
3   Inform patient of the need for him to tell any doctor, dentist or nurse in his future contacts that he is on steroid therapy.
4   Be sure he knows that steroids are unique drugs prescribed in a dosage specific for him and that no one else should use his medications.

GUIDELINES: The Patient Receiving Steroid Therapy—Clinical Assessment, Surveillance and Health Teaching

Objective

To detect early signs of side effects from steroid therapy.

Nursing Action	Reason
Infection Control	
1 Encourage patient to avoid crowds and the possibility of exposure to infection.	Because steroids may affect the circulating blood—resulting in decreased eosinophils and lymphocytes, increased red cells and increased incidence of thrombophlebitis and infection.
2 Utilize exercise schedules to prevent stasis.	
3 Be aware that cardinal symptoms of inflammation may be masked.	
4 Instruct all persons coming in contact with this patient to wash hands thoroughly and practise meticulous asepsis.	
Diet and Metabolism Considerations	
1 Determine whether the patient needs assistance in dietary control.	1 Because steroids may cause weight gain and an increase in appetite.
2 Administer a high protein, high carbohydrate diet.	2 Because steroids affect protein metabolism, there may be negative nitrogen balance.

Nursing Action	Reason
3 Encourage patient to take steroids with milk or food.	3 Because steroids cause an increase in secretion of gastric hydrochloric acid and have an inhibiting effect on secretion of mucus in the stomach, they may aggravate an existing peptic ulcer.
4 Be on guard for early evidence of tric haemorrhage such as melaena, blood in vomitus.	
5 Check urine for evidence of glucose.	5 Because steroids precipitate gluconeogenesis and insulin antagonism, which results in hyperglycaemia, glucosuria, decreased carbohydrate tolerance.

Possible Bone Complications

1 Be on the alert for the possibility of pathologic fractures. Stress safety measures to prevent injury.	Because steroids affect the musculoskeletal system, causing potassium depletion and muscular weakness. (Steroids cause increased output of calcium and phosphorus, which leads to osteoporosis).
2 Administer a diet high in calcium and protein.	
3 Recommend a programme of activities of daily living, normal range of motion for the bedridden.	

Electrolyte Disturbance

1 Restrict sodium intake and increase potassium intake. a. Lemon juice is high in potassium and low in sodium. b. Avoid saline as a diluent in preparing injectable medications.	Because mineralocorticoid differs from other steroids, resulting in sodium retention and potassium depletion: oedema, weight gain.
2 Check blood pressure frequently and weigh patient daily.	
3 Observe for evidence of oedema.	

Behavioural Reactions

1 Watch for convulsive seizures (especially in children).	Because steroids may alter behaviour patterns, increase excitability and affect the central nervous system.
2 Avoid overstimulating situations.	
3 Recognize and report any mood deviating from the usual behaviour patterns.	
4 Report unusual behaviour, haunting dreams, withdrawal or suicidal tendencies.	

Nursing Action	Reason
Stress Reactions	
1 Recommend that the patient carry at all times an identification card indicating that he is on steroid therapy and including the name of his doctor and hospital and instructions for emergency care.	Because steroids affect the hypothalmic–pituitary–adrenal system, this in turn affects the individual's ability to respond to stress.
2 Advise patient to avoid extremes of temperature, as well as infections and upsetting situations.	
Safety Measures	
1 Admonish the patient to avoid injury; stress safety precautions.	Because steroids interfere with fibroblasts and granulation tissue, there is altered response to injury, resulting in impaired growth and delayed healing.
2 Observe daily the healing process of wounds, particularly surgical wounds, in order to recognize the potential for wound dehiscence.	

5. Disorders of the Pituitary

THE PITUITARY

The *pituitary gland* is called the master gland of the endocrine system because it controls hormone production of the other endocrine glands. It lies in the sella turcica at the base of the brain and is connected to the hypothalamus by the hypophyseal (pituitary) stalk.

1 *Anterior lobe*—produces at least seven hormones, six of which primarily affect the other endocrine glands and also control the posterior lobe.
2 *Posterior lobe*—believed to be responsible for storage of the antidiuretic, oxytocic and vasopressor hormones produced in the hypothalamus.

HYPERPITUITARISM

Hyperpituitarism results from an excessive amount of growth hormone secreted by the pituitary gland.

Predisposing Factors

1 Overactivity of the eosinophilic portion of the anterior lobe of the pituitary.
2 Effects of a benign adenoma (tumour).

Types of Hyperpituitarism

Gigantism

Hyperfunction of the pituitary, causing a generalized increase in size, particularly in the long bones of children before the epiphyseal lines close.

Acromegaly

1 Excessive secretion of growth hormone after epiphyseal closure, causing a chronic disease characterized by enlargement of bone, cartilage and soft tissues of the body.
2 Causes:
   a. Increase in size and function of a portion of the anterior lobe of the pituitary gland.
   b. Eosinophilic tumour of the pituitary gland.

HYPOPITUITARISM (SIMMONDS' DISEASE, PITUITARY CACHEXIA)

Hypopituitarism is pituitary insufficiency resulting from destruction of the anterior lobe of the pituitary gland.
   Panhypopituitarism (Simmonds' disease) is total absence of all pituitary secretions.

Clinical Manifestations

1 Extreme weight loss.
2 Atrophy of all organs.
3 Loss of hair.
4 Impotence; amenorrhoea.
5 Hypometabolism; hypoglycaemia.
6 Coma; death.

Cause

Total destruction of the anterior lobe of the pituitary by trauma, tumour, haemorrhage.

DIABETES INSIPIDUS

Diabetes Insipidus is a disorder of water metabolism caused by deficiency of vasopressin, the antidiuretic hormone (ADH) secreted by the posterior pituitary.

Aetiology

1 Unknown.
2 Secondary causes—head trauma, neoplasm, surgical removal or irradiation of pituitary gland.

Clinical Manifestations

1   Marked polyuria—daily output of 5–25 l of very dilute urine; appearance of urine like that of water, with a specific gravity of 1.001–1.005.
2   Polydipsia (intense thirst); 4–40 l of fluid daily; patient has a craving for cold water.

Diagnosis

Fluid Deprivation Test.

Objective

To restrict water intake and observe changes in urine volume and concentration.

1   Fluids deprived for 8–12 hours or until 3% of body weight is lost.
2   Plasma and urine osmolality studies are determined at beginning, during and end of test—inability to increase specific gravity and osmolality of urine is characteristic of diabetes insipidus.

Treatment and Nursing Management

Objectives

To replace vasopressin (usually a lifelong therapeutic programme).
To search for and correct underlying intracranial pathology.

1   Give antidiuretic hormone, vasopressin tannate (Pitressin Tannate)—reduces urinary volume for 24–48 hours.
    a. Warm vial—medication is in oil and warming makes administration easier.
    b. Shake bottle vigorously before administering drug—active hormone settles to the bottom of the oil.
    c. Give in evening—maximum results obtained during sleep—or
2   Give vasopressin by topical application to the nasal mucosa (lypressin nasal spray [Syntopressin])—drug absorbed through the nasal mucosa into the blood.
    a. Nasal insufflation administered by one or two sprays in each nostil as directed.
    b. Watch for chronic rhinopharyngitis.
3   Administer chlorpropamide (Diabinese)—reduces urine volume.
    a. May be used as an antidiuretic in *mild* cases to potentiate action of vasopressin.
    b. Warn the patient of possible hypoglycaemic reactions.
4   Weigh patient frequently.
5   Support the patient undergoing studies for a cranial lesion (See Chapter 1, Volume 3, Neurological Conditions).

PITUITARY TUMOURS

Types of Pituitary Tumours

1   *Chromophobe adenoma*—tumour of the anterior pituitary gland of adults.
    a. Comprises 90% of pituitary tumours; produces no hormones but can destroy rest of pituitary gland.

b. Produces failing vision, optic atrophy, bilateral hemianopia, enlargement of sella turcica and endocrine disturbances.

2 *Eosinophilic adenoma*—endocrine secretion of tumour produces gigantism in children and acromegaly in adults.

3 *Basophilic adenoma*—gives rise to so-called Cushing's syndrome with features largely attributable to hyperadrenalism—masculinization and amenorrhoea in females, girdle obesity, hypertension, osteoporosis and polycythaemia.

HYPOPHYSECTOMY

Hypophysectomy is removal of pituitary gland.

Indications

1 Primary neoplasms (tumours) of the pituitary gland.
2 Diabetic retinopathy.
   a. Used to halt progress of haemorrhagic diabetic retinopathy and to prevent blindness.
   b. Also reduces insulin requirements.
3 Palliative measure for relief of bone pain secondary to metastasis of malignant lesions of breast and prostate; alters hormonal milieu of body to create a hormonal environment hostile to continued growth of neoplasm.

Methods of Pituitary Ablation (Removal)

1 Extirpative hypophysectomy—done by transfrontal, subcranial or transsphenoidal approaches.
2 Hypophyseal stalk section.
3 Implantation of radioactive yttrium.
4 Radiation x-ray—proton irradiation from a cyclotron.
5 Destruction with cryosurgery (freezing).

Management

The absence of the pituitary gland alters the function of many parts of the body.

1 The patient may need substitution therapy with adrenal steroids (hydrocortisone) and thyroid hormone.
2 Menstruation ceases and infertility occurs almost always after total or nearly total ablation (removal).
3 See p. 580 for treatment of diabetes insipidus.
4 See Volume 3, Chapter 1, Neurological Conditions for nursing management of the patient undergoing cranial surgery.

6. Disorders of Purine Metabolism

GOUT

Gout is a disease caused by excessive accumulation of uric acid in the blood and eventual deposition of uric acid crystals in various tissues.

1 *Uric acid*—end produce of purine metabolism.
2 *Hyperuricaemia*—persistent elevation of urates in the blood.
3 *Tophi*—deposits of urates in the tissues about the joints or on the ear; development of tophi related to duration of disease, degree of hyperumicaemia and renal function status.

Underlying Considerations

1 Hereditary factor present—mode of genetic transmission not established.
2 Males are predominantly affected; peak incidence between 30 and 50 years.
3 Potential inciting agents—rich food, overindulgence in alcohol, physical and emotional stress, acute infection—may contribute to temporary disorganization of homoeostatic mechanisms of body as well as bring about factors that alter uric acid level in body.

Types of Gout

1 *Primary*—basic problem appears to be a genetic defect in purine metabolism.
2 *Secondary*—hyperuricaemia is produced by increasing breakdown of nucleic acids in certain diseases (such as blood dyscrasias) or because of interference with renal excretion.
   May be precipitated by prolonged ingestion of diuretic agents, trauma, treatment of myeloproliferative diseases.

Clinical Manifestattions

1 Sudden onset of severe pain in one or more peripheral joints—may be accompanied by intense inflammation, swelling and tenderness.
   a. First joint of great toe is susceptible; later, other joints of foot are affected.
   b. Joints of feet, ankles, knees, wrist and elbow commonly affected.
2 Fever 38.3–39.4°C (101–103°F).
3 Attacks involving the same joints tend to recur; variable lengths of time between attacks.

Diagnosis

1 Sudden attack of severe pain in one or more peripheral joints in a previously healthy male.
2 Therapeutic response to full course of colchicine.
3 Elevation of serum uric acid.
4 Identification of uric acid crystals in synovial fluid—obtained by arthrocentesis (aspiration of fluid from a joint cavity).
5 Elevated erythrocyte sedimentation rate and white blood count—in acute attack.

6   X-ray findings—presence of tophi and radiographic evidence of urate deposits in bone (late manifestations).
7   Other diagnostic features:
   a. Positive family history for gout.
   b. Unexplained proteinuria and hypertension.
   c. Passage of renal stones.
   d. Patient taking thiazide for non-gouty conditions.

Treatment and Nursing Management

Objectives

To relieve acute discomfort.
To prevent the development of chronic gouty arthritis, renal calculi and renal damage.

Acute Attack of Gout

1   Give colchicine *early* in attack—suppresses inflammatory manifestations of acute gout; useful in establishing diagnosis since it gives dramatic relief if patient has gout
   a. An initial dose of colchicine is given and is followed by doses every 2–3 hours until the pain disappears and gastrointestinal symptoms develop (nausea, vomiting, abdominal cramping, diarrhoea).
   b. Colchicine produces diarrhoea—stop drug temporarily until diarrhoea subsides. Give medication to relieve diarrhoea.
   c. A maintenance dose of colchicine is given as soon as diarrhoea stops as a prophylactic agent against recurrent gouty arthritis.
   d. Colchicine may be given before and after surgery to patients with gout—reduces the incidence of acute attacks of gouty arthritis precipitated by operative procedures.
2   Alternative forms of therapy.
   a. Phenylbutazone (Butazolidin) or oxyphenbutazone or indomethacin (Indocid) are other drugs given during the acute stage of gout—these drugs reduce the fever and have an anti-inflammatory effect.
   b. Give these drugs with meals or with milk since they are ulcerogenic.
3   Give analgesic for severe pain until specific drug is effective.
4   Encourage the patient to stay on bed rest for 24 hours after acute attack—early ambultion may precipitate a recurrence.
5   Advise the patient to avoid high purine foods (Table 5.4).
6   Encourage large fluid intake to maintain a high 24-hour urinary volume—urinary urate excretion increases 24 hours after introduction of uricosuric drugs and may lead to stone formation.

Chronic Gouty Arthritis

1   Give drug (uricosuric agent)—acts on renal tubule to inhibit urate reabsorption and thereby increases urinary excretion of urate and lowers the serum urate level; prevents formation of new tophi and reduces size of those already present.

Table 5.4. Low Purine Diet*

Purines are derived from ingested food and from the breakdown of body proteins. Purines are also synthesized in the liver. A low purine diet is seldom used but it is advocated that patients with high blood uric acid levels avoid foods highest in purine content and also avoid alcohol.

Foods Highest in Purines	Foods High in Purine	Foods Lowest in Purine
Sweetbreads	Meat	Fruits
Anchovies	Poultry	Vegetables (except those listed)
Sardines in oil	Fish	
Liver (calf, beef)	Lobster, crabs, oysters	Most breads, cereals and cereal products
Kidneys	Meat soups and broth	
Meat extracts	Beans, dried	Milk
Gravy	Peas, dried	Cheese
	Lentils, dried	Eggs
	Spinach	Fish roe
	Oatmeal	Nuts
	Wheat germ and bran	Fats
		Sugars, syrups, sweets
		Gelatin
		Milk and fruit desserts
		Vegetable and cream soups

* Foods listed from Church, C F and Church, H N (1975) Food Values of Portions Commonly Used, 12th edition, J B Lippincott.

Purines are derived from ingested food and from the breakdown of body proteins. Purines are also synthesized in the liver. A low purine diet is seldom used but it is advocated that patients with high blood uric acid levels avoid foods highest in purine content and also avoid alcohol.

    a. Probenecid (Benemid).
    Side-effects—headache, gastrointestinal disturbances, skin rash.
    b. Sulphinpyrazone (Anturan)
    Side-effects—gastrointestinal disturbances (including peptic ulcer), skin rash, haematological side-effects.
    c. Give after meals or with antacids if there are gastric side effects.
2 Or give allopurinol (Zyloric), a xanthine oxidase inhibitor—interferes with final stages of conversion of the products of purine metabolism to uric acid (inhibits formation of uric acid).
    Dosage based on serum urate determinations.
3 Encourage large fluid intake to maintain a high 24-hour urinary volume—urinary urate excretion increases 24 hours after introduction of uricosuric drugs and may lead to stone formation.
    a. Maintain an alkaline urine in patients with a history of stone formation.
    b. Give sodium bicarbonate or citrate solutions.

Health Teaching

Instruct the patient as follows:

1   Take colchicine as prescribed as a prophylactic measure against acute attack.
2   Take uricosuric agent (see above) or allopurinol—to prevent further deposition of uric acid in joints.
    Colchicine and uricosuric agents may be given in combination for indefinite periods of time.
3   Avoid specific foods (or alcohol) known to precipitate an attack. See table, above.
4   Maintain a high fluid intake to maintain high urinary volume—minimizes urate precipitation in urinary tract.
5   Avoid fasting (to lose weight or when on alcoholic spree)—fasting has been found to increase the serum uric acid level.
6   Avoid crash diets—rapid reduction of weight may increase the serum uric acid level; slow weight reduction reduces the serum urate level without inducing an acute attack.
7   Recognize the warnings of an impending attack. Start therapy promptly.

FURTHER READING

Books

Bloom, A (1978) Diabetes Explained, 3rd edition, MTP Press
Drury, M I (1979) Diabetes Mellitis, Blackwell Scientific
Lee,, J and Haycock, J (1978) Essential Endocrinology, Oxford University Press
Mason, S A (1976) Health and Hormones, Pelican
Mason, S A (1976) Hormones and the Body, Pelican
Oakley, W G, Pyke, D A and Taylor, K W (1978) Diabetes and its Management, 3rd edition, Blackwell Scientific
Thomason, J A (1976) An Introduction to Clinical Endocrinology, Churchill Livingstone

Articles

Ayres, O (1979) Living with diabetes, Nursing, 12: 532–534
Barnett, A H et al. (1980) The mini pump methods of diabetic control during minor surgery under general anaesthesia, British Medical Journal, 78–79
Cook, K A (1979) Diabetics can be vegetarians, Nursing, 9: 70–73
Felstein, I (1980) Ten faces of disguised diseases, Nursing Mirror, 150: 34–35
Fletcher, C (1980) Personal paper—one way of coping with diabetes, British Medical Journal: 1115–1116
James, I (1979) Tailoring the insulin to the patient's needs, Geriatric Medicine, 9: 79–80, 83
Kelly, B A (1979) Nurses' knowledge of glycosuria testing in diabetes mellitus, Nursing Research, 28: 316–319

Mahon, S (1979) Consciousness and diabetes, Nursing, 8: 363–364

Roberts, A (1979) Systems of Life 50. Hormones and homoeostasis, Nursing Times, 75: Supplement, 1 February 1979

Roberts, A (1979) Systems of Life 51. The energy supremo 1: The control system, Nursing Times, 75: Supplement, 1 March 1979

Roberts, A (1979) Systems of Life 53. The energy supremo 3: Failures of control, Nursing Times, 75: Supplement, 3 May 1979

Roberts, A (1979) Systems of Life 56. The adrenal glands 1, Nursing Times, 75: Supplement, 2nd August 1979

Roberts, A (1979) Systems of Life 57. The adrenal glands 2: Disorders of glucocorticoids, Nursing Times, 75: Supplement, 20 September 1979

Roberts, A (1979) Systems of Life 58. The adrenal glands 3. Aldosterone and abnormalities of adrenal sex hormone production, Nursing Times, 75: Supplement, 25 October 1979

Roberts, A (1979) Systems of Life 59. The adrenal glands 4: The hormones of the medulla, Nursing Times, 75: Supplement, 15 November 1979

Roberts, A (1979) Systems of Life 60. The pituitary gland 1: Physiology and disorders, Nursing Times, 76: Supplement, 6 December 1979

Roberts, A (1980) Systems of Life 61. The pituitary gland 2: Hypopituitary, growth and development, Nursing Times, 76: Supplement, 3 January 1980

Roberts, A (1980) Systems of Life 62. The pituitary glands 3: The posterior pituitary and water homoestasis, Nursing Times, 76: Supplement, 7 February 1980

Thom, M H and Studd, J W (1980) Procedures in practice—hormone implantation, British Medical Journal: 848–850

Thomas, B J and Powell, H E (1980) New perspectives on the dietary management of diabetes, Journal of Human Nutrition, 34: 70–73

Tunbridge, W M (1979) Acromegaly, Nursing Times, 75: 110–112

Voke, J (1979) Pituitary gland—master of the endocrines. Nursing Mirror, 149: 26–28

Wilkes, E and Lawton, E E (1980) The diabetic, the hospital and primary care, Journal of the Royal College of General Practitioners, 30: 199–206

INDEX

The Index covers all three volumes of *The Lippincott Manual of Medical-Surgical Nursing*. The figures printed in **bold** type before each entry or group of entries indicate the volume in which that page number or numbers will be found. The page numbers in italic indicate a figure, and page numbers followed by 't' indicate a table.